Jim Crow in the Asylum

Studies in Social Medicine

Allan M. Brandt, Larry R. Churchill, and Jonathan Oberlander, *editors*

This series publishes books at the intersection of medicine, health, and society that further our understanding of how medicine and society shape one another historically, politically, and ethically. The series is grounded in the convictions that medicine is a social science, that medicine is humanistic and cultural as well as biological, and that it should be studied as a social, political, ethical, and economic force.

A complete list of books published in Studies in Social Medicine is available at https://uncpress.org/series/studies-social-medicine.

Jim Crow in the Asylum

Psychiatry and Civil Rights in the American South

....

KYLIE M. SMITH

The University of North Carolina Press Chapel Hill

© 2026 Kylie M. Smith
All rights reserved
Set in Charis by Westchester Publishing Services
Manufactured in the United States of America

Library of Congress Cataloging-in-Publication Data
Names: Smith, Kylie, 1968– author
Title: Jim Crow in the asylum : psychiatry and civil rights in the American South / Kylie M. Smith.
Other titles: Studies in social medicine
Description: Chapel Hill : The University of North Carolina Press, [2026] | Series: Studies in social medicine | Includes bibliographical references and index.
Identifiers: LCCN 2025022657 | ISBN 9781469689197 cloth | ISBN 9781469689203 paperback | ISBN 9781469689210 epub | ISBN 9781469689227 pdf
Subjects: LCSH: African Americans—Mental health services—Southern States—History | African Americans—Mental health—Southern States—History | Racism in medicine—Southern States—History | Racism against Black people—Southern States—History | Mentally ill—Care—Southern States—History | Psychiatric hospitals—Southern States—History | BISAC: MEDICAL / Health Policy | SOCIAL SCIENCE / Disease & Health Issues
Classification: LCC RC451.5.B53 S65 2026 | DDC 362.2089/96075—dc23/eng/20250812
LC record available at https://lccn.loc.gov/2025022657

Cover art: *Court for Women, Showing Group of Patients, Searcy Hospital, Mt. Vernon, Alabama*, 1954. Annual Report to the Board of Trustees. Courtesy Reynolds-Finley Historical Library, the University of Alabama at Birmingham.

This book is freely available in an open access edition thanks to TOME (Toward an Open Monograph Ecosystem)—a collaboration of the Association of American Universities, the Association of University Presses, and the Association of Research Libraries—and to the generous support of Emory University and the Andrew W. Mellon Foundation. Learn more at the TOME website, openmonographs.org. To view the MANIFOLD edition of the book, see http://jimcrowintheasylum.com.

This work is licensed under a Creative Commons Attribution-NonCommercial-NoDerivatives 4.0 International Public License. To view a copy of this license, visit https://creativecommons.org/licenses/by-nc-nd/4.0/legalcode. *Note to users*: A Creative Commons license is only valid when applied by the person or entity that holds rights to the licensed work. This work may contain components to which the rightsholder in the work cannot apply the license. It is ultimately your responsibility to independently evaluate the copyright status of any work or component part of a work you use in light of your intended use.

For product safety concerns under the European Union's General Product Safety Regulation (EU GPSR), please contact gpsr@mare-nostrum.co.uk or write to the University of North Carolina Press and Mare Nostrum Group B.V., Mauritskade 21D, 1091 GC Amsterdam, The Netherlands.

For all the patients and descendant families

How and why does one write a history of violence?

—Saidiya Hartman, "Venus in Two Acts"

Contents

List of Illustrations, ix

Prologue, 1
Mrs. Hurston's Letter

Part I
Creating Jim Crow in the Asylum

1 Promoting Mental Health at the Tuskegee Institute, 17

2 Enabling Segregation, 38

3 Diagnosing Difference, 66

Part II
Performing Jim Crow in the Asylum

4 Negotiating Daily Life, 91

5 Exposing Southern Snake Pits, 126

Part III
Ending Jim Crow in the Asylum

6 Planning Community Mental Health, 157

7 Mobilizing Grassroots Activism, 179

8 Enforcing Civil Rights, 205

Aftermath, 233
Mrs. F.'s Letter

Appendix 1. Power and Politics in the Psychiatric Archives, 249
Appendix 2. Theorizing the History of "Black Madness," 259

Acknowledgments, 269

Notes, 273

Bibliography, 307

Index, 323

Illustrations

Figures

1.1 Staff of the Tuskegee Mental Hygiene Clinic, 1950, 19

1.2 Portrait of Dr. Prince Barker, 1959, 23

2.1 Map of Milledgeville State Hospital, Georgia, 1965, 45

2.2 Colony farm at Central State Hospital, Georgia, 1904, 47

2.3 Searcy Hospital, Mount Vernon, Alabama, 1935, 49

2.4 The Jemison Plantation, Northport, Alabama, 1933, 51

2.5 Mississippi State Hospital staff, 1950, 55

4.1 "News from Coloured Folks," *The Whit*, 1951, 96

4.2 Dayroom at Searcy Hospital, 1949, 116

4.3 State Farm Colony, Alabama, 1948, 118

4.4 Patients working a field, Alabama, 1946, 120

5.1 Front page, *Delta Democrat-Times*, 1949, 135

7.1 Portrait of John LeFlore, c. 1942, 181

7.2 Letter from John LeFlore to Governor Persons, 1953, 182

7.3 Clipping from *The Southern Courier*, 1967, 198

8.1 Memo from Governor Wallace to Superintendent Tarwater, 1965, 223

Tables

3.1 Psychotic disorders diagnosed on first admission, 1956, 72

3.2 Chronic brain syndromes diagnosed on first admission, 1956, 75

3.3 Use of electroshock therapy in Alabama state hospitals, 1956, 83

Jim Crow in the Asylum

Prologue
Mrs. Hurston's Letter

In January 1965, Mrs. Claudette Hurston of Vicksburg, Mississippi, wrote the following letter to the secretary of the Department of Health, Education, and Welfare (HEW) in Washington, DC:

> Dear Sir
>
> I have written the president also.
>
> I have a desperate problem, I don't have any alternative.
>
> I have a violent, mentally ill eleven years [sic] old son.
>
> For five years I have gone through every step in the state to get help.
>
> They haven't given me anything but the runaround I am afraid.
>
> I can't handle my son, Thomas anymore.
>
> He's a danger to himself, my smaller children, and everyone else around as well.
>
> He disturbs the whole neighborhood.
>
> Five years I have [been] begging and going through everything to get help from this state.
>
> Five months ago I found out the hospital I had applied [to], Ellisville State Hospital, has taken out all the negro children and it's not any place here for negro children.
>
> A judge here made out a court order for him to go to Whitfield State Hospital for adults.
>
> It's been five months [since] he was in jail and he can't take care of himself and I had to go get him.
>
> He fell on the heater and burnt his arm terribly during a nervous fit.
>
> He throws anything he gets his hands on at the other children and myself.
>
> Sir, I can't keep him here anymore and he can't stay in jail (I had to let him go back) because he will die from lack of attention.
>
> Please help if you can sir.
>
> It's a matter of life and death now.

> I waited until he got too large and sick thinking the state would help me.
>
> Please let me hear from you right away.
>
> Thank you so much
>
> Mrs. Claudette Hurston

Mrs. Hurston's letter lives in the files of Senator John Calhoun Stennis as part of the Mississippi Political Collections at Mississippi State University in Starkville. It's in a folder labeled Public Health Service (PHS) 1965, which for the most part contains correspondence between the senator and the PHS as he sought to keep abreast of funding grants made to various state health services.[1] There is also a good deal of correspondence with constituents, most of them concerned about the new Medicare entitlements and how their access to care would be affected by the requirement for hospitals to be racially integrated. Stennis answered each of these letters, agreeing with people's outrage about medical integration and thanking them for their support. Stennis received a copy of Mrs. Hurston's letter forwarded from Allen Menefee, assistant chief of the Mental Retardation Branch of the Chronic Diseases Division within HEW. Menefee replied to Mrs. Hurston, expressing his concern and dismay, and referred her to Dr. Dorothy Moore, the coordinator of mental health and mental retardation planning in Mississippi. Menefee cc'd Dr. Moore on his reply as well as Senators Stennis and Eastland and all of Mississippi's representatives. Written in red pencil on the side of Stennis's copy are the words "No Reply."

When I came across Mrs. Hurston's letter in the archive file, my first instinct as a historian was to treat it at face value as a letter in an unrestricted file that was mine to use as I saw fit, a letter that told me a particular story in the words of the writer herself. I therefore decided to start this book with a verbatim reproduction of that letter to center Mrs. Hurston's words, unmediated by me. Then, in 2021, when I explained to my Digital Monograph Writer's Workshop colleagues that I was going to start the book with that letter and have it speak for itself, someone suggested that I should do more than that. "Why don't you look her up?" Pat said, and I was a little shocked at the suggestion. It seemed like some kind of ethical transgression to go beyond the confines of the letter, an intrusion on personal privacy, as if using the letter verbatim was not such an intrusion. The idea to track Mrs. Hurston down had not really occurred to me—it was not really how I was trained—but the possibility of it, the idea that doing so might actually be the only ethical to do, played on my mind until finally, I took the leap.

Late in 2021, I googled "Claudette Hurston, Vicksburg Mississippi" and immediately, there she was, via two links to an obituary. I knew it was her straightaway—she had lived and died in Mississippi, had five children, had lost a son called Thomas. According to the Jackson Memorial Funeral Service, "Mother Hurston" had passed away in March 2018. She had been an active member of a number of churches, but her funeral service was held at Refuge Temple in Jackson. I thought that might be my best point of contact. On Tuesday, October 26, 2021, I emailed Pastor Mark Gilbert at Refuge Temple, explaining who I was and that I had a letter from Mrs. Hurston I would like to share with her family, and asking if it would be possible to speak to any of them. Within half an hour I had a reply from Pastor Gilbert. He explained that he did not know Mrs. Hurston personally, as he started his work at the church after her passing, but he had certainly heard of her and her civil rights activism. He told me that one of her other sons was in fact still an active part of the church, having been a deacon there for thirty years. He had passed on my information to Deacon Hurston, who said he would be happy to speak with me. I gave myself an hour or so to write down some notes and questions, and then I called Deacon Hurston in Jackson. He was willing to talk but was at work, so we scheduled a time for the next day. When I called the next morning, I took a minute to explain what my book was about and how and where I had found his mother's letter. I did not record our conversation—throughout this project I have been cognizant of how a recording device can act as a barrier to open discussion—but using the notes I took, I will try to repeat his story as he told it to me.

The first thing I did was ask Mr. Hurston if he would like me to read his mother's letter to him. He said he would, and I did, slowly, trying to give her words the space they deserved. When I finished, there was silence for a moment, and then, unprompted, Mr. Hurston began to speak in his lovely deep voice. He said he remembered the incident in his mother's letter. Thomas, his older brother, "was born a normal child." Then, when he was about six, Thomas contracted measles. He had a particularly bad case with an extremely high fever. Their mother was at work when the fever accelerated, and Thomas ran outside to the tap at the side of the house, soaking himself with water. When his temperature continued to accelerate, he was taken to the hospital, but it was already too late; the measles had caused irreparable brain damage. Ronald remembered Thomas coming home, not being able to talk anymore, and how frustrated he was at people not understanding him. He was angry for a long time, and would get upset and irate, taking his anger out on the rest of the family. Ronald remembered the terrible burden for their mother, who couldn't handle Thomas by herself. Their father was in the air force and often not home. In addition to Thomas and Ronald, she had three other children: Ronald's twin brother Donald and two girls, one older and one younger. As Mrs. Hurston's own letter reveals, she spent five long years trying to get help, and being repeatedly ignored or rebuffed, until the state saw fit to imprison an eleven-year-old with brain damage.

At this point my conversation with Ronald turned toward his mother, whom he remembers with great love and respect. He explained that at the same time she was dealing with Thomas and taking care of her young children, she was attending Hinds Community College at night to get an associate's degree in stenography, becoming extremely proficient in shorthand. She applied to work at the US Postal Service (USPS) and sat for the entrance exam. Her score was the highest in the state of Mississippi, but she was not offered a job. She immediately filed a complaint with the Equal Employment Opportunity Commission and was eventually employed by the Postal Service, where she became the first Black stenographer. She joined either the National Postal Workers Union or the United Federation of Postal Clerks—Mr. Hurston couldn't remember which one—and eventually became the union secretary. She worked for thirty years at the USPS and the union, actively working to secure people their rights as federal workers, especially in the context of the civil rights movement.

I asked Deacon Hurston if his brother ever got any help or made any improvement. Ronald thinks that he was initially admitted to Whitfield—I know from my research that a new unit for Black developmentally disabled people was opened on the grounds of the Mississippi State Hospital in Whitfield in 1963, which held more than 800 people and had a long waiting list at the time of Mrs. Hurston's letter. Ellisville was the state school for disabled children, designated for white children only at the same time as the new unit at Whitfield was opened, so that all the Black children were moved to Whitfield. But Whitfield was an adult hospital and no place for children. After some resistance on the part of the State of Mississippi, which Mrs. Hurston alludes to in her letter, the unit at Whitfield was desegregated in 1968, at which time Ellisville was also integrated. Ronald told me that Thomas was moved to Ellisville, where he was given a lot of medication, which calmed him down. I asked Ronald what Mrs. Hurston had thought about Ellisville: Was she happy with the care there, did Thomas improve, were they able to visit him there? Mr. Hurston was forceful in his reply: "She was not happy with Ellisville; she didn't like it at all." Mrs. Hurston continued to advocate for Thomas, eventually securing a place for him at Brookhaven, a group home community, where he continued to improve and was able to come home on weekends. Thomas was never able to talk again, but he was calmer, Ronald remembered. He said that he enjoyed seeing his brother. I asked Ronald how he felt about the impact of Thomas on his own life. He thought for a moment, then said that he did not think he could answer that question. That answer has stuck in my mind, as I wonder what it signals about the way that Black families and patients processed trauma in the midst of state neglect and abuse.

Thomas stayed at Brookhaven until he became ill in 2013. After surgery, he developed an infection and was in the ICU at the University of Mississippi Medical Center in Jackson. As he recovered, he developed blood clots, but the medical center couldn't (or wouldn't) keep him, and he was released. He was sent back to Brookhaven, but the clots worsened. He was admitted to King's Daughters Medical Center, where he died on March 29, 2013.

I said to Ronald that his mother must have been devastated, and he told me she was. It was very sad, he said, because Thomas seemed to be doing better after the surgery, but by the end of the week, he was gone. We talked about the impact of the many traumatic experiences that his mother had experienced with her oldest son; we talked about the role of her faith and the church community for healing and support; and we talked about the influence she had on all her children, two of whom (Ronald and Donald) went on to work for the USPS themselves (they are both now retired). Their two sisters are both professionals, one working for the state, another for an insurance company.

I told Ronald I would send him a copy of his mother's letter, and also this version of our conversation for him to check for accuracy. I added that when I returned to Jackson, I'd like to buy him a cup of coffee, and he said that both he and Donald would enjoy talking to me more. Because of COVID and other life interruptions, it would take two long years before I was able to get back to Mississippi, but in March 2024, I finally met Ronald, his wife Pamela, and Donald Hurston in person. We had lunch at the Cracker Barrel in Pearl, just south of Jackson, and not far from the Whitfield institution itself. Over breakfast, we talked about everything from federal politics to water pollution. The Hurston brothers shared many memories of their family and photos of their mother, Thomas, and their own children and grandchildren. They were also incredibly generous in showing me the printed booklets from both Thomas's and Mrs. Hurston's funerals. The booklets were full of photos of multiple generations of the Hurston family, smiling and hugging—so many beautiful people it made me teary. It struck me how much love and warmth were captured in the photos, and I felt that warmth in their interactions with one another and also in their kindness and generosity toward me. As I drove home to Atlanta the next day, it struck me how much strength there was in this closely knit network of friends, family, and community, stretching back to Vicksburg in the 1960s and beyond, and how—despite so much trauma and struggle—they retained compassion and care for one another through kinship and faith.

Thomas Hobart Hurston was born on November 8, 1955, and died on March 29, 2013. Mrs. Claudette Hurston was born on September 26, 1934, and passed away on March 30, 2018, at the age of eighty-four. They are both laid to rest in Jackson, Mississippi.

· · · · · ·

The story contained in Mrs. Hurston's letter, and the process and consequences of me finding it, are central to the framing of this book. The dilemma Mrs. Hurston faced exemplifies the story I'm trying to tell: that psychiatric and disability services in the South were actively shaped by a virulent white supremacy—operating in the shadow of the plantation—which ultimately led to a failure to provide meaningful services. Her letter names those services in Mississippi directly: Ellisville is the state hospital for developmentally delayed children; Whitfield is the large state hospital for mentally ill adults; and then, there is the jail. These services formed a network of confinement where people were transferred between school, hospital, and prison—often all three within a lifetime. In these constant mobilities, I saw not only the instability of psychiatric categories but also the obvious overlap between conceptions of disability, mental illness, and criminality, as well as the active ways that a commitment to racial segregation left the states' Black families without support—both at the time and for decades to come.

Mrs. Hurston's letter also reveals the systemic and functional problems within Mississippi's mental health system, symptomatic of other systems in the South—especially in the context of the civil rights movement: a long history of racial segregation; a general disdain for any kind of social welfare programs; a refusal to accept community mental health money, which became available in 1963; and a general overcrowding and underfunding of the state hospital system. Mrs. Hurston wrote her letter in 1965, when hospital facilities were being racially integrated due to the Civil Rights Act of 1964 and the nondiscrimination clause of the new Medicare and Medicaid Act of 1965.[2] It was because of her awareness of these legislative changes and her belief in the power of them that she wrote her letter, demanding that the state uphold the law. Mrs. Hurston's words speak to the broad impact of the movement toward hospital integration and the way that states like Mississippi sought to avoid it.

This is the precise legislative and policy moment that I initially thought this book would be about. I started with an interest in exploring how the Community Mental Health Act (1963), the Civil Rights Act (1964), and the Social Security Amendments (Medicare and Medicaid Act, 1965) combined to interrupt Jim Crow in the asylum and create the conditions for the mental health disparities that exist today. In the last ten years of researching the history of American approaches to mental health, I saw the extent of the damage that had been done through racially segregated psychiatric systems. The legacy of that damage is evident every day where I live in Atlanta—in the violence of the police who shoot first, ask questions never; who arrested the Black man in the Starbucks that time because he made someone uncomfortable; who let Lashawn Thompson and others like him die in Fulton County Jail from lack of care. It is evident in the little tent cities that appear and disappear and reappear under the I-75/I-85 flyover when you come off I-20 to head south, or under the bridge that crosses the Chattahoochee just north of the sparkling silver shopping malls of Buckhead. It is evident in the creation of first-class facilities like Skyland Trail, which are designed to help kids with mood or affective disorders but require a second mortgage to afford, while the Black kids get diagnosed with behavioral problems and kicked out of school. It is evident in the politics of Georgia, where the refusal to expand Medicare or Medicaid deprives people of basic services; where entire medical systems can close down because they don't make enough profit; where medical residents go to train at Grady because they can see things there they'll never see in their lives again, only to disappear into the comfort of suburban practice in Peachtree Corners. And it was evident in 2021 and 2022, when the Georgia House and Senate published a series of recommendations and bills that finally sought to address the crisis in mental health services because a white politician had a son who ended up in jail due to untreated symptoms. In a classic case of interest convergence, Representative Jones (who had not given a damn about mental health before) lamented that his son had not been able to get care that would have kept him out of the jail system, and then constructed and passed a House bill that mentioned race or disparities not one time and doubled down on the use of police as first responders.

This constant dissonance in legislation has direct links to the longer history of mental health policy and to the violence of white supremacy at the intersection of disability and Blackness. But documenting that history has been more difficult than I anticipated, and that difficulty has shaped the content and structure of this book. My research had originated in the legal cases that demonstrated the centrality of health care to civil rights activists like John LeFlore and the NAACP, the Legal Defense Fund, and the Medical Committee for Human Rights.[3] I wrote that part of the book first, originally thinking that I would trace the impact of that activism forward into the present, but it soon became obvious that I needed to explore what the institutions had been like for Black patients before the Civil Rights Act. Finding Mrs. Hurston's letter became a pivotal moment because it made clear that I needed to work backward to try to understand the conditions that had existed for patients and families well before they became the subject of civil rights activism. I needed to try to understand what ideas and practices had sustained the creation and perpetuation of hospitals in ways that seemed to mimic the original plantations on which they had been built, and how those ideas were enabled by psychiatry itself. Plenty of scholars have made the argument that prisons are a continuation of the plantation system, and rightly so.[4] Prisons replicate plantation relations in obvious ways, particularly in the South because they exist in the same places that had once been plantations, because the majority-Black population they house are not free, because they rely on forced labor, and because they are surrounded by rhetoric about the inherent badness and criminality of the Black person.

It soon became obvious to me that Southern psychiatric hospitals worked in this way as well. This was obvious immediately in the first set of records I encountered—the court case *Marable v. Alabama Mental Health Board*. This case was combined with a HEW and Department of Justice case against the state of Alabama for maintaining segregation.[5] Housed in several hefty boxes at the National Archives and Records Administration in Atlanta, this court case drew on an investigation documenting the use of patient labor; horrific living conditions; a lack of meaningful treatment; and abuse, violence, and neglect. One of the investigators went so far as to declare Alabama's hospitals no better than "Southern plantations." If people in the 1960s thought they resembled plantations, then I needed to take this claim seriously.

To help think through this link between plantations and asylums, I turned to the scholarship and debates within slavery studies, all of which informed my thinking in one way or another. I have set out some of these theoretical concepts in more detail in appendix 2, but I want to discuss three particular ideas here that have helped to frame the analysis in the chapters that follow: "the wake," "social death," and "the Jim Crow routine." The idea of "the wake" comes specifically from Christina Sharpe's work, which, building on Saidiya Hartman, explores the myriad ways that the "afterlives" of slavery continue to ripple throughout modern society, shaping the lived experience of Black Americans.[6] The wake manifests across domains, not just in this thing called "racism" and its creation of Blackness as "other" but in the ways that racism, as anti-Blackness, is embedded in restricted access to social opportunity and manifests in health, in confinement, in systems of care. Sharpe's concern is to explore "how slavery's violence emerges within the contemporary conditions of spatial, legal, psychic, material, and other dimensions of Black non/being as well as in Black modes of resistance."[7] Therefore, all institutions that contain and confine the Black body need to be understood as existing in the wake of the plantation system, which also shapes the way that Black Americans see and understand themselves and how they can react. This seems like a particularly pertinent tool for a critique of psychiatry, not simply because psychiatry was a practice shaped on and by the plantation but because it continues to define the possibilities of acceptable personhood and constrains the way we understand responses to trauma and its legacy.[8]

Sharpe also raises the specter of death in relation to the wake. Intersecting with the idea of "necropolitics," Sharpe makes the point that being Black means always living in the wake of the history of death attendant to slavery.[9] The question then becomes, "How do we attend to physical, social, and figurative death and also to the largeness that is Black life, Black life insisted from death?"[10] In the history of psychiatry, how do we account for a practice of confinement that is at its essence predicated on the belief that some people are less than human? Suggesting that psychiatric hospitals exist in the wake of the plantation therefore raises the question of social death, and to what extent can or should this idea be applied to Black patients in psychiatric hospitals as opposed to enslaved people on the plantation? I could write about the psychiatric experience without reference to the concept of social death—there are enough critiques of psychiatry as a form of social control out there already that make similar claims.[11] But thinking about social death adds an extra analytical tool when it comes to understanding the particular significance of the confinement of Black patients in the South. I am drawing primarily here on Orlando Patterson in his groundbreaking study of slavery, but the concept has been used by others in analyses of the prison system.[12] There are obvious parallels between the modern prison and the psychiatric systems that make this comparison feasible and show the ways that social death has been a continuous and defining aspect of Black life in the wake of slavery. In the analysis to come, I explore the ways that the afterlife of social death as a legacy of slavery lived on in the asylum through the violence and lack of due process around "capture" and admission; the lack of access to rights and protections of the law; removal from family and subsequent dehumanization; the length of time that confinement could last without access to law or appeal; the banality of everyday life, where plantation ideas about the Black body-mind were enacted through lack of therapy and treatment as punishment; and, most obviously, through the violent, forced, and extractive labor to which Black patients were subject.

There has been some debate about the application and consequences of the concept of social death: that it does not sufficiently account for agency or resistance, for survival or life itself, that it adds to dehumanization and revictimization.[13] These are valid critiques if that is all that is said about either plantation or asylum relations, but an analysis of the everyday practices and relationships within the plantation/asylum system can demonstrate the way that social death was both enacted and refigured.[14] At the same time, it is absolutely necessary to document and to lay bare the ways that relationships under Jim Crow replicated and continued the patterns of social death that had been established by and in the wake of the plantation system. To put psychiatry into conversation with slavery is not to say that the asylum is just the plantation but to make clear that the same forces that characterized white supremacy in its most brutal form reverberated a century later, now remade and disguised as therapy. If patients were not slaves exactly (although parts of this book argue that they were treated like them), they were also not entirely free. This is the reality of psychiatric confinement. My goal in this book has been to try to avoid victimization and dehumanization, and to avoid the treatment of the Black body-mind as yet more spectacle. Instead, I strove to clearly document the way that white supremacy continued to work through psychiatric power.[15] Understanding how Black patients, families, communities, and activists responded to the threat of social death posed by inhumane psychiatric practices is the through line of my argument.

A focus on "how" psychiatric power played out in the specific time and place of the mid-twentieth-century South is best evoked not just with theoretical reference to Foucault but with analysis of everyday practices in what Stephen Berrey has called "the Jim Crow routine."[16] In his detailed analysis of everyday life in civil-rights-era Mississippi, Berrey argues that Jim Crow structures were replicated, enforced, and reshaped in an active performance by both Black and white actors. It is not simply that relations of power existed, and were submitted to, but that they were enacted and contested every day in multiple different ways and were shaped by the ways that Black people tried to navigate and negotiate them. At the same time, the threat of both social and literal death, either through incarceration or at the end of the lynching rope, meant that Black folks understood the very real constraints that shaped the possibilities of their resistance, and that they acted accordingly—not out of timid submission but out of a will to live.

One other argument that I try to make throughout this book is that the problem with psychiatry is not that it has been unfortunately racist because of already existing social structures or individual bias, but that it is inherently racist in its origins—that the problem is actually what I am calling "the internal racism of psychiatry." Yes, I am interested in how psychiatric power worked at the intersection with race relations in terms of the structures of segregation, but I am also concerned with how practices within institutions exposed this internal racism of psychiatry. Therefore, this is a book that is deliberately about Black patients only. Terrible things happened to white patients and still do, and I found a great deal more evidence in the archives about white patients than I did Black ones. It would in fact be easier to write a book about the experience of white patients and then discuss how it compared with that of Black patients, but that comparison would be problematic, as it would automatically defer to the power of the archive, privileging the stories that have been deemed worthy of keeping and telling. I am deliberately choosing not to center white stories here as the default position against which the experience of the "other" is measured. I avoid stories about white patients to let the experience of Black patients exist outside the framework of white normalcy, outside the exercise of comparison. Determining whether Black people or white people were treated better does not make any of it acceptable.

Similarly, I am often asked if the Southern institutions I write about are comparable to or any worse than Northern institutions, and while they are probably not, I am not sure what point that comparison serves either. I am not interested in comparisons that make a case for it being better or worse somewhere else, only in trying to excavate what it was like for the most marginalized of the marginal. In this sense, I am informed by Foucault's idea that the point of any historical analysis of psychiatry is to explore *how* that power worked in a particular time and place. Rather than comparing North and South, I am interested in comparing like with like—that is, looking at institutions across the South and teasing out the differences and similarities of experience specific to local contexts using the three neighboring states of Georgia, Alabama, and Mississippi.

As in slavery studies, there has been pressure in the history of psychiatry to find ways to center the patient experience and to read resistance and agency into those stories.[17] This is an important shift in focus and one I try to follow here, but there are challenges and caveats. The possibilities of that approach for this book were limited by the politics and power of the archive, by what stories were originally considered worth recording and keeping, and by the way in which those stories were interpreted. It is also an effect of what artifacts have been kept or made available to the public; these choices are everywhere in this book. This is not the definitive story of three states and their institutions; rather, it is a multitude of stories about the people who inhabited those institutions and how they lived and died in them—stories that stand in for all the stories that are not documented, the stories that I cannot tell.

Putting this argument/book together has not been a straightforward process. I have set out some of the specific challenges posed by the archival sources for this project in appendix 1, but I want to make the point here that these challenges were not just an afterthought or a technical glitch to be worked around. Rather, they became the very foundation for the structure of this book, which has become as much about the process of negotiating the sources as the content they contained. The major challenge was the gaping silence in the archives. This was so endemic that at times I thought of giving up completely. I doubted my ability to say anything meaningful in the face of them. As Trouillot has argued, "Silences enter the process of historical production at four crucial moments: the moment of fact creation (the making of *sources*); the moment of fact assembly (the making of *archives*); the moment of fact retrieval (the making of *narratives*); and the moment of retrospective significance (the making of *history* in the final instance)."[18] If the Black person was not even a person in the context of Southern power in the mid-twentieth century, if the very nature of that personhood was the grounds for contestation over rights, then there was already little chance that the formal archive would have considered the Black "mental patient" a worthy subject of assemblage.

This is especially the case when proper documentation would lay bare the blatant inequities that would challenge the myths of "separate but equal" and the allegedly benign paternalism of segregation (it was not benign). But this silence also reflects the fact that—segregation was about invisibility, and this truth continued into the archive, where the Black noncitizen was relegated to the margins in a kind of archival social death. These people were of no matter in real life, why would it be any different in the archival space? If history is written by the victors, this is particularly the case when it comes to the assemblage of the psychiatric archive, in which both the formal structures of psychiatry and the governments it operates within are interested in creating a particular image of their practices—ordered, fair, procedural, rational—and these are the parameters by which things are deemed worthy of filing in the acid-free folders in the acid-free boxes, the organization of which is part of the ongoing colonial project.

These silences, and my attempts to read between them, have overtly framed the content and structure of this book. It is not a seamless history of "the facts" as they happened, with sources tucked neatly into footnotes, and I cannot pretend otherwise. I was forced to build a story around certain key documents and the sources that did exist, and so I am overt about that process and about my role in interpreting those sources. This approach raised several ethical questions about my own positionality.[19] I am a white person, not American, writing about what was done to Black people by white people in the American South. I am writing about the way white supremacy worked in psychiatry in an attempt to expose the harms of that racism, which live with us still. And if I wanted to just write the history of the policies, then I probably would not think about ethical questions at all. But I am not that kind of historian, and this is not that kind of book. My desire to try to say something about why this history matters to the people who lived through it means that I must pay attention to the harms I may cause by not considering my positionality.

Publishing this book in an open access format does not necessarily solve all my ethical dilemmas, and in some ways, it creates new ones. Given that the book will be freely available to anyone with an Internet connection (and therefore also potentially searchable and scrapable by AI bots), I have to think seriously about the possible afterlives of a digital project both in terms of sustainability and preservation and in terms of future use, over which

I have no control. These are deep ethical questions about what historians owe to the dead when traditionally we may not have thought we owe them anything. Despite my precautions, I cannot avoid the fact that I am a white academic who stands to benefit in some way from the reproduction of the violence and abuse suffered by Black people in the past. Documenting this history is just the first step in a possible act of reparation.[20] But my best hope is that the people whose history this is will see and read this book and will let me know what I have missed and what I got wrong, and might be willing to tell me their story.[21] In that sense, this book is not the end of this history nor is it a definitive one. It is merely a gesture toward the enormity of what I cannot possibly know, the scraping of ice off a massively submerged iceberg.

It is my contention in this book that this iceberg is a form of white supremacy that replicated plantation relations, which were both re-created and reinforced by American psychiatry. My goal here is to take what looks like psychiatric practice not at face value but to place it more clearly in the longer history of the specific time and place in which it was occurring in order to argue that what we see is about more than just psychiatric science, and to deliberately look for continuities between past colonization and plantations and present-day forms of control and confinement. Looking at the way psychiatry was enacted in the South allows for a closer examination of the way that racism was both intrinsic to psychiatric practice and actively enabled by that practice. I am also trying to argue that the nature of Southern society actively shaped the way that psychiatry was practiced *there*; that there are specific continuities that need to be unpacked that continue into the present; and, in the same vein, that there are continuities in the ways that Black families, communities, and patients sought to disrupt the banality of oppression. In other words, there were always possibilities for different choices and decisions, and always the potential for an antiracist psychiatry.

To that end, I start the book with the story of the Tuskegee Veterans Administration Hospital (TVAH), which employed the only Black psychiatrists working in the South. The attempt of the TVAH to provide mental health care in Macon County, Alabama, shows these tensions inherent to psychiatry at the intersection with race and racism in acute detail, offering a clear view into the struggles of Black doctors trying to help Black patients in a white-controlled state.

Part I **Creating Jim Crow in the Asylum**

1 Promoting Mental Health at the Tuskegee Institute

> There is ... no such natural phenomenon as a "Negro personality" or "basic Negro personality" except as a hazy, dubious concept which is based almost entirely on his ability to be readily identified by color or features. While "personality" may be resumed in broad categorical compartments for convenience, it is in fact an integrative blend of a host of attributes, the outstanding feature of which is the uniqueness of behavior which characterizes the individual. Race (genetics) is only one of these attributes.
>
> —Dr. Prince Barker, "Psychoanalysis of Groups"

Dr. Barker well knew that essentialist (and false) ideas about the nature of the Black personality were at least one of the rationalizations that administrators used to justify and maintain segregated psychiatric facilities in the South well into the twentieth century.[1] At the time of the passing of the Civil Rights Act in 1964, Georgia, Alabama, and Mississippi were all still running racially segregated psychiatric systems and showed no intention of ending that practice. In fact, the more progress was made toward civil rights in these states, the more some of them doubled down on what they considered their right to run segregated health-care systems. In the chapters that follow, I look at how a network of confinement, of social and literal death, of abuse, violence, and neglect, was created in the American South, where psychiatry worked to uphold white supremacy.

But in line with the thinking that I set out in the prologue, I have tried to subvert this colonial process in my own writing and in the stories I chose to tell. For this reason, instead of fitting in the approach of Black psychiatrists as an afterthought or as a comparison with that of white physicians, I begin with a look at the Tuskegee Institute in Alabama. To start with Tuskegee is to study the usual process of the history of psychiatry in reverse and to actively decenter white psychiatrists. What white psychiatrists thought about the nature of the Black psyche is telling—and it was powerful. But it was not honest or factual; rather, it was part of the active lies and deception that white supremacy, white America, needed to tell itself about the alterity of Blackness in the aftermath of slavery. While Fanon was writing about sociogeny in the 1950s in the context of the Algerian liberation movement, Black psychiatrists were grappling with similar issues in their own practice in the United States.[2] Most of those psychiatrists worked at the Tuskegee Institute, and their writing about the intersection of race and psychiatry reveals many of the same tensions and concerns that had interested Fanon.

I did not set out to write about Tuskegee in this book. I thought I was writing about asylums in the form of the big state hospital system run and controlled by white people, asylums that operated in the wake of the plantation and formed part of a network of confinement of Black disability. Tuskegee never seemed to fit that bill, until of course I realized that it did. Once I found the material about this hospital, and thought about what it signified, I realized that it was not just part of that system—it was central. Symbolically, Tuskegee was the lens through which the white-run system could be understood because it was at once both its opposite and its reflection, the Black mirror image to the white fantasy. Through Tuskegee, I could see the full impact and violence of segregation—a microcosm of every harm done and at the same time its antidote. It was all the themes of this book distilled into one place, a glimpse into an alternative reality and the potential for a different future, shimmering just out of reach, as if I were Alice through the looking glass.

In fact, it was only when I found the material relating to a small mental health clinic at Tuskegee that the pieces of the rest of the story fell into place. Housed at the Reynolds-Finley Historical Library at the University of Alabama at Birmingham is a collection of *Alabama Mental Health*, a magazine published by the Department of Mental Hygiene beginning in 1949. It contained page after page of stories about the importance of mental health care and the stressors of daily life, all aimed at white people until the sudden appearance of a photo and story about Tuskegee. "Tuskegee Clinic . . . Of, by and for the People" proclaimed the headline on page 1 of the magazine in November 1950. "Every Saturday morning you'll find them mighty busy helping troubled people. . . . From all over Macon County and sometimes from counties nearby, people come—delinquent children, 'nervous' college students, alcoholics, quarreling parents, jobless husbands, ailing wives. They know that the clinic is theirs, regardless of age, sex or ability to pay."[3]

Featured in the accompanying photo (figure 1.1) were Dr. Eugene Dibble, director of the John A. Andrew Memorial Hospital (on the grounds of

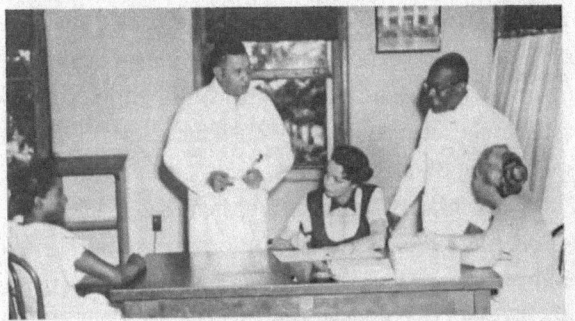

Tuskegee Clinic . . . Of, By And For The People

Every Saturday morning you'll find them mighty busy helping troubled people. For in the Mental Hygiene Clinic in Tuskegee they crowd a lot into the one day each week they are open. From all over Macon County and sometimes from counties nearby, people come — delinquent children, "nervous" college students, alcoholics, quarreling parents, jobless husbands, ailing wives. They know that the clinic is theirs, regardless of age, sex or ability to pay.

Left to right: Patient from Macon County; Dr. H. E. Dibble, Director of John A. Andrew Memorial Hospital; Mrs. Vera Chandler Foster, Social Worker; Dr. P. P. Barker, Psychiatrist; and Mrs. B. B. Walcott, Executive Secretary of the Mental Hygiene Society.

FIGURE 1.1 Tuskegee Mental Hygiene Clinic, *Alabama Mental Health*, November 1950. Courtesy of the Reynolds-Finley Historical Library, University of Alabama at Birmingham.

the Tuskegee Institute), which housed the clinic; Dr. Prince Barker, chief of the Neuropsychiatric Service at the Tuskegee Veterans Administration Hospital, just down the road from the institute, and the clinic's consultant psychiatrist; Vera Chandler Foster, a social worker at the clinic and at the Tuskegee VA Hospital; and Bess Bolden (B. B.) Walcott, executive secretary of the Tuskegee Mental Hygiene Society. According to the article, the society had been formed in 1941 with two distinct aims: "to study the facilities in the various states for the care of the colored mentally ill and . . . to make the Tuskegee community and the outlying county areas mental-hygiene conscious."[4] While these goals had been challenged by the advent of World War II, the members of the society had persisted, and they had finally been able to establish a regular Saturday morning clinic beginning in 1949. The clinic was running on volunteer labor, but the article reported that "the State Public Health Department is now considering a grant to the Tuskegee Clinic to expand its services not only to Macon County but to the state as a whole. The work and plans of the clinic has [sic] been approved and the money will be granted if the present budget will allow it. This clinic is the only one in the state set up specifically to serve our colored people. It certainly deserves our interest and support," wrote the editor.[5]

Over the next few years, *Alabama Mental Health* continued to report on the activity of the clinic, but I found few mentions of it in the state archives. The Tuskegee University Archives were much more forthcoming and revealed a complicated and interesting history. The story of the clinic not only captures a moment when Black clinicians sought to build an active alternative to white-run approaches to mental health but also reveals the complex set of relationships between the state government, the Tuskegee Veterans Hospital (TVAH), the Tuskegee Institute, and the local community. These relationships in turn provide a unique lens through which to view the development of psychiatric services in the South after World War II, which centers the perspective of Black clinicians.

Scholarship about Black psychiatrists and mental health services, especially in the postwar period, has tended to focus on Northern or borderland hospitals or clinics, often where most of the care and administration was still undertaken by white people.[6] In contrast, the Tuskegee clinic was fully run and staffed by Black clinicians, and those clinicians spanned both the North and the South, often traveling north to undertake further study or internships and bringing that knowledge back to Tuskegee. The ways they engaged with psychiatric ideas and practices, and applied those ideas in their local practice, can reveal a great deal about the possibilities for, and limitations to, an antiracist psychiatry.

Focusing on the people and practices of the Tuskegee Mental Hygiene Clinic also demonstrates the way that Black intellectuals needed to navigate Jim Crow segregation and the role that psychiatric discourses played in that process. The clinic existed *because of* the South's totalizing racial segregation, and its physicians were aware of that fact. They understood that segregation was a double-edged sword for them—it allowed a measure of autonomy and facilitated Black leadership, but it also placed them outside many opportunities for professional growth and funding, and potentially at the margins of rapidly evolving psychiatric thinking.

They were also aware of the ways that these evolving discourses and practices could themselves be inherently racist and deployed in the arguments about segregation, at the same time as they offered the promise of scientific solutions to real mental health problems. They were also reminded, at least daily, of their position as Black medical men in the violent and segregated South. As Susan Reverby has shown, this tension between their reality as Black men and their education and training as scientists permeated all the health work that emerged from the place called Tuskegee.[7] This tension lay at the heart of the institute and the TVAH's involvement with the untreated syphilis study, and it also existed in their approach to psychiatric work. In the same way that we need to understand the syphilis study, we need to understand the mental health work at Tuskegee as more than a simple victim–complicit partner binary. But most importantly, we need to understand the work of Black psychiatrists like Dr. Barker as an attempted corrective to the racism inherent in psychiatric discourses and practices in the South.

In his attempt to bring psychiatric services to the people of Macon County, Barker was attempting to take seriously the anxieties and stressors of Black patients and to situate them in the very real context of life in the segregated South. In doing so, he tried to create a viable alternative to the state hospital system, which was overwhelmingly controlled by white people and based on racist and eugenic ideas about the alleged inferiority of the Black psyche—ideas that were used to justify continued segregation.

Contesting Racism in Southern Psychiatry

Long after Northern states had begun to make attempts at hospital integration, segregation persisted in the South. It proved hard to dislodge not just because of long-running racist attitudes about the Black psyche but because of the structural arrangement and organization of the various systems and the policies that supported them. These structures and policies acted as part of a broader network of confinement, in which psychiatry and various forms of incarceration were interchangeable. They also reflected long-held beliefs that stretched back to the days of the plantation. The fear of the "Negro insane" and the persistent belief in differences between Black and white psyches had shaped the origins of the asylum and been reinforced through various reform movements. The so-called father of modern psychiatric institutions, Thomas Kirkbride, made it clear that integration "is not what is wanted in our hospitals for the insane," and Kirkbride and his peers reacted violently to the limited integration practiced by renegade John M. Galt, superintendent of the Eastern Lunatic Asylum in Virginia.[8] These debates had shaped the way that the state hospitals in Alabama, Georgia, and Mississippi were built and expanded, and thus also shaped the way that Tuskegee physicians and Black Southerners interacted with the mental health system.

The Tuskegee Mental Hygiene Clinic was located at the center of this complicated network, which was designed to replicate and reinforce segregation. Operating from the John A. Andrew Memorial Hospital at the Tuskegee Institute, the clinic was only 40 miles from the state capital of Montgomery; 200 miles northeast of Searcy Hospital, just outside Mobile; and about 170 miles southeast of Bryce Hospital in Tuscaloosa. Bryce and Searcy were the only other public mental health facilities in Alabama, and they were deeply, indelibly segregated.[9] From 1909, most of Alabama's Black patients were admitted directly to Searcy Hospital, while Bryce continued to take the state's white patients. Children with a physical or mental disability were admitted to the Partlow School and Hospital, which was located on the grounds of Bryce at Tuscaloosa and took both Black and white children but kept them entirely separate from each other. In Mississippi, by comparison, Black patients were only admitted to Whitfield Hospital, twenty miles southeast of Jackson, but were confined to one-half of the campus. In Georgia, Black patients were admitted to the massive Central State Hospital in Milledgeville and confined to run-down buildings at the rear of the campus. I will explore in more detail how these particular hospitals worked in chapter 2.

The other major system providing institutional mental health care across the South was the Veterans Administration. The Tuskegee VA Hospital was one of the few places in the country, and the only place in Alabama (or the broader South), that would employ or train Black physicians and psychiatrists. But this, too, was shaped by debates about segregation and conflicting ideas about who should be in charge of providing care to Black patients.[10] The NAACP had originally opposed the idea of a veterans hospital dedicated to the care of Black patients only, especially when located "in the lynching belt of mob-ridden Alabama," and both the NAACP and the National Medical Association (NMA) were disappointed and outspoken about the early compromises that placed white professionals in charge of both management and everyday care of patients at the new facility in Tuskegee.[11] White support for the facility was initially based on concerns for the white community, who argued, "The negro insane are a danger and they are much more liable to be a danger to white than to negro."[12] But that support was also premised on the demand for managerial control of the institution, out of an insistence that any white person who worked there could not be under the supervision of a Black manager.

Despite the NAACP's opposition, the NMA recognized the reality of a lack of services for Black veterans in the South, as well as a lack of training op-

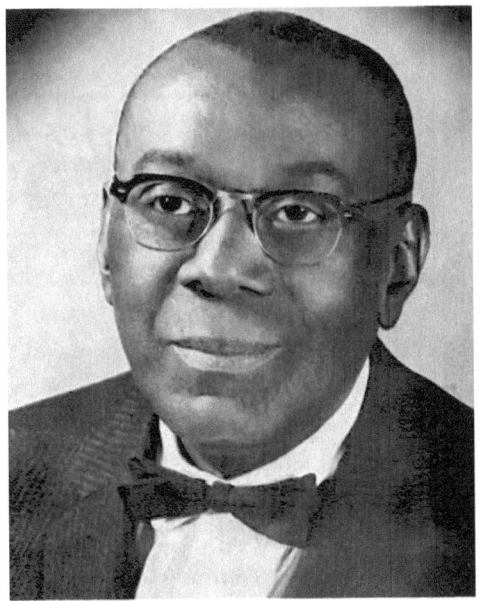

FIGURE 1.2 Dr. Prince Patanilla Barker, 1959. Photo from Retirement Celebration Program, box 18, file 2, Correspondence: Dr. Prince Barker, Dibble Papers.

portunities, and argued that it was better to compromise initially and push for change later. Their tactics worked; within four years, the Tuskegee VA Hospital was managed and staffed entirely by Black physicians, nurses, attendants, and laborers. This initial segregation was a double-edged sword, however. While it meant a guarantee of jobs at Tuskegee for Black practitioners (which, the NAACP argued, was too high a price to pay), the existence of Tuskegee as a separate Black-only institution meant the possible marginalization of both clinicians and patients.[13]

Yet the TVAH was also home to some of the best-trained psychiatrists, Black or white, in the country. The first cohort who arrived in the 1920s were trained by renowned neuropsychiatrist Solomon Carter Fuller at the Boston University School of Medicine.[14] They were Toussaint Tildon, who had just graduated from Harvard Medical School; Simon Overton Johnson, who had received formal psychiatric training at both the London National Hospital and the famous Salpêtrière in Paris; and George Branche, who received his psychiatric training at the Boston Psychopathic Hospital.[15] In 1924 the team was joined by Dr. Prince Barker (figure 1.2), who graduated from Howard Medical School; interned at both Freedmen's Hospital and St. Elizabeths in Washington, D.C.; and then studied further at the Northport VA in New York and at Columbia University.[16]

Barker was an active scholar, like many of the Tuskegee clinicians, publishing his early work on neurosyphilis and the importance of understanding the connection between neuropsychiatric symptoms and medical/surgical problems.[17] He engaged with the neuropsychiatric work emerging from the war effort to consider the use of insulin shock therapy for the treatment of returned soldiers at the Tuskegee VA Hospital, presenting this work at the American Psychiatric Association meeting in 1941.[18]

In his writing, Barker was always careful to avoid unproblematized racialization of illness, and he actively campaigned against the idea that there was anything biologically or psychologically inferior or even different about the Black race. In his work on insulin shock treatment, for example, he argued that it was contraindicated for most of the patients because of the danger it posed to people with arteriosclerosis. If that disease was prevalent at the TVAH, it was not because of anything inherent to "the Negro race" but was more likely attributable to the social conditions under which Black veterans had lived since youth.[19] These were conditions marked by poverty and racial hostility, which shaped the lives of Barker's patients long before he encountered them. Barker went so far in this article as to argue that in fact not nearly enough attention had been paid to these environmental influences on the "Negro personality," and that white social scientists had a tendency to make assertions about a group of people about whom they knew nothing.[20]

Barker took up these thoughts again in a short article critiquing the highly influential work of white psychiatrists Abram Kardiner and Lionel Ovesey in their book *The Mark of Oppression: A Psychosocial Study of the American Negro*. His sharp critique of the book took aim at the methods, assumptions, and conclusions that Kardiner and Ovesey drew from their small Northern sample. For example, Barker argued that "racial personality, basic or otherwise, is probably as erroneous an assumption as racial vulnerability or immunity to disease. This has been disproved for the Negro. The only disease, that comes to mind, to which the Negro seems genetically susceptible is sickle cell anemia. This increased susceptibility to tuberculosis seems, for example, due not to race genetically considered, but to his relatively unfavorable economic status and to the fact that he has been more recently exposed, and has not had as long a time as the Caucasian to build up immunity."[21] He also argued that the authors' findings of "a lack of spontaneity" in their Black subjects needed to be understood both in the context of the power relations of the study itself and as an effect of life in America's stifling "bi-racial system."[22] More than anything, he argued, Black patients were human beings. Informed by these ideas and his interest in psychotherapy as a treatment method, Barker turned his attention to providing services to local residents around Tuskegee. In order to do so, however, he needed to engage with the potentially problematic underpinnings of mental hygiene.

Negotiating Eugenics and Mental Hygiene

When Barker opted for a mental hygiene approach to outreach work, he was also engaging with the longer history of eugenics. Eugenic thinking was central to the development of the New South in the early twentieth century and was responsible for a complex network of policy and medical practices designed to eradicate so-called social problems along race, ethnicity, and class lines.[23] These policies had particular consequences for approaches to Black mental health. The intertwining of eugenics with public health practices in the South led to the easy conflation of feeble-mindedness with criminality. Combined with hierarchies at the intersection of race, class, and gender, the new conceptualization of disability enabled a shift away from a concern with rehabilitation, as historian Gregory Dorr has argued, to the idea that "those with physical or mental impairments (were) less as a class to be rehabilitated and more . . . a dangerous group in need of control."[24]

This was particularly evident in states like Alabama, where the superintendent of the children's state school and hospital, William Dempsey Partlow, continually advocated for the broadening of eugenic sterilization laws. Partlow argued that "feeble-mindedness" was hereditary and needed to be bred out like disease from cattle.[25] He urged the state to create a special bureau for "mental hygiene and eugenics," unproblematically blending the two concepts together.[26] As late as 1935, Partlow tried to pass a state law that would allow the mandatory sterilization of all institutionalized people considered mentally deficient, as well as a host of others, including imprisoned criminals with "sexual perversion" and people with "constitutional psychopathic personalities."[27] The Alabama House and Senate passed the bill in 1935, but Governor Bibb Graves vetoed it, fearing the risks from surgery. Nevertheless, Partlow was happy to report that he had already sterilized more than 200 boys and girls at the "state school" that came to bear his name.[28]

The wide net that Partlow, and others like him, sought to cast was based on a very broad definition of "deficiency," which reflected the nature of psychiatry in the early twentieth century. Even though most physicians and psychiatrists differentiated (sometimes crudely in this earlier period) between mental illness and mental deficiency, attitudes toward treatment and care of both were underpinned by eugenic thinking to the extent that they were perceived as inheritable disorders—through either genetics or family patterns of behavior—which led to unethical and involuntary forced sterilizations.[29] These attitudes were compounded in places where "mental illness" and "mental deficiency" were treated in the same space, which was usually the case in the South because of the reliance on single large institutions. For the Black patient, this was particularly problematic because of the existing tendency to conflate Blackness with intellectual and emotional inferiority (and therefore disability). This made it particularly easy for white supremacists to make a case for eugenics when Blackness and madness were posed as a threat to white society.[30] If social segregation and Black codes worked to control the threat of miscegenation in everyday life, then the network of confinement created by institutions like prisons and psychiatric hospitals were designed to take care of everyone else.

Beyond its association with eugenics, however, mental hygiene as a movement always had community-based initiatives at its core. In its origins, it was designed to address the social conditions that could be considered precursors to mental illness, and therefore its practitioners ostensibly recognized the environmental stressors that were believed to contribute to mental illness.[31] While it may still have been "eugenic" in that its supporters also believed that the onset of illness was often related to underlying genetic weakness or poor lifestyle choices, it was not the same as formal eugenics because practitioners argued that society was as much to blame, and that given the right skills and tools, people could be treated for mild mental health issues before they became acute, requiring hospitalization.

This was especially the case when dealing with children, and it led to the development of the child guidance movement, which sought to educate parents about the "correct" way to bring up a healthy, happy child—one particularly fit for American middle-class life.[32] In this sense, mental hygiene and child guidance were intricately linked with white, patriarchal, heteronormative patterns of behavior and set rigid limits of the idea of "normal," from which Black people were almost automatically excluded.

Despite its historically problematic connotations, however, the idea of mental hygiene proved a useful vehicle for Tuskegee physicians and coincided with the general principles that had informed the racial uplift work of the institute.[33] The ideology of racial uplift meshed well with mental hygiene because it enabled a framework for an understanding of the social elements that structured African American mental well-being and focused on the impact of racism, stress, and anxiety rather than on racial difference. In this way, "positive eugenics," racial uplift, and mental hygiene can be understood as ways that Black clinicians sought to resist the totalizing rhetoric of racial inferiority. Rather, it often became a tool of Black liberation.[34] Black psychiatrists at Tuskegee engaged with public health because they believed in the science and because they wanted to take advantage of anything that could improve the lives of local Black communities.[35]

But they also applied these concepts in particular ways. They engaged with the evolving sciences of psychiatry and psychology in a manner that took Black mental health seriously.[36] And they used those ideas to argue that the "Negro problem" was not one of their making, and neither was it one of built-in genetic pathology. Rather, the "psy-sciences" (psychology, psychiatry, and psychotherapy) could be used by Black clinicians and Black patients to help deal with the very real stress of everyday life in the segregated South and to explain mental health issues as the consequence of structural issues, not genetic inferiority.[37] If studies by white people that sought to understand the nature of the Black psyche did so purely to reinforce already existing prejudices and assumptions of difference and inferiority rather than to provide actual help to the people who needed it, Black psychiatrists themselves tried to do something entirely different.[38]

The motivation to help people deal with social pressures was clearly evident in Barker's work on mental hygiene. In 1946, he wrote explicitly about the benefits of mental hygiene for all people, regardless of skin color, and for understanding the dynamics of human relationships as both individuals and groups.[39] He explicitly made reference to the impact of race relations in the United States, where "we as Negroes are naturally interested in how adverse group tensions react on Negro mental health."[40] Mental hygiene was therefore a broad framework through which to understand the psychodynamics of human relationships and to take seriously the stress and anxiety caused by those relationships.

Rather than blaming individuals for weakness, Barker argued that "no personality is so strong that it may not need some of the good offices of mental hygiene."[41] The added benefit of a mental hygiene approach for Barker was that it was applicable and useful outside "the old state hospitals" and provided a more humane approach to the "mild mental or nervous disorders" that could be treated before they required hospitalization. He also argued that mental hygiene could help to break down stigma about mental health and illness because it could demystify the science of psychiatry and make it clear that there was no such thing as good or bad people, just illness like any other.[42]

In Barker's work, psychodynamic and somatic approaches coexisted, as he sought to combine neuropsychiatric science with Freudian analytical insights. But there is a tension in this eclectic approach as it was used in the Mental Hygiene Clinic, which brought the Tuskegee psychiatrists into conflict with the state department of public health and demonstrated the limits of their ability to create alternative spaces for mental health care.

Creating Alternative Spaces

World War II had interfered with the momentum for the outpatient clinic, but the end of the war brought with it new energy—and new money—for mental health work. In 1946, Congress passed the National Mental Health Act, which enabled an appropriation for the establishment of the National Institute of Mental Health (NIMH). The need for a coordinated approach to mental health work and for more research had been made obvious by the impact of war on American society through the vast amount of "combat neurosis" and postwar anxiety. In the 1940s and 1950s, psychiatrists became experts on the state of the nation's emotional and mental health, now posed as a security risk and thus a concern for practitioners and legislators alike.

Beginning in the late 1940s, the NIMH combined with the GI Bill to make various funding schemes available for the education of psychiatrists, psychologists, and nurses, as well as the advancement of related research. However, most of these new initiatives remained closed to Black clinicians, frustrating many aspiring professionals. This situation was further cemented by the passing of the Hill-Burton Act in 1946. Co-sponsored by Senator Lister Hill of Alabama, Hill-Burton allowed for continued construction of segregated medical and psychiatric facilities with federal money provided that "equal" services, or access to them, were made available for Black patients.[43]

In this swirl of activity, which demonstrated clearly that Black psychiatrists were on their own, the Tuskegee group gathered to take up the issue of the Mental Hygiene Clinic again. In September 1947, Tuskegee Mental Hygiene Society president Sarah Howell distributed a memo throughout the Tuskegee community inviting anyone with an interest in mental health to attend a meeting with the society's executive committee. The aim of the meeting was to discuss a proposal for a regular outpatient Mental Hygiene Clinic to be held at the John A. Andrew Memorial Hospital (or the John A., as it was often called) with the cooperation of the hospital's director, Dr. Dibble.

In the memo, Howell wrote that the establishment of the clinic "will be a definite contribution to the health of this community. . . . This request is being addressed to those whom we feel will recognize the importance of this contribution and the obligation inherent upon us to contribute our special talents to the amelioration of human suffering."[44] This is an important recognition of the impact that mental health concerns were having on the local Black community. Initial clinics were sporadic, however, due to a lack of infrastructure and support staff, and as volunteers, there was only so much Barker and his colleagues could do. It is also not clear what the initial commitment from Dibble was; given the desire to have the clinic at the John A. rather than onsite at the VA, it was imperative that Dibble, who moved across both institutions, was able to support the clinic physically and financially.

Barker began negotiations with Dr. Jack Jarvis from the state's Division of Mental Hygiene, who seemed friendly to the Tuskegee Mental Hygiene Society. Their correspondence demonstrates that Barker and Jarvis both knew that someone would need to be paid to run the clinic properly rather than it relying on unsupported volunteer labor from the TVAH, and the Alabama Department of Public Health indicated it was willing to pay for a medical or psychiatric social worker with a master's degree. But Jarvis made it clear that if the state was going to pay, it would make the social worker an employee of the state health department, subject to its rules, regulations, and policies—policies that discriminated against Black employees.

But more than a year later, no formal agreement had been reached. A memo from Dibble to Barker and the Mental Hygiene Society in the spring of 1949 revealed some of the underlying tensions between the institute and the state department. Dibble wrote that he believed that running the clinic on a volunteer basis initially was preferable to taking money from the state, and he went on to say that even though both the VA and the US Public Health Service (USPHS) were willing to support the clinic, "it is further believed that if we can get something started on our own, without any help from the state or federal government, the clinic would be under the control of a private hospital rather than under the control of any agency."[45] This is an interesting comment from Dibble, given what we now know about his cooperation with federal agencies like the USPHS in relation to the Tuskegee syphilis study.[46] Perhaps here we see an admission that cooperating with the US Public Health Service is a poisoned chalice for the Tuskegee Institute, and it certainly indicates Dibble's hesitance to work with the Alabama state government.

As director of the state's new efforts to provide community-based outpatient preventive mental health care that had *no* plan for Black communities, Jarvis must have known that the group at Tuskegee was his best and only chance of getting a clinic happening for the Black community. However, in all his proposals he continued to insist that the state have complete control over hiring, while the Tuskegee group wanted someone already known to them. The group also argued for a medical social worker rather than a strictly psychiatric one (these were very rare in the Black psychological workforce).

The state department eventually prevailed, but with a compromise. From August to December 1950, Dibble met repeatedly with Jarvis, and in February 1951, an agreement was made to supply funds for a full-time social worker and a stenographer; to pay for supplies, equipment, and travel; and to reimburse the VA psychiatrists for their time. However, the institute continued to rebuff Jarvis's suggestions for who to employ, continuing to prefer people with connections to the local community rather than bringing in outsiders. The continued attempts of the VA and the institute's clinicians and management to control their own practices was consistent with community expectations, as they sought to rebuff attempts from the white physicians and bureaucrats in the state government to interfere with Tuskegee's hard-fought autonomy.

Service to the local community was the first and primary motivation of the Tuskegee group, but the impact of that service has been difficult to quantify. No one I spoke to at Tuskegee had a distinct memory of the clinic, although they did remember some names, especially B. B. Walcott for her work with Black disability organizations and the Red Cross, and Vera Chandler Foster, as the wife of the Tuskegee Institute's president. There is no single set of records related to the running of the clinic, and the archives of the Veterans Administration Hospital, where they may exist, are not available to the public. A search of the state health officer's files at the Alabama Department of Archives and History did not reveal any real trace of the clinic at all, meaning that if Jarvis kept his correspondence with Dibble and Barker, it is not in the state archives now. There are, however, copies of regular reports submitted by the social workers who ran the clinic, and they demonstrate the breadth of community and outreach work undertaken, as well as the ways that individual community members engaged with the clinic.

Beginning in March 1951, the first social worker, Vera Chandler Foster, submitted regular reports to both the state government and Dibble, detailing the ways that the clinic was making itself available on Monday and Wednesday afternoons, attended by rotating physicians from the TVAH and by herself as social worker. In the first month alone, she conducted forty-eight interviews with patients and families, and referred people to the psychiatrist only when the issue was beyond her scope. She wrote, "It is usual that the larger number of patients are seen by the social worker, inasmuch as history-taking is routine; also a considerable proportion of problems are amenable to case-work treatment without referral to a psychiatrist."[47] She reported that patients who could afford it paid fifty cents for their attendance at the clinic, and that she had worked with a number of students at the Tuskegee Institute as a kind of counseling service as students prepared to undertake professional internships. She reported, "In this connection one fourth (five) of the twenty students sought the social worker's assistance with a variety of emotional problems related to sex, marriage and family relationships. One student indicated a desire for psychiatric help upon his return from internship."[48]

Foster and Barker also conducted extensive public outreach and education activities. In April 1951 alone, they gave multiple talks, including at a local teachers meeting about the relevance of a mental health program for schools; showed the film *Palmour Street* and spoke about children's well-being to three separate PTA groups; spoke to the Tuskegee Women's Club about "government and family life"; distributed leaflets at the Tuskegee Institute Food Show (which had 2,800 attendants) titled *Emotional Nutrition for Good Mental Health*; ran a study group on the "psychiatrists evaluation of religion in the present crisis for professional persons interested in human relations"; and ran an exhibit during that year's weeklong Clinical Society meeting.[49]

While the clinic, especially the social worker, spent a great deal of time and energy undertaking preventive outreach and education work, especially as part of National Mental Health Week, the psychiatrists also saw themselves as responsible for active treatment of people with symptomatic illness. From its inception, the proposed budget for the clinic included psychological tests and a sum for the purchase of an "electric shock machine."[50] The inclusion of an electroshock machine speaks to the particular ways that the Tuskegee psychiatrists understood their role and the purposes of the clinic, which went far beyond education and outreach work. The VA psychiatrists, fully trained in a myriad of approaches, would have seen no reason why they were not entitled to act to the full scope of their authority in the clinical setting, and the inclusion of electroshock reflects an attempt to set their own therapeutic and clinical agenda. It could also be surmised that in doing so, the clinic psychiatrists were deliberately working to provide services in the outpatient setting that would normally only be available with hospitalization as a way to circumvent that hospitalization. But this approach quicky brought them into conflict with the state department of public health.

In 1952, the clinic's new social worker, Ethel Harvey, attended a meeting of the state mental health services in Birmingham run by Mary Belle Roberts, the state's chief psychiatric social worker. On her return, Harvey wrote a memo to the Tuskegee Mental Hygiene Society stating that the thinking of the state program was that "the main emphasis on the program's clinic services should be children. The time should not be spent on those children who are pathologically inferior. . . . Those persons needing intensive therapy are not the kind of the patients to be seen in our mental hygiene clinics at present. Generally, there should be no physical treatment in our clinics, all treatment should be purely psychotherapy. It was the thinking of the group that electroshock should be a part of the state hospital system."[51] Harvey herself did not comment on the use of the term "pathologically inferior"; given the role of positive eugenics in racial uplift work (including at Tuskegee), it would not necessarily be shocking for her to accept that idea. Roberts reiterated the state's position in a letter to Barker dated December 22, 1952. She argued, "It has been the position of the State Department of Public Health that shock treatment is the responsibility of a hospitalization program, rather than a mental hygiene clinic. The in-take policies for the mental hygiene clinic have been conceived as a preventive rather than a curative approach to mental health problems. Many communities have found it necessary to think in terms of hospitalization programs and hospital extramural services for some kinds of mental illnesses"[52]

For Black communities, of course, the idea of hospitalization was a last resort. Regular citizens could not be admitted to the TVAH, but would have been committed to Searcy, the one and only psychiatric hospital taking Black patients. The TVAH psychiatrists were well aware of the nature of state hospitals and fully cognizant of the lack of treatment options and potential for abuse of Black patients. Admitting people there was to be avoided, and the use of electroshock by the clinic's physicians can be understood as an active attempt to create an alternative space for treatment outside the state hospital.

At the same time, the state's insistence on the delineation between preventive and treatment work demonstrates a kind of paternalism inherent to the state's approach to the Black physicians, who by virtue of their Blackness could not possibly be considered more competent than the state's white physicians (even when they obviously were). But it also demonstrates the state's belief in its sole authority to administer somatic treatments to Black bodies. Outside the Tuskegee VA, there was not a single Black clinician applying an electroshock machine to Black patients. The administration of a painful and violent technology by white clinicians to Black patients, and the state's insistence that it was the only entity authorized to undertake the practice, was a symbolic and literal reminder of the power of the state to exercise control over Black bodies.

The physicians of the Tuskegee clinic also interacted with other institutional spaces in Alabama in ways that demonstrate attempts at and limits to psychiatric autonomy and authority. Beyond the weekly outpatient clinic, the VA psychiatrists were also involved with the nearby Alabama Industrial School for Negro Children, also known as Mt. Meigs. Mt. Meigs was located about twenty-five miles west of Tuskegee on the road to Montgomery, and had been initially established by Margaret Murray Washington, Booker T. Washington's third wife, but came under the purview of the state of Alabama from about 1911. While its staff and superintendent were a mix of white and Black, it reported to the state departments of education and public health.[53]

Barker had been trying to forge a relationship with the industrial school for some time and had been rebuffed, but in 1952, Ethel Harvey managed to convince new leadership in the state department of public health that the Tuskegee Mental Hygiene Clinic should visit Mt. Meigs to run in-service training for staff there and also assess some of the children. The details of these visits are patchy in the official records, but two clinical notes in the papers of Eugene Dibble tell us something about the ability of the VA psychiatrists to intervene in the developing school-to-prison pipeline system.

For example, one note states, "A student from Mt. Meigs Industrial School for Negro Children has been evaluated in the Mental Hygiene Clinic and it is recommended that this 16-year-old child 1. receive long term close supervision when discharged from the industrial school [and] 2. that she receive care and education for [the] mental deficient."[54] The second note concerns an eighteen-year-old woman, "a student of Mt. Meigs industrial school for negro children," who had been evaluated by the Mental Hygiene Clinic from May 20, 1954, to August 5, 1954. The note states, "It is our conclusion that this person is mentally retarded and that her sexual delinquency is dependent upon her poor intelligence status. It would seem to us that this girl will need prolonged institutional care for her own self-protection, but she could be assigned vocational tasks commensurate with her limited intellectual capacity. Diagnosis 1. Mental Deficiency[,] 2. Sexual Deviation (promiscuity)."[55] Unfortunately, for an eighteen-year-old, that institution would most likely have been Searcy Hospital. There are no other notes about these or any other children, but in these two notes and the relationship between the TVAH and Mt. Meigs, there are several tensions playing out.

First there is the tension between the TVAH and the state in that Alabama public health officials were reluctant to have Black physicians present at Mt. Meigs at all. Barker's attempts to have TVAH psychiatrists visit Mt. Meigs demonstrates his concern that the care provided to "students" there was not therapeutic or versed in psychological methods. And the consistent refusal of the state to allow access to the TVAH psychiatrists can be understood as both racial and professional gatekeeping. In the same way that the Mental Hygiene Clinic was scolded for its use of electroshock, the TVAH psychiatrists were not initially welcome at Mt. Meigs because of assumptions that Black clinicians could not possibly bring any new knowledge or practices. But more importantly, Black clinicians could not be allowed to see, or to interfere in, the discipline that white authorities felt was theirs to mete out to wayward Black youth.

Later in the 1950s, public concerns about the conditions at all the state's industrial training schools eased the path for Tuskegee physicians a little, and they continued to provide both psychological and medical consultative services well into the 1960s.[56] But the situation at Mt. Meigs also raises questions about the extent to which Black physicians were able to meaningfully challenge the punitive nature of that institution and its link to further institutionalization. While in the case of the sixteen-year-old, the clinicians were able to recommend continued outpatient services, the eighteen-year-old was consigned to further institutionalization because of "sexual delinquency." In that recommendation, there is tension between the professional and social identities of the physicians, in that sometimes Black psychiatrists were psychiatrists first, activists second. Their clinical training and the nature of prevailing scientific knowledge and practice meant that the "out of control" disabled Black body was still perceived as needing to be confined, echoing the eugenic practices of previous decades.

Nevertheless, Barker continued his attempts to bring psychoanalytic and preventive mental health approaches to his outreach work. He had support from influential white Northerners in this endeavor. For example, during the annual Clinical Society meeting in 1954, Dr. Karl Menninger—one of the founders of the Winter Veterans Administration Hospital in Topeka, Kansas—paid the Tuskegee physicians a visit. Menninger spent a few days at Tuskegee, dining with Dibble and Barker and giving lectures and talks at the Clinical Society gathering. He also had a private discussion with Barker about the latest thinking in psychoanalytical methods and later offered them a doctor who might visit to help train TVAH staff in group psychotherapy for the inpatient population. Menninger also offered the possibility of rotating some Tuskegee staff with Winter VA staff for a few months at a time so that the two groups could learn from each other and so the Winter VA could support the work Barker and others were trying to do at Tuskegee.[57]

Menninger himself was stunned and impressed by what he saw at Tuskegee, and he told the federal VA so in a long letter dated April 13, 1954, which he copied to Dibble. The letter was addressed to Admiral Joel T. Boone, chief medical director of the VA, and Menninger was gushing in his praise. "I scarcely know where to begin my report," he wrote. "Tuskegee is one of the most amazing phenomena I have ever seen."[58] He extolled the level of skill and training and the vast amount of community service the Tuskegee psychiatrists sought to provide in very difficult circumstances. He admired their enthusiasm and commitment to new ideas, but he also noted the difficulties they faced, which all stemmed from segregation. Although he noted that relations with the Montgomery VA were cordial and "progressive," and that the Tuskegee VA did take white patients, he lamented the fact that the Tuskegee clinicians were ostracized from formal professional associations. They were also not permitted to undertake rotations at other VAs, nor did white consultants ever spend time at Tuskegee—apart from certain physicians from Emory University in Atlanta, which bothered Menninger because "the theory and practices of the group at Emory are in considerable disfavor among large numbers of the psychiatric profession, and the staff at Tuskegee know this."[59] Menninger offered his own staff as residents or interns and followed through on his offer to Barker of rotations to the Winter VA.

But Menninger's comments ultimately came to nothing. Admiral Boone himself visited Tuskegee in November 1954, but Dibble kept no record of their conversation in his files. Dibble and Menninger continued to maintain a casual correspondence, and in 1959, Dibble wrote, "We have not moved as fast as we would like in psychiatry. The prospects are that we are not going to get a career resident coming back this year, and we hope that the stimulus that we so much needed in psychiatry will be provided and the problems will be licked."[60] Dibble wrote this as major reform and spending efforts were underway across the South through the Mental Health Training and Research Program of the Southern Regional Education Board, but there was no seat at this table for anyone from Tuskegee.[61] As usual, white systems promised much and delivered little, proving Dibble's initial distrust well founded. Inertia at the state level, a deepening resistance to desegregation following the *Brown v. Board of Education* decision, and the utter failure of the American Psychiatric Association to address the racism and segregation within its own structures impeded any possibility of major structural change in Southern psychiatry.

Dr. Prince Barker retired from Tuskegee in 1959 and published a short article in the *Journal of the National Medical Association* in 1962, looking back over his experience in Macon County. He noted the way that Tuskegee psychiatrists, despite their exclusion from so many professional opportunities, had developed treatment programs that "paralleled progress elsewhere in neuropsychiatry."[62] From insulin shock to psychosurgery to ECT, followed by the advent of psychotropic medication, "scores of patients previously inaccessible, were rendered available for a variety of therapeutic measures."[63] The TVAH itself ran a program based explicitly on the concept of a therapeutic milieu, "non-authoritarian, permissive, and with the entire organization geared to provide the best therapeutic atmosphere for patient improvement."[64] An overt commitment to these principles put the Tuskegee VA well in advance of most other public institutions in the United States at this point in time, and definitely positioned the TVAH as the best possible place for treatment for Black patients in the state of Alabama.

Barker was particularly proud of the active attempts being made to more fully integrate both Black and white patients and clinicians at the TVAH. "No insuperable problems have been encountered. Desegregation of staffs by the Veterans Administration outside the South has opened opportunities hitherto closed to Negroes. . . . An integrated Tuskegee . . . is a pending reality. History has seldom traveled a longer road in 38 years," he concluded.[65] These comments would prove telling, however, given the lengths to which the state government in Alabama would go to maintain segregation in the state hospital system, and their continued failure to support the Mental Hygiene Clinic at Tuskegee in the wake of the Community Mental Health Act of 1963.[66]

On their own, individual efforts at Tuskegee had not been enough to ameliorate the racism that continued to pervade attempts to provide mental health care for Black Alabamians. Yet in an analysis of the work of Barker and the Mental Hygiene Clinic, there was a moment when despite the challenges, Black psychiatrists, social workers, and nurses—some of the most well-trained people in the country—worked to carve out a space for meaningful mental health care for Black patients. In the work of the clinic and the ideas of its clinicians, Black psychiatrists attempted to stay abreast of the latest thinking and clinical practice, and to provide alternative forms of care outside the asylum walls. The Tuskegee group stands out as a psychological oasis in the Southern racist desert, but it also demonstrates the debilitating and alienating effects of segregation. For patients caught in the state system, the situation was dire.

2 Enabling Segregation

> So far the peckerwoods have given me no trouble, but that doesn't fool me. This is an insane asylum and one must act as if one were among maniacs. They are likely to become violent at any time. . . .
> Incidentally, Mississippi boasts of having the world's largest and finest insane asylum!!! It is indeed palatial and is jammed with Negroes.
> —George Schuyler to Louis T. Wright, October 2, 1935

If the psychiatrists at Tuskegee were working hard to ameliorate the racist tendencies of the psychiatric system in the South, other Black thinkers were more pessimistic. Schuyler was a satirist, and this letter was possibly also satire.[1] But this communication with Wright, who was well established as a surgeon at Harlem Hospital at the time, demonstrates the tensions in trying to understand the relationship between Black communities and psychiatry. As a Black journalist and novelist, Schuyler's work was not just critical of white supremacy but also at times critical of the way Black people seemed to be complicit in their own oppression.[2] He had less than generous thoughts about the Black folks of Mississippi, and in the rest of his letter he bemoans their tendency to defend or want to stay in the South. Satire or not, his point about white violence is important and reminds us of the true nature of Jim Crow relations, especially as it intersects with psychiatry. Many times during the research for this book I encountered a rhetoric of hatred and violence spewing from the pens of white people arguing for the continued oppression and isolation of their Black neighbors. Schuyler's letter speaks to this broad atmosphere of simmering rage that pervaded "the closed society" and reminds us that segregation, while posed as natural and desired by all, was in fact a deliberate and determined tactic of white supremacy aimed at the oppression and exploitation of the Black body, maintained by the violence of the gun and the lynching rope.[3]

Psychiatric spaces and practices were not exempt from this violence; in fact, it shaped almost every aspect of daily life in the institution, as did the unquestioned fact of segregation. The idea that Black and white bodies and minds, especially disabled ones and especially in the intimate setting of the hospital, needed to be segregated was linked most obviously to eugenic hysteria about "feeble-mindedness" and race mixing. But it was also linked to the desired impact of segregation as a social structure, which ensured that Black people were excluded from the full rights of citizenship and health itself, enduring vastly inferior medical services.

Segregation in the asylum was not a perverse anomaly but a deliberate tactic working exactly as it was designed: to create and maintain health disparities, to provide the justifications for lack of spending, and to reify social categories as science. These issues were made worse by the internal racism of psychiatry itself, a field long complicit in the creation of ideas about the Black psyche as a form of savagery and a eugenic threat to the dominance of white society.[4] Segregation proved itself as enduring inside the psychiatric hospital as it was outside, and so psychiatry became another force of oppression to be endured by Black patients.

Southern politics and racist psychiatry combined to maintain and reinforce segregation and its attendant practices within psychiatric facilities in Alabama, Mississippi, and Georgia. In this chapter, I use official sources—including annual reports and American Psychiatric Association (APA) inspections—to unpack the tactics and impact of segregation. Long-running ideas about the alleged difference and inferiority of the Black psyche were used to justify segregation, ideas that were not seriously challenged by the growth of modern psychiatry. Geography and physical spaces were also used to keep Black patients separate from white, creating the conditions for abuse, neglect, and violence. The way these spaces functioned reinforced to outsiders, both funding bodies and the broader public, that the insane or disabled Black person was safely confined, while making sure that not too many tax dollars were spent on them. These spaces of confinement also reiterated to the Black patient that they were on the lowest rung of an already dehumanizing system and that opportunities for resistance would be limited. Those opportunities were even more limited by the methods of commitment and continued confinement, which seemed to be based on laws and policies but were in actual fact arbitrary and capricious. The principle that commitment to psychiatric institutions should be bound by due process of the law was continually undermined by the way the law itself was a tool of white supremacy, especially in the Jim Crow South before the Civil Rights Act of 1964.

Justifying Segregation

The justifications for segregation within medicine and psychiatry are legion and complex. These justifications are inseparable not only from the fear of race mixing (which would lead to eugenics) but also from the fear of Black people flourishing post-Reconstruction. Scholars have long argued that the deliberate failure of Reconstruction, the re-inscription of Black codes, and Jim Crow laws arising out of *Plessy v. Ferguson* were deliberate and malicious policies designed to ensure the continued oppression of the freed Black person in new forms.[5] That is, if Black schools and hospitals were not funded adequately, it was not so much out of benign neglect but a deliberate attempt to ensure that Black communities did not have access to the things that free white people used to ensure their position at the top of the ladder. Public education and medical systems were generally vastly underfunded in the South, but when it came to services for Black communities, underfunding of education, lack of access to health care, lack of stable and safe employment, and lack of housing opportunities were deliberate tactics. Underfunding did exactly the job it was supposed to do, re-creating plantation type labor and social relations in ways that kept freed Black people at the mercy of white supremacy and racial capitalism.

These forms of oppression also worked discursively as a form of gaslighting: segregation was posed as the normal way of things, desired by all. This "common" desire, it could be argued, was demonstrated by the fact that the Black community was actively building institutions for itself (Tuskegee, for example). Of course, that argument would need to deliberately ignore the fact that Black communities built their own health-care facilities because they were generally excluded from white ones and understood that any care they received in them was substandard.[6] Even when funded by philanthropies, Black institutions often struggled to provide for their communities adequately, not because of inferior training or talent but because of deliberate underfunding. The gaslighting about the impact of segregation was reinforced by government policy itself. That is, if there was any insinuation about inferiority, that was not the fault of white society but of Black people themselves, an idea enshrined into law by the judgment in *Plessy v. Ferguson*. As Justice Brown wrote, "We consider the underlying fallacy of the plaintiff's argument to consist in the assumption that the enforced separation of the two races stamps the colored race with a badge of inferiority. If this be so, it is not by reason of anything found in the act, but solely because the colored race chooses to put that construction upon it."[7] This disingenuous rhetoric refashioned pre-emancipation ideas about Black life in ways that blamed Black people themselves for both their real-life material conditions post-slavery and the ways they felt or thought about themselves in a highly racialized society.

Ideas about racial difference and the alleged inferiority of the Black body-mind, which permeated American psychiatry, can be traced directly to the plantation. Scholars of race and medicine have made clear the connections between the construction of racial biology as inferiority and the justification for slavery.[8] In the history of psychiatry, this has taken a particular form in the racist construction of the "Black personality" as alternately childlike, savage, or criminal. Scholars have documented in detail how Black people's resistance to enslavement, as well as their behavior in freedom, was easily constructed as "mental illness."[9] Yet at the same time, Black people were not generally considered potential patients in the establishment of the first state hospitals because of equally racist ideas that the enslaved person did *not* experience mental illness, either because they were too happy or simple by nature or because they were too well cared for by the institution of slavery itself.[10]

These racist ideas were particularly heightened in the two decades prior to emancipation. In her book *Mad with Freedom,* historian Elodie Edwards-Grossi has documented the way that the construction of arguments about the 1840 census positioned psychiatry as foundational to debates about abolition.[11] Falsified or erroneous census data was used to argue that the free Black person was adversely affected by their encounters with so-called civilization and should therefore remain enslaved, which was positioned as a form of paternalistic protection rather than a tool of extractive capitalism and violent oppression.

From there it was easy for physicians like Samuel Cartwright to argue that the enslaved person who escaped or resisted forced labor was therefore suffering from invented mental illnesses like *drapetomania* or *dysaesthesia aethiopica.*[12] It was also the case that enslavers' economic interests were served by rhetoric that argued that mental illness was rare among enslaved people, given that they were not considered people but chattel for whom soundness of mind and body was paramount for market value.[13]

This complex of attitudes and self-interest meant that the enslavers and psychiatrists could twist ideas about psychological difference to whatever cause suited them at the time. Even when proven wrong, the census data continued to inform the segregationist and racist policies of politicians and psychiatrists from emancipation through Reconstruction. For most of psychiatry, the census data served merely to confirm what was already believed: that the Black person was not cut out for Western civilization.

Psychiatrists were therefore able to have it both ways. That is, if slavery had rendered the Black person's alleged natural savagery muted and contained, freedom supposedly revealed their also naturally inferior intellect and unchecked promiscuity and violence. This latter categorization of Black behavior when insane was then used as justification for segregation within emerging psychiatric institutions.

The existence of segregation in psychiatric institutions is not in itself surprising. As historian Wendy Gonaver and others have demonstrated, segregation was utterly foundational to the wave of psychiatric hospital building that occurred from the mid-nineteenth century, and those who did not abide by it, like John M. Galt in Virginia, found themselves quickly ostracized by the professional associations linked to the emerging psychiatric profession.[14] The often-cited "heroine" of psychiatric history, Dorothea Dix, showed no concern or interest in the welfare of the few Black patients she may have seen, and their interests were never part of her appeals to state governments for psychiatric reform.

The same is true of the father of the modern psychiatric hospital, Thomas Kirkbride.[15] In the context of psychiatry, this needs to be understood not so much as benign oversight but the active repudiation of the idea of Black psychology itself—the belief that there was no illness to be cured because Black patients were not capable of complex emotional or affective lives, and if they were institutionalized, it was because their behavior was seen as a threat to white society in some way. In this sense, for psychiatry, the Black patient was never fully human, and this belief laid the foundation for not just institutional segregation but the way the Black person would be treated as a patient.

The end of slavery did not bring with it the desire or the structures to create an integrated society, and decisions like *Plessy v. Ferguson* made it even easier to reify segregation in ways that created spaces where the Black patient could be neglected or abused. With the rise of eugenics in the late nineteenth and twentieth centuries, the scientific and nation-building discourses of race purity and race protection served again to reinforce and legitimize segregation as everyday practice. The blatant inequalities it created were met with either a shrug of indifference or the active violence of eugenic thinking.[16] In Georgia and Mississippi, segregation was accepted, normal, and sometimes vigorously defended until at least 1964, and in Alabama, until 1969. It did, however, take slightly different forms in each state, and these forms can tell us something about local politics and its impact on psychiatric practice in the South.

Segregated Spaces

Knowledge about how segregation worked is limited by the availability and transparency of the sources. In the 1950s and early 1960s, official documentation primarily took the form of reports submitted either annually (Alabama and Georgia) or every two years (Mississippi) to the governor or state body. In Georgia, the hospital reported initially to the Department of Public Welfare and later to the Department of Public Health. In Alabama and Mississippi, the hospitals did not technically report to any centralized government department but rather to a board of trustees, which also made finding the actual documents in the first place difficult.[17] This situation varied by state and also changed over time as a result of various exposés, political reshuffles, and reform movements, which also means there is no single set of records clearly marked for each hospital; in other words, records are scattered across numerous collections and groups. Nevertheless, it is possible to get an overview of each of the three state systems, give some basic background, and set out the way that segregation was operationalized through the annual reports and the writings of some institution's superintendents. What follows is the story of the three state systems, not as a complete chronology but rather as a teasing out of their similarities and differences and a consideration of what these comparisons signify about local politics and attitudes.

The oldest of the hospitals under study in this book is Central State Hospital (CSH) in Milledgeville, Georgia.[18] Central State was established in 1842 on 170 acres located halfway between Augusta and Macon. CSH took only white patients at first because of the prevailing idea that slavery protected the Black person from mental illness, but it was forced to construct a single building for "colored patients" after the Civil War, when the failure of Reconstruction saw the breakdown of Freedmen's Bureau hospitals and general concerns about the presence and behavior of freed people grew.[19]

At no point was there any question of Black patients inhabiting the same spaces as white ones, and administrators of Central State argued that a separate facility would be preferable, and somewhere other than Milledgeville. As hospital superintendent Thomas F. Green wrote in 1870, this was the solution "manifestly desired by the colored citizens generally and would be more satisfactory to them."[20] By perpetuating the notion that segregation was preferred by Black people themselves, Green sidestepped the real issue of white violence and the underlying unfairness of segregation. It was, however, a moot point, as the Georgia legislature was not interested in spending that kind of money on the Black insane; instead, they were admitted to hastily and poorly constructed buildings on the Milledgeville campus.

Plagued by underfunding, the original campus became ever more sprawling. Overcrowding was a constant. By the 1950s, the hospital had grown to over 3,000 acres—including a self-sustaining farm, post office, railway station, dairy, mattress factory, shoe shop, and printing press—and a total "on the books" patient population of more than 12,000. By all reports, this makes this one hospital in Georgia likely the largest psychiatric hospital in the world at the time.

Tracking segregation at CSH is particularly difficult because of the silences in the annual report and the lack of clear demarcation between Black and white sections. In terms of the physical plant, this is exacerbated because of the way the buildings were named. That is, they were not identified by patient population but by the names of people who had been significant to the hospital at some point. This tactic worked as a kind of deliberate obfuscation, as a map from 1966 demonstrates (see figure 2.1).[21] The map (and the Annual Report) gives no indication of who was in what building, and the only mention of race is the label "Colored Women's Prison," identifying a building that sits on the curve of Lawrence Road, leading down to the swamp.

The main focus of the CSH campus was always the Powell Building (a big white building with a dome, which seems to be a standard feature of large rural institutions). Situated at the top of a rise overlooking a pecan orchard, with a curving driveway and a fountain out front, this building was named after the superintendent who ran the hospital from 1879 to 1907, actively reinforcing segregation in both buildings and in the everyday distribution of resources.[22]

Several huge buildings—Ingram, Holly, Kemper, Bostick, and Washington—made up the "back wards"—so far removed from the main part of campus that they were quite literally out of sight and out of mind. The naming of some of these buildings was also significant—the Ingram Building, for example, was named after Joe Ingram, a Black ex-patient who became a significant employee and was often touted as a symbol of CSH's progressivism.[23] From conversations with people who used to work at Central State, I learned that all the buildings down Lawrence Road housed Black patients only, at least until 1964.[24]

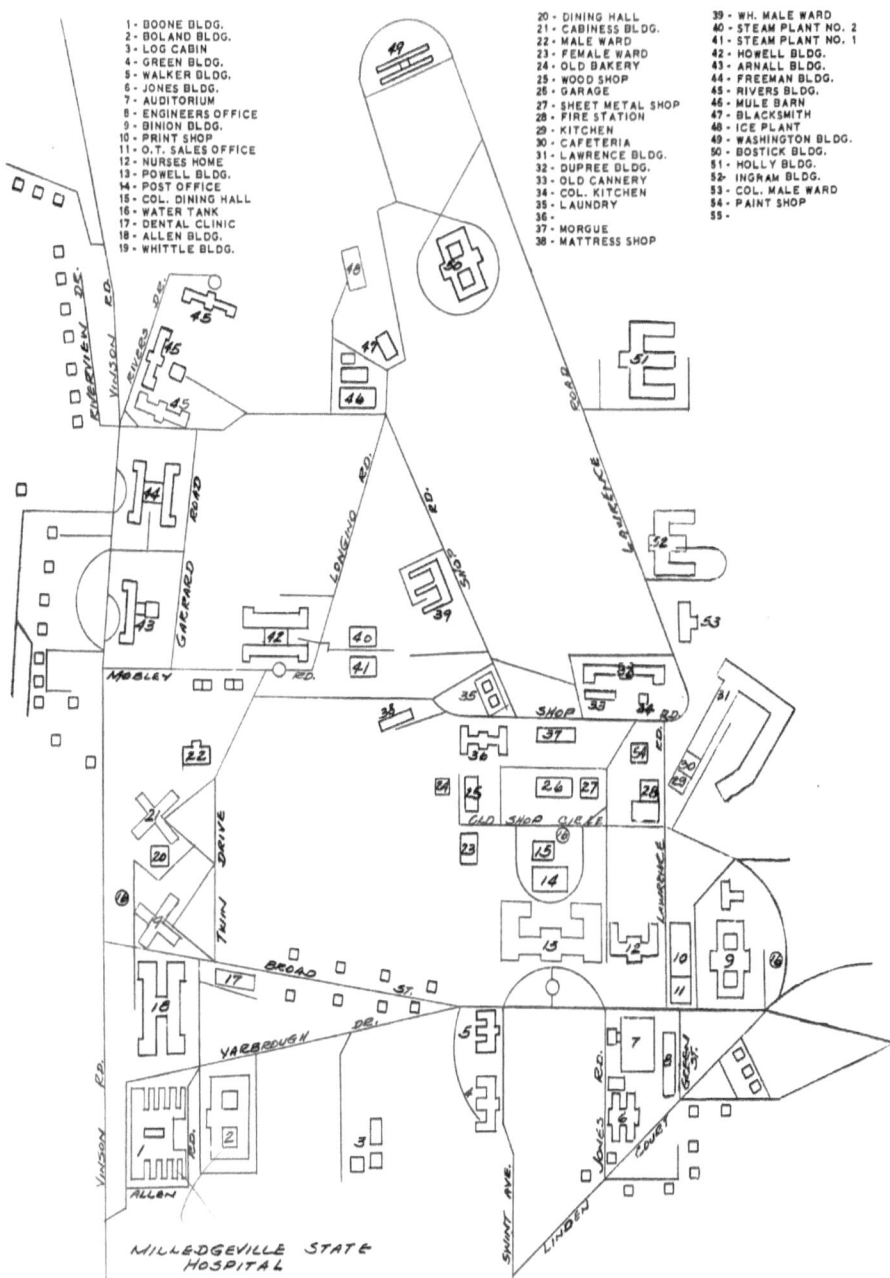

FIGURE 2.1 Map of Milledgeville State Hospital (CSH) campus, 1965. Director's Administrative Records, 1964–1969, RG 26-24-35. Courtesy of Georgia State Archives.

Segregation was carefully maintained in death as much as in life. At its height, CHS maintained six cemeteries, with Jasmine Ridge for the Black patients and Cedar Lane for the white patients being the two largest. At Jasmine Ridge, graves were marked by numbered brass symbols; after integration, the cemetery was never maintained. When the state sold a portion of the CSH grounds to the Georgia Department of Corrections, excavators mowed over the brass plates. Some of them are still in place at the original site but are not easily accessible to the public, while others were recovered and are now arranged in a corner of the Cedar Lane Cemetery, which is a beautiful sprawling garden marked with headstones and statues for the white patients.[25]

Other indications of the ways that services for patients were separate and *not* equal are scattered throughout the annual reports from the 1950s. For example, at the front of each annual report was a listing of the names of the various division heads. In 1956, there are listings for W. T. Berry as "Supervisor, White Male Service" and for M. M. Bonner as "Supervisor, Colored Male Service." Further down is listed Vera Knowles, RN, as "Supervisor, Colored Female Service," but the white women seemed to have no designated service supervisor. We might surmise that this role fell to Myra S. Bonner, RN, the director of nurses and nursing services. These women are significant because they speak to the important role of nurses in providing direct care to psychiatric patients and the way that nursing as a profession itself dealt with segregation.[26]

The Georgia Nurses Association was one of the last state associations in the United States to allow Black nurses to join (in 1968), making it hard for Black women to train or practice as nurses in Georgia.[27] But Central State Hospital did employ and provide training for nurses. It ran its own psychiatric nurse training school from 1907 to 1947, which admitted white women only, and had affiliations with several university and hospital-based nurse training schools across Georgia. White student nurses lived on-site for three-month rotations while training, and then moved on to another affiliation or employment elsewhere. The Colored Female Service was run and staffed by Black nurses who also lived on-site but they had already been trained elsewhere (usually Grady Hospital's School of Nursing in Atlanta).[28] There is evidence in the earlier annual reports that the hospital employed Black attendants to work in the Black service and that accommodations and pay for Black nurses and attendants was substandard. The overall director of nursing was a white woman.

In this same annual report from 1956, the superintendent, Thomas Peacock, demonstrated the ways that segregation worked as an unquestioned

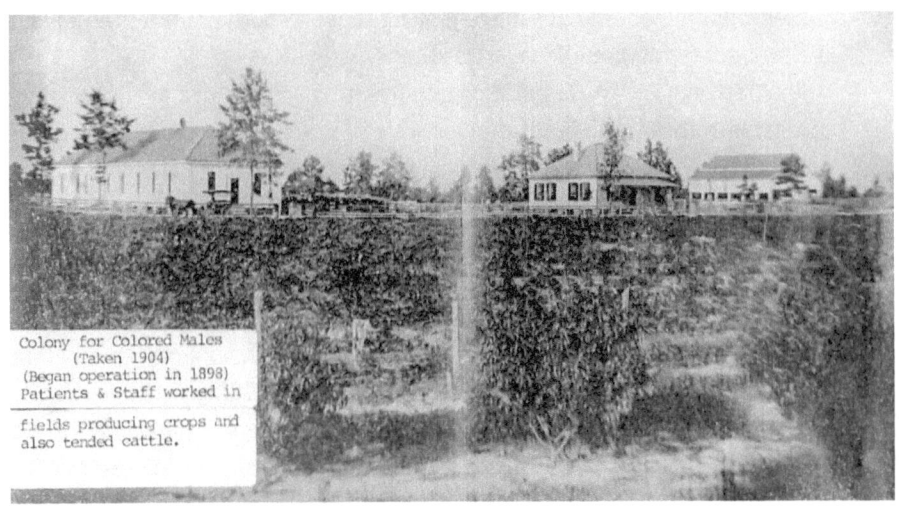

FIGURE 2.2 Colony for Colored Males, 1904, Central State Hospital, Milledgeville, GA. Georgia Department of Behavioral Health and Developmental Disabilities.

norm, at the same time revealing the pressure that came with the growing number of Black patients being admitted. In his recommendations to Judge Kemper, the director of the Public Welfare Department to which CSH reported, Peacock listed four items specifically related to the construction of new accommodations for Black patients: "Medical and Surgical Department for Colored Division. Recreation Hall for Colored Division. New dormitory type building for Colony 2. Completion of improvements begun at Colony 1."[29] Peacock's request for an entire medical and surgical department and a recreation hall for the Black patients meant that they did not currently have those facilities, while the white patients most certainly did. The lack of a recreation hall was part of a broader segregated occupational therapy department, which also included crafting, industrial, and semi-agricultural pursuits.

The "colony" requests were related to full-scale farming enterprises, which used Black patients as labor. The annual report was markedly silent about this aspect of its segregated practices, but whenever the word "colony" is used in relation to psychiatric hospitals, it is referring to farming enterprises away from the main location that were worked primarily by Black patients.[30]

These colony farms (see figure 2.2), occurring in the wake of the breakdown of the plantation system and the creation of small farms and

Enabling Segregation   47

sharecropping, would have made perfect sense to both administrators and the broader (white) public in particular.

In Alabama, Bryce Hospital originated in Tuscaloosa as part of a wave of asylum reform in the mid-nineteenth century driven by white Northern psychiatrists and reformers concerned with the custodial nature of America's psychiatric institutions. According to Alabama's "official" medical historian, Howard Holley, Bryce Hospital was a model of psychiatric progressivism, adopting techniques from genteel "retreats" like the York Retreat in England and the Friends Hospital in Pennsylvania.[31] These techniques, of course, were never meant to apply to the Black body, and before the Civil War, Bryce took no Black patients at all. Built on the Kirkbride model, it became an ever sprawling campus on the southern side of the Black Warrior River, and a little too close to the town of Tuscaloosa for comfort.

In the aftermath of war and the failure of Reconstruction, the issue of "the colored insane" became a more pressing problem for institutions across the South. In the 1890s, the then superintendent of the Tuscaloosa campus, James T. Searcy, expressed concern about the growing number of Black patients, which he associated unproblematically with an increase in insanity among freed people. "The causes of insanity," he wrote in his 1894 annual report, "are all interwoven with the habits of the person extending through the years, and are affected by the habits of his family, and of his race, extending through generations."[32] Like most medical men at the time, Searcy argued that this alleged increase in insanity among African Americans was an effect of incompatibility with Western civilization now that people were emancipated but forced to fend for themselves. When the population at Bryce Hospital tipped over 1,100, Searcy advocated for a separate facility for Black patients, and was eventually given a site in Mount Vernon, 33 miles north of Mobile and about 170 miles south of Tuscaloosa, quite literally in the middle of nowhere.

The Mount Vernon site was not, and never had been, a hospital. It was originally the Mount Vernon Arsenal—a civil war barracks, transferred from the US government to the state of Alabama in 1895 (see figure 2.3). In 1900, the state government agreed to renovate it as a hospital "solely for the care, treatment and custody of insane patients," and it was placed, along with Bryce Hospital, under the direction of one board.[33] Originally intended for between 400 and 500 patients, the Mount Vernon campus had the benefit of 1,600 acres of land for farming. Dr. Searcy died in 1919, and the Mount Vernon hospital was named for him a year later.

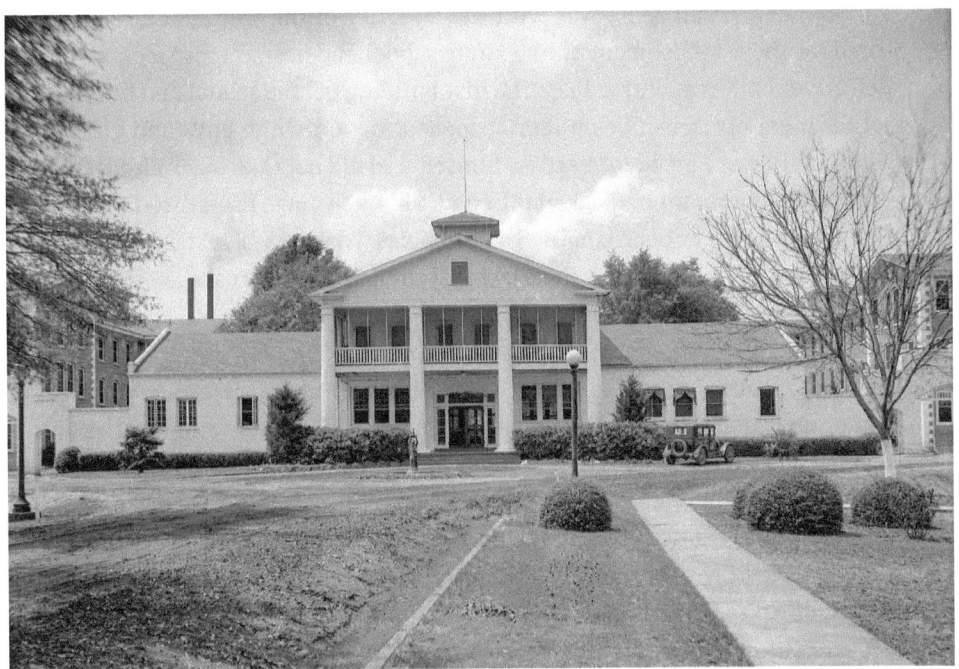

FIGURE 2.3 Mount Vernon Arsenal Administration Building, Old Saint Stephens Road (County Road 96), Mount Vernon, Mobile County, AL. Historic American Buildings Survey, E. W. Russell, photographer, April 2, 1935. Library of Congress Digital IDhhh al0618.

Writing about Dr. Searcy in his "brief history" of the Alabama mental health system, James Sidney Tarwater, a future superintendent of the Alabama hospitals, wrote, "The Negro population of Tuscaloosa was grieved at his death, and paid tribute to the man who had done so much for them by establishing the hospital at Mt. Vernon."[34] Tarwater himself was an ambiguous figure in the history of Alabama's mental health system. To claim that local Black families were happy about the creation of a hospital that confined and removed their family members more than 170 miles south was at best disingenuous, but it demonstrates his long-running complicity with the rationale and justification for segregation.

In his article, Tarwater also reported on the work of Searcy's successor, William Dempsey Partlow, a notorious eugenicist. As Tarwater pointed out, the laws governing the "Alabama Insane Hospitals" did not make specific provision for what were then called "mental defectives," explicitly stating that the hospitals were for the treatment of "insanity" only. But this distinction was at times both hard to make and nearly impossible to sustain.

Enabling Segregation 49

Partlow, concerned as he was with the integrity of the white race, advocated for the establishment of a separate school and hospital for "mentally defective" children, and in 1923, the first building of "the school and hospital for mentally defective children" opened for 160 white boys and girls. The facility was named for Partlow himself and did not take Black children until 1944. Before then, Black children would likely have been cared for in their community or been confined at Mt. Meigs (Alabama Industrial School for Negro Children), where the Black psychiatrists from Tuskegee tied to provide what care they could.

The ever-increasing population and the pressure it put on existing buildings and resources was a source of constant concern for Tarwater, who became superintendent of both Bryce and Searcy in September 1950. When he took over, there were 6,000 patients at Bryce and Searcy, and the state appropriation amounted to less than $1.50 per patient per day.[35] The hospitals had also recently been the subject of a Senate investigation about conditions following a fire, and Tarwater toured the facilities with Senator Patterson in 1948. This committee made some recommendations for improvements of the buildings, but had no problem with the way segregation was working or the conditions that it rendered for Black patients.[36]

While it is hardly surprising that the white people who ran Alabama in the 1950s were not troubled by segregation or the dire conditions that it produced for Black patients, it is worth noting that the American Psychiatric Association had little to say on the matter either. In 1958, the Central Inspection Board of the APA visited the two facilities and made recommendations for improvements. The final report, totaling more than 320 pages, contained extensive details about the nature of the facilities at that point in time, and was a damning indictment of the physical plant.

The inspector noted that the entire facility in Mobile was contained within the original wall that encircled the old forty-eight-acre military fort. Many of the original buildings were not fit for purpose and constituted fire traps, and the area inside the wall was crowded because of the "hodgepodge" nature of construction that had taken place in order to fit all the staff and patients within the existing space. The report detailed the way that white and Black employees were kept separate and that accommodations for Black staff were noticeably substandard. The wards for patients were often fire traps with inadequate plumbing, and the whole facility was chronically overcrowded. The inspector noted that "most of the wards at this hospital are lacking in day room space. . . . Too many of them have large dormitories (10 to 88 beds) in which the patients both sleep and sit. The toilet and

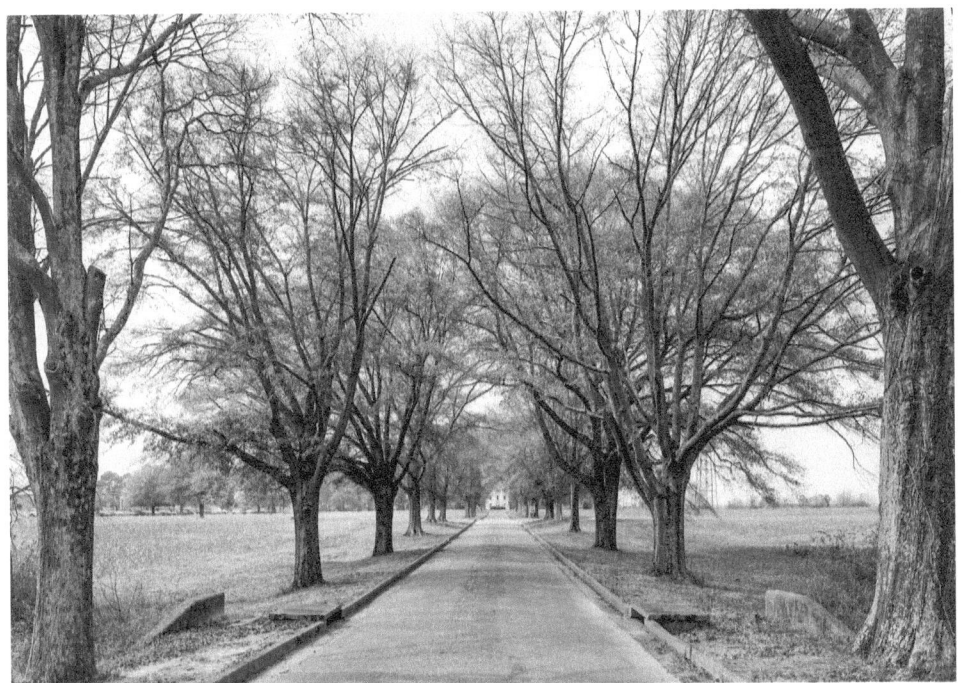

FIGURE 2.4 Robert Jemison plantation, Byler Road, Northport, Tuscaloosa County, AL, 1933. Library of Congress, www.loc.gov/item/al1023/.

bathing facilities are also inadequate. More space, more privacy and more fixtures are needed. Complete remodeling will be necessary on most wards. . . . Overcrowding amounts to approximately 550 beds. This should be relieved as soon as possible as it interferes with the treatment and proper care of the patients."[37]

The report also made mention of the extensive farming operations (which I will explore further in later chapters) but recommended that they be expanded beyond the walls of the original fort, as they were causing hygiene problems. As a result, the state acquired more land north of the original Bryce Hospital in Tuscaloosa, which it made into a "new hospital for the admission of Negroes from the North and North-Central counties."[38] This facility was known in various sources as either the Bryce Treatment Center #2 or the Jemison Center, named after major planter and enslaver Robert Jemison Jr., a prominent person in the history of Alabama who owned the land on which the new center was built (see figure 2.4).

Jemison was instrumental in the construction of the original Bryce Hospital site in Tuscaloosa. He used enslaved architect and bridge engineer

Horace King to build a bridge across the Black Warrior River to Northport, and from there expanded his plantation holdings to include the site on Byler Road.[39] Jemison had four children, and one of his descendants, another Robert Jemison Jr., would serve as vice president of the board of trustees of the Alabama Mental Hospitals.

While the nature of segregation was particularly stark in Alabama in that it operated distinct and entirely separate locations based on race, this was not the case in Mississippi. Segregation at Whitfield worked in a way that reflected a very particular performance of Jim Crow in that state. Here, Black and white people lived in the same physical spaces but in ways that maintained relationships of deference and subservience. White dependence on free or cheap Black labor was reframed as caretaking and maintained by both segregation and violence. This racist paternalism informed the design and redesign of the mental health system in Mississippi. The original asylum in Jackson, built in 1855 on the site of the current University of Mississippi Medical Center, had become badly crowded and neglected. Black patients were admitted, but they were rare.

In 1882, a second facility—East Mississippi State Hospital (EMSH)—was built in Meridian. Initially, EMSH admitted both Black and white patients, but less than ten years later a decision was made to send the Black patients back to the run-down facility in Jackson. This made the brand-new Kirkbride-style EMSH a white-only facility, meaning that middle class and rural white patients were admitted to better conditions while the poor white and Black patients remaining in Jackson endured ever-worsening conditions. This rapidly deteriorating, fire- and flood-ridden Jackson facility was the "palatial" facility that Schuyler mentioned in his letter to Wright. A new hospital was needed, and the state government appropriated 3,300 acres from an old penal colony about fifteen miles southeast of Jackson to establish the new Mississippi State Hospital—or "Whitfield," as it became known.

In terms of construction, the state opted for the newer cottage model rather than a Kirkbride-style single building for the new center. This design meant that buildings could be smaller and more spread out, and people more easily segregated by race. The buildings for the initial hospital were erected in 1925, but due to various legislative issues and lack of infrastructure funding, the first patients were not moved in until 1935.

The initial campus was also firmly centered around the idea and practice of agriculture. A report written by F. J. Hurst from the Mississippi State Extension Service ran in both the *Jackson Daily News* and the *Commercial*

Appeal in October 1938 and clearly spelled out the dual function of farming at Whitfield, where most of the work was done by patients. Government appointed superintendent Dr. Charles Mitchell argued that "work in the open is not only highly essential to the physical well-being of the patients, but their labor is necessary in the production of an adequate food supply and the proper feeding of the big population of the institution." The article called the state farm "magnificent" and "one of Mississippi's finest diversified farms."[40] Both articles ran with photos of patients working, and the version that ran in the *Commercial Appeal* appeared under the headline "Mississippi Hospital's Farm Cares for Patients."[41] But Mitchell was a government appointee, and the hospital was quickly beset by political problems and internal corruption. The farmland deteriorated under bad management, and the conditions of the buildings declined rapidly under the strain of habitation and neglect as a result of diverted resources for World War II.

In 1947, an internal investigation (which I discuss in more detail in chapter 5) led to demands for change, and the government advertised for and employed its first externally trained and independent medical director, Dr. William Jaquith.[42] Jaquith is a complex and significant figure in Whitfield's history, especially because he was superintendent until his retirement thirty years later. He is the main source of information about Whitfield, in both his official correspondence, such as the biennial reports, and in his publications, personal collection, and newspaper appearances.

One of the most informative pieces about Whitfield came later in Jaquith's life, when he was interviewed by the *Clarion Ledger* on the eve of his retirement from Mississippi mental health services in 1979. In this article, Jaquith remembered what it was like when he first arrived:

> When I first came I was appalled at what I saw. . . . I almost left immediately, I was so upset with the total picture. Things were terrible. It made grown men cry. It was shot with politics. All jobs were up for grabs when the administration changed. I was the only physician for 10 buildings and 800 patients. The buildings were in a terrible state of disrepair. The war years had ravaged them. Raw sewerage ran on the floor from the broken plumbing fixtures. Sewage had leaked through the ceiling into food stuffs and caused an outbreak of dysentery. The first night I was there I was called to see an elderly patient in the senile ward. When they turned the lights on thousands of rats jumped out of the patients' beds. I was called late one night to see a patient who had died and got there in a

few minutes after receiving the call. The roaches and silverfish were eating at his eyes. The patients slept on handmade mattresses, sacks stuffed with hay. The hospital also made the caskets—four planks nailed together. There were rats and vermin everywhere.[43]

Jaquith noted that the patients had an incomplete diet, with the total caloric intake less than 800 calories a day, and that many patients suffered from malnutrition. This particularly bothered him, having been a naval surgeon in the Pacific during World War II, and the state of the hospital struck him as a visceral reminder of a prisoner-of-war camp. At the time of his arrival, the state appropriation amounted to a measly ninety-eight cents per patient per day, and the white attendants were paid fifty-five dollars a month, the Black employees a mere forty-five dollars. Outside the untrained attendants, the entire professional and clinical staff and directors were all white (see figure 2.5).

In all of Jaquith's writing and reporting, there is no attempt to obfuscate or hide the nature and extent of segregation, and Jaquith's openness about it reflects the accepted state of affairs, serving the twofold purpose of assuring the (white) taxpayers of Mississippi that Black patients were being kept entirely separate and in their place, while at the same time placating paternalism by demonstrating how they were being cared for. Yet there were times when Jaquith clearly expressed the need for better conditions for Black patients, and over the next few years he made several concerted attempts to provide better services for them, including employing a young psychological intern and occupational therapy students from nearby Tougaloo College.[44]

In 1955, Jaquith personally appointed the hospital's first Black physician, Dr. Charles Washington, who had also graduated from Tougaloo College and then medical school at Howard University. Dr. Washington was returning to Mississippi as part of a deal with the state that paid medical students' tuition in return for five years of service. While Washington had no specific psychiatric training beyond his regular medical school classes, he stated that he was glad to be at Whitfield and looking forward to the work he might do there.[45] Dr. Washington's appointment signaled an interesting paradox in that Jaquith could be seen as both progressive and conservative at the same time: progressive in that he was one of the first, if not the first, to appoint a Black physician in a state hospital in the South, and conservative in that Dr. Washington was appointed to care for the Black patients only. At no point would Dr. Washington have had any contact with white

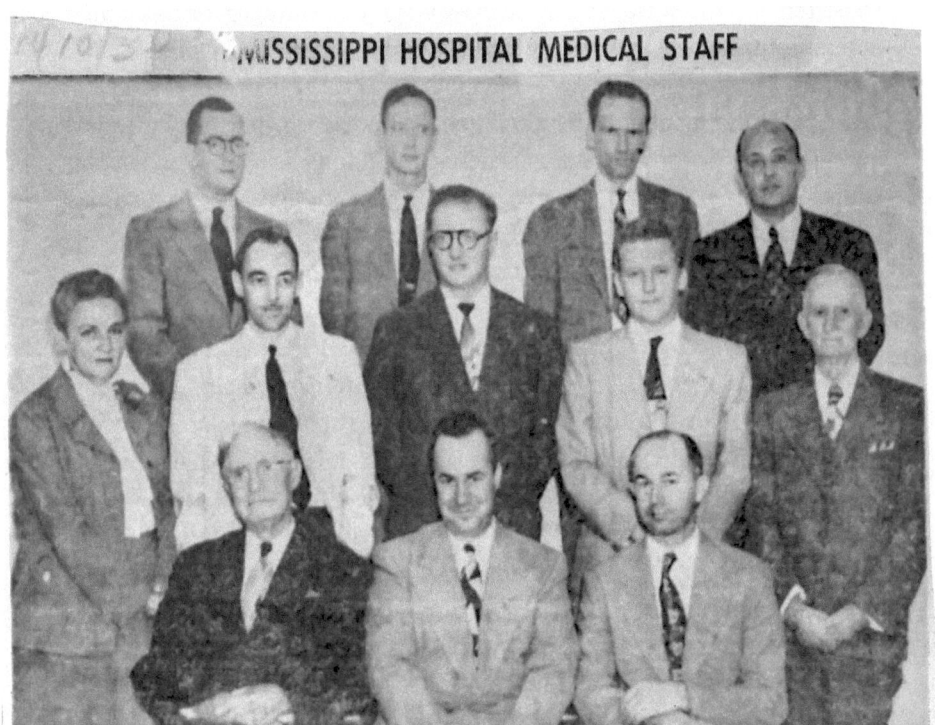

Mississippi Hospital medical staff meets regularly four times a week to diagnose and discuss patients. They are, left to right, seated, Dr. B. J. Marshall, in charge of Negro service; Dr. W. L. Jaquith, director; Dr. F. A. Latham, clinical director. Second row: Dr. Sara R. Dean, Dr. F. M. B. Slater, Dr. C. S. Woodward; Dr. W. J. Spann, and Dr. P. B. Williamson. Third row: Dr. J. H. Fry, Dr. W. W. Dreher, Dr. Vincent J. Daly (first full-time psychologist on the staff) and Dr. A. J. Santangelo. Not shown are three dentists and six consulting specialists who visit Whitfield each week and are on call.

FIGURE 2.5 Mississippi State Hospital medical staff, 1950. Clipping from Dr. Jaquith's scrapbook. Courtesy of the Archives and Records Services Division, Mississippi Department of Archives and History.

patients, and there was no attempt to employ another Black psychiatrist until the 1960s.

Ultimately, segregation was an indelible, unquestioned, and enduring fact of life at Whitfield. The campus was divided down the middle, with one set of buildings for Black patients to the west of the main drive, and another for white patients on the eastern side, clustered around a picturesque lake. The first report that Jaquith supplied to the Board of Trustees of Mental Institutions was published in April 1951 and set out clearly the way that Whitfield ran two entirely separate services, one for white patients and one for "colored." There were separate receiving wards where people were initially admitted for observation and diagnosis, and then "the colored service"

Enabling Segregation 55

consisted of four "cottages" for Black women, two cottages for Black men, and an infirmary, epileptic and disturbed cottages for each gender, and a convalescent cottage for Black men. The white service was largely the same, with more cottages for each gender (four each) plus the infirmary and epileptic, disturbed, and convalescent buildings for both genders, but white patients of both sexes also had access to a "re-educational" unit, which was not part of the colored service.

There were also entirely separate hospital buildings on each side of the campus, a white and Black general hospital, and a white and Black tuberculosis (TB) hospital, where both sexes were admitted together. A note at the end of this section explained that the buildings called cottages "house the chronically mentally ill patients," while "the Re-educational wards house the chronically mentally ill, but [they are] able to enjoy the privileges of an unlocked building. . . . The Convalescent buildings house those patients who are almost ready to leave the institution. All cottages, the disturbed buildings, the epileptic buildings, the infirmaries, the TB hospitals are locked buildings."[46] This system meant that Black women were confined at all times, having no re-educational or convalescent building, though Black men in their convalescent building may have had some more freedom.

These distinctions speak clearly not only to the prevailing social hierarchy but also to gendered ideas about patient behavior and vulnerability. There was one alcohol and narcotic building, which was also locked, but this was for "all patients (white) being treated."[47] This was a new building, erected in 1950, at a cost of $750,000. It housed 200 beds, open to white people only, and its cost represented an extraordinary figure considering that the total income for the year ending 1951 was $2,146,529, giving Jaquith a budget of $1.51 per patient per day.

The discrepancy did not go unnoticed at the time. On November 29, 1952, the *Jackson Daily News* ran a small article about Representative Harry Applebaum from Yazoo County calling for the abolition of the facility. Applebaum labeled the ward a "summer resort for drunks" while "right across the way they have what I call a tomb of the living . . . poor old people who are crammed into wards like they are barracks."[48] If Applebaum was referring to the conditions for white patients as a tomb, I can only imagine what they might have been like for Black patients on the other side of campus.

There is some evidence that Black and white patients were able to mix at times outside the formal structures of segregation, but this was rare and quickly shut down. For example, in the 1955–57 report, there is a small section titled "Confectionary," in which the director reported on the establishment of a small canteen: the "modern, brick building . . . serves both white and negro patients and families as well as employees."[49] Here, people could buy treats and other supplies beyond what the hospital furnished, which helped break up the monotony of the daily fare. The canteen raised more than $96,000 a year, and some of the profits were used for the recreation fund, which purchased equipment for recreational activities.

But its potential as a site for racial mixing was quickly dissolved when a small trailer was placed on the Black section of the campus ostensibly to save "the negro patients long walks from the negro section of the hospital to the main canteen."[50] The plan was to eventually replace this trailer with a brick veneer canteen for Black patients on their side of the campus, allowing the present canteen to be "converted into an all-white canteen with a small order lunch room in conjunction."[51] As was often the case, when Black patients were moved to their own section or facilities, the spaces they vacated were upgraded to suit the expectations of white patients.

Formally, Whitfield maintained separate kitchens and dining halls for Black and white patients, and separate live-in accommodations for Black and white staff. There is a particularly telling example here of how segregation affected not just the patients but the staff, and placed pressure on the facilities overall. Whitfield employed around 400 live-in Black people as attendants (not as trained nurses or physicians) but necessarily separated them on the campus into dormitories. Jaquith's report from 1951 documents five dormitories and a dining hall dedicated to white employees, but this was not the case for Black employees. They had two dormitories only, one for men and one for women, and no dining hall at all.

In fact, Jaquith noted that "the hospital is very much overcrowded at this time, especially the infirmaries, where the old and senile are housed. The negro section of the hospital is overflowing, and we have had to open up basement space for the overflow. Two of our negro patients' buildings are used for housing quarters for the employees. There is no relief in sight at the moment to transfer negro mental defectives."[52] Jaquith appealed to the legislature to build a cafeteria for Black attendants and staff in repeated reports, which also spoke to the way that segregation was actively reinforced throughout the 1950s.

In the 1953–55 report, he remarked, "The colored employees are in dire need of a cafeteria. At the present time, with approximately 400 colored employees, these employees occupy a portion of the patients' Dining Hall. It is necessary that the patients be fed in shifts. The Dining Hall assigned to colored employees is so small they also must be fed in shifts. We need this space in the Dining Hall urgently for patient care. For the sum of $40,000.00 we believe that a now empty space in the institution could be converted into a colored employees' dining hall, and we make this recommendation." This cafeteria was finally opened in 1958 "with modern equipment and facilities," serving four meals daily to an average of 357 people.[53]

But Jaquith also regularly pointed out that with wages so low and conditions so bad, it was to be expected that staff morale was low and turnover was high, exceeding 900 people a year. These factors created a situation in which the hospital was forced to employ a great many untrained and unskilled people, which had implications for patient care.[54] This is not to say that all employees lacked compassion or were abusive or violent, but a lack of formal training in therapeutic techniques in an underfunded and overcrowded facility, at a time when mental illness and disability were so badly stigmatized, overlaid with racial hierarchies, created conditions in which Black patients were particularly vulnerable.

Conditions in all these hospitals deteriorated throughout the 1950s due to over-admissions and overcrowding, enabled by inconsistencies in commitment processes, which relied on obscure legal technicalities and, in Mississippi, provided no legal protections.

Pathways to Commitment

The sheer size of these institutions raises questions about the processes by which so many people were admitted and how this was justified. These are not easy questions to answer due to the amount of silence in the official sources and differences in the way information was recorded across states. There is also silence due to what has been kept in each state and how, the politics of which I have set out more specifically in appendix 1.

Nevertheless, in this section I try to lay out the ways that each state admitted people and recorded information about them. I differentiate here between the actual processes as they occurred versus the processes as they were recorded. This differentiation in my interpretation is not just an arbitrary decision based on my personal politics or theoretical orientation (although it is also that) but a conclusion that stems from various conversations with people who have worked in, lived near, or prosecuted the state systems under study here. There is also more than enough evidence in sources beyond the official state records (some of which I set out in chapter 3) to support the idea that what states said they did versus what they actually did are two largely different things.

This disparity between theory and practice is exacerbated where psychiatry intersects with racism in the context of massive resistance to evolving civil rights movements in the South. In this sense, the regular tension between psychiatry and race is amplified because of broader social and racial tensions, in which the Black person is already seen as a threat, subject to violence, disrespect, and incarceration with no due process. It would be a mistake to assume that psychiatric hospitals were exempt from these problems, or that they were islands of benevolence in an otherwise raging sea of racism. And if local politics did not already create problems for Black patients, the internal racism of psychiatry itself surely did. These problems are clearly displayed through the way states reported their official admission processes.[55]

Specific admission processes for each patient are impossible to document because it would require access to individual records that do not exist or have been lost. In Georgia or Alabama, it would also require access to probate court or local county court records, which have become impossible to access without being a direct descendant.[56] In Mississippi, the admission process becomes even more obscure, as it was medical as opposed to legal—that is, there was no requirement for admission to occur via a court. Admission processes in all three states were technically covered by verbiage in each state's code, which evolved over time. In the mid-1950s, each state had a paragraph or clause in their respective state code, or in other documents, that set out the formal process for admission and commitment to the relevant state institutions.

Mississippi's admission processes were set out in Chapter 342 of the state code—Senate Bill No. 19, which was updated in 1950—and was unchanged until at least 1964, when Dr. Jaquith published them as a separate document called *Admission Laws for State Mental Hospitals of Mississippi*. In his preface to this 1964 document, Jaquith wrote that the revised 1950 laws were "modern and workable. There is little or no stigma attached to our present admission laws and very little legal action is needed except in exceptional cases. While these laws may be not [be] termed ideal by many people as they do not contain a purely voluntary clause, the admission procedure is so simple as to almost amount to a voluntary admission in the vast majority of cases."[57]

In the document, Jaquith summarized the legalese of the state code to explain that there were two routes of admission, but the difference between them was minor and rested on the willingness of the patient. In the ideal situation, the patient or family of the patient would have two physicians conduct an examination—any physician known to the family was acceptable. If the two physicians agreed that admission was warranted, they would both sign a statement to that fact, or they could sign an admission blank from the hospital, which many physicians kept a supply of in their office. Then the patient would be brought by the family (or themselves) to Whitfield for admission and observation. Jaquith pointed out that "the two physicians who sign the admission application are in no way held liable under the law if they act in good faith." If the patient was "hostile to admission," the family or friends could appeal to the local chancery clerk, who would then summon the two physicians and the patient for "a sanity hearing." If these physicians felt admission was warranted, they would sign the same forms, and the patient would be brought to the hospital by law enforcement, "or by his family if they so desire and this is practicable."[58]

Jaquith noted that often the physicians in this situation did not feel admission was warranted, and the person would be released by the court. Patients admitted under a court order had this admission recorded by the court, but if they were subsequently released by the hospital as either not insane or treated successfully, then that release was also recorded by the court. Patients who were admitted "voluntarily" by family and physicians did not have their admission or discharge recorded by the court. Jaquith also made it clear that only the admitting physicians at the state hospital could determine the nature of the person's illness and whether they should be committed for treatment or not—this process came at the end of a period of observation the length of which was not specified by law.

Jaquith was right to comment that these processes were less than ideal, resting as they did on a tenuous differentiation between voluntary and involuntary commitment, the word of physicians not trained as psychiatrists, and an indeterminate observation period. Even if final admission was the decision of Whitfield doctors, the nonlegal route to admission was surely subject to exploitation and abuse by families, neighbors, and law enforcement, and gave patients no protective oversight from the court (such as it may have been). The rationale for a nonlegal method of admission was in fact to avoid the stigma and official recordkeeping of the court process, not for the patient's sake but for the family's. And without a record in the court of provisional admission or subsequent commitment to Whitfield, patients could easily get lost in the system—dropped at the door and no longer a problem for the family.

This scenario would certainly have been exacerbated for indigent or single Black patients who could have easily been committed with no family notification. In conversations I have had with mental health lawyers from Mississippi, it was not uncommon for the highway patrol or other law enforcement to bring a patient to Whitfield with the signatures of two physicians on the back of a speeding ticket. These kinds of cases would, years later, require extensive habeas corpus petitions to secure release.[59]

In contrast, both Alabama and Georgia used a legal process for admission. The best summary of the admission processes in the 1950s in Alabama is contained in the 1958 inspection report by the American Psychiatric Association, which set out the intricate details around the kind of contract entered into between the institution and the county courts. Much of the legal process here was designed to ascertain the patient's ability to pay for their admission and treatment, and to secure a bond between the county court and the institution for that payment and for the expenses incurred by the death of a patient if required.

Relatives or friends could recommend to the county probate judge anyone they believed required admission, and the probate judge would initiate an investigation. The judge would then examine witnesses, at least one of whom needed to be a physician, either with or without a jury, and with or without the presence of the prospective patient, as the judge saw fit. The judge would then issue two "certificates of mental disqualification," one to go with the patient to the hospital and one lodged with the court. The law clearly stated that "a person shall be judged insane who has been found by a proper court to be sufficiently deficient or defective mentally to require that, for his own or others' welfare, he be removed to an insane hospital for restraint, care, and treatment. Whether the person's mental abnormality is sufficiently grave to warrant such procedure is always the question to be decided by the court."[60] The superintendent technically had the ability to refuse admission once a patient was delivered if the hospital was too crowded, but it was often the case that other political pressures were brought to bear to force the superintendent to accept a patient.[61]

In Georgia, which used a similar legal process, the ability to have friends or relatives committed without any real psychiatric oversight led to a rapid growth in the amount of people committed to Central State Hospital after the 1940s, especially under the direction of superintendents like Thomas Peacock, the "king of Georgia eugenics."[62] Commitment procedures and definitions of insanity were covered by the Georgia Health Code, Chapter 88-5, which was more expansive in its definitions than Alabama's. Whereas Alabama's code explicitly stated that the state hospitals were for the admission of "insane" people only, and not those with learning or development disabilities, Georgia's code acted like a veritable catchall. It defined "mentally ill person" as anyone "who is afflicted with a psychiatric disorder which substantially impairs his mental health; and because of such psychiatric disorder requires care, treatment, training, or detention in the interest of the welfare of such person or the welfare of others of the community in which such person resides and shall include, but not be limited to, any mental retardation, alcoholism, or drug addiction when due to or accompanied by mental illness or mental disease, or, in the case of any mental retardation, when the mentally retarded person is incapable thereby of making a satisfactory adjustment outside of a psychiatric hospital."[63]

Under this code, voluntary patients over the age of eighteen could admit themselves, or be admitted, to Milledgeville, and they would be assessed there for mental illness and discharged as necessary. However, it was noted that even in the case of voluntary patients, the superintendent retained the right to not discharge people whom he believed a threat to themselves or others. Section 88-504 of the code specified that a voluntary patient could request a discharge in writing and thus be entitled to discharge within fifteen days of the receipt of that request. If the superintendent thought that the person was not well enough to be discharged, he could then lodge a certificate with the probate court to have the patient retained as "involuntary." Both the patient and the next of kin were supposed to be notified of this change in status.

Section 88-513 of the code specified that the patient had the right to appeal their continued detention at the court through which their commitment was processed but would require another physician and an attorney to testify that they were no longer mentally ill. Involuntary commitment followed a process similar to Alabama's, but two physicians and an attorney were required to argue the case in front of the court. If the judge believed that the person required committal, the person could be detained immediately either in their own home or in another "suitable facility"—including the county jail—to wait for transportation by the sheriff to Central State Hospital.[64] Once admitted to Central State, the person needed to be assessed and diagnosed "as soon as practicable," which in a hospital the size of Central State could be anywhere from days to weeks, to possibly never for some.[65]

It is one thing, however, to have a written legal or medical admission procedure and quite another to have followed it to the letter in every single case. In the absence of access to the formal legal records of commitment, I cannot say with any certainty that due process was ever followed. But there is plenty of evidence in the archives and elsewhere to indicate that it was not. There are numerous letters in the archives from family members begging for their relatives to be moved or released or admitted in the first place, all of which indicate that legal due process was not in play. Many letters from (white) family members trying to have someone committed are accompanied by a plea from the governor to the superintendent to "just let them in for a while"; one letter I found in Georgia from as late as 1989 was from Senator Culver Kidd asking Dr. Gates to admit someone's wife because the divorce settlement would be easier.[66] Of course Dr. Gates refused, but in the earlier period with which this book is concerned, that resistance was less likely and less supported by either custom or practice, and I have no doubt that the law as it was written was rarely, if ever, applied to Black families. The silence in the official archives, the impossibility of accessing them, and the breadcrumbs I have been able to find are, I would argue, evidence of laws and codes decidedly not adhered to.

If the processes for commitment varied across the three states, so too did the amount of people who ended up confined. As the only state hospital at the time in Georgia, Central State in Milledgeville was notoriously overcrowded, and in the 1956 annual report, Superintendent Peacock reported that the hospital had a grand total of 14,058 patients "on the books."[67] More than 7,000 of the inpatients in 1956 were white (3,339 men, 4,035 women), plus 2,077 Black men and 2,393 Black women, making a total of 4,470 Black people confined on-site at Milledgeville. The percentage of Black patients being admitted was about 37 percent in a state with a 39 percent Black population, as recorded in the 1960 census.[68] In Alabama, the 1956 annual report recorded a total "on the book" patient population of 8,051, with 7,197 inpatients. Of these, 5,007 were white (2,393 men, 2,614 women), and 2,913 were Black (1,395 men, 1,518 women). The percentage of Black patients being admitted here was 40 percent in a state with a 30 percent Black population.[69] And most of these patients were physically located in Mount Vernon, where they were out of sight and out of mind.

Frustratingly, Mississippi's recordkeeping is less than detailed. In the first official report submitted by Dr. Jaquith in 1951, the director recorded the total patient population from 1922 (1845) to 1952 (4412) but rarely publicly broke these statistics down by race. In the 1953–55 biennial report, he reported, "Some study must be given to the alleviation of the crowded conditions that exist in the Negro section of this institution. At this writing, 2,440 of our patients are Negroes. The crowded conditions on these wards are not complimentary to the institution. There has been no new construction for Negro patients since the institution was opened in 1935. A study of the Negro section of the institution should be made and plans for [an] additional patients' building should be brought forth during this session of the Legislature, if we are to continue our present service to our Negro population."[70]

Yet from this point on, there is no official breakdown of admission statistics by race. It is impossible to tell whether they kept those records or chose not to report them. This could have been an act of deliberate obfuscation in order to hide how many Black patients they were admitting in comparison to white (whether it was more or less, there were implications either way). Or it may have simply been enough to report that Black and white patients were physically separated and placed in a cottage with those most like themselves for ease of patient management. Perhaps this came from being chronically understaffed, or perhaps it was an effect of a different kind of segregation in Mississippi that also fell across class lines.

The vast disparity between the white wealthy and the rest of society might have created a kind of flattening effect when it came to the admission of the mentally ill to Whitfield, which received payment for services from only about 100 patient families. If you were white and wealthy with a mentally ill family member in Mississippi, it was highly unlikely you would admit that person to Whitfield if you had an alternative. In this sense, then, the poor white and the Black person may have had more in common when it came to admission to Whitfield than in other arenas of Mississippi life. The omission is also striking because it speaks to a covert recognition of the lie of biological racial difference. In Mississippi, the stakes were about miscegenation and re-creation of relations of deference and servitude, rather than any kind of science. This thinning of the color line at the intersection with psychiatry is particularly telling, revealing the extent to which Jim Crow was indeed a performance in Mississippi in different ways than in Alabama or Georgia.[71]

Using official records like publicly available annual reports demonstrates something about the way Jim Crow in the asylum was justified and operationalized, and the extent to which segregation was posed as a seemingly natural and normal way of life. When the official reports accounted for that segregation, they did so in order to assure policymakers and legislators that the norms of Southern life were being maintained in the asylum, and that all possible measures were being taken to keep Black patients away from white patients. This practice was a performance of the Jim Crow routine in that it did actually keep Black patients away from white patients, thus reassuring the white public and family members, but it also served to reinforce ideas about the supposed risk posed to white fragility by the "mad"

Black person and enabled practices based on the so-called eugenic threat and danger of the Black patient when confined with white patients. It reminded the white public and legislature that no unnecessary tax dollars were being spent on "those people," which therefore limited the possibility of compassionate care for Black patients.

In the very real sense, segregation (and less spending) enabled a literal performance of white supremacy, which placed the Black patient at greater risk of unlawful confinement, neglectful care, and abusive treatment, while maintaining a public veneer of benevolent paternalism. But official reports in themselves were problematic, as they demonstrated the political and account-keeping purposes they served but told very little about everyday practices or the lives of the people who were admitted. Laws such as state codes also served a political and social purpose. They gave the appearance of color blindness in that there was no stated difference in the routes of admission and commitment for Black versus white patients, yet this race-neutral language hid the reality of violent policing behind the letter of the law to which everyone supposedly had access (when they most definitely did not). Later in this book I will tease out some of the ways that this was not the case in reality.

But hospitals and asylums were not prisons; they relied on medical justifications for confinement. Diagnosis was essential to this process, and treatment was the stated aim. In the 1950s, the diagnostic and treatment practices of American psychiatry were dynamic and rapidly evolving, but they were also inherently racist. If segregation in the asylum hid behind the custom and practice of Southern life codified by law, the actual practice of psychiatry—the implementation of diagnosis, the approach to treatment—were equally problematic and hidden behind the fiction of science. The implications of the internal racism for psychiatric practice within Southern asylums is the subject of chapter 3.

3 Diagnosing Difference

United States Department of Justice
National Training School
Washington D.C.

November 8, 1966

The boy in question is . . . a 17 year old Negro boy from Savannah, Georgia. . . . It has been strongly felt by various members of the staff that he represented an extremely disturbed boy. He has been aggressive, provocative to his peers and assaultive. . . . He has been obsessed with the thought of committing suicide. . . . From my examination of him I would describe him as a functionally retarded boy with brain damage associated with epilepsy, with manifestations of psychosis. . . . My diagnostic impression, at this time, is chronic brain syndrome associated with convulsive disorder with psychotic reaction. I would recommend that he be transferred to the Milledgeville State Hospital . . . as soon as possible.

Sincerely yours,
Harding W. Olson MD.
Consulting Psychiatrist
National Training School for Boys

Dr. Olson's letter to Dr. Charles Bush, director of the Hospital Services Branch in the Georgia Department of Public Health, reads like a veritable menu of diagnostic classifications, ranging from retardation to epilepsy to brain damage to psychosis.[1] Olson's letter is important because it speaks to many of the problems facing Black patients caught in the psychiatric network of confinement and reveals the way that psychiatric diagnosis was an inherently racist practice. In this example, multiple diagnoses are stacked on top of each other, labels like "aggressive" and "paranoid" are unproblematically applied and disconnected from the social forces that might have caused them, and personality disorders coexist with organic issues. This diagnostic miasma was symptomatic of the internal racism of psychiatry, where behavioral issues were linked indelibly to race and culture as deprivation.

The young man in Olson's letter clearly suffered from traumatic brain injury due to untreated epilepsy, but in a move typical of psychiatrists when dealing with Black patients, Olson shows no hesitation in also blaming the boy for his own behavior. Elsewhere in the letter, Olson argued that the boy's attempts at suicide were "attention getting maneuvers" and that "he is extremely embittered and at times shows definite paranoid trends." While he noted that the young man came from a "very deprived background with an absent father, a mother who died in 1960, and a grandmother who is limited in her resources," he also argued that the boy "is unable to see himself as having anything to do with the constant difficulty he gets into with peers and staff. Through his consistently demanding behavior he evokes a rejecting attitude on the part of others which causes him to be even more embittered. Even his suicidal ruminations tend to have a manipulative quality about them."[2] Olson prescribed a heavy dose of Thorazine (75 mg, 3 times per day) and anticonvulsants for his epilepsy and requested that the young man be transferred to the Chatham County Jail in Savannah and then admitted via the probate court to Central State Hospital (CSH) in Milledgeville. There is a scrawled note on the first page that the young man was "admitted," but no further details are attached.

This chapter is an attempt to try to understand the way that diagnosis and treatment were enacted in the South at the intersection with race. To do so, I am forced to rely on the available diagnostic and treatment data presented in annual reports from the state hospitals, which presents several complex problems. Understanding diagnoses in the past is always a fraught and ethically treacherous enterprise—the reports we have as sources can be suspect, as can our interpretation of them, and the data they contain is never complete.[3] In all three states, the published annual or biannual reports are only useful for an analysis at the large group level; due to the lack of individual patient records, it is not possible to analyze how any one person was committed, assessed, diagnosed, treated, cured, or discharged, or even how they died. My goal, therefore, is to explore the ways that the newly released *Diagnostic and Statistical Manual* (*DSM*) was being interpreted and implemented across these states; to tease out similarities and differences; and, as a result, to demonstrate the way that a supposedly neutral and scientific process like diagnosis was in fact highly political.

The first section of this chapter explores the context for the development of the first version of the *Diagnostic and Statistical Manual (DSM-1)*, analyzing the ideas that informed it and considering the implications of those ideas for racialized diagnostic practices. In the second section, I focus on the implementation of the *DSM* a few years after its release in 1952 by analyzing a snapshot of data from Georgia and Alabama.[4] While the *DSM* contained dozens of diagnostic categories, my analysis here focuses on the three major categories attributed at first admission: schizophrenic reactions, chronic brain syndromes, and mental deficiency.

An analysis of the application of diagnostic criteria shows how it reflected prevailing social ideas about race and gender, demonstrating that diagnoses were not stable criteria. But it also shows that many of the disparities and discrepancies in diagnosis today had their foundation laid at this early stage of *DSM*-related classification. Stereotypes about differences between Black and white psyches were reinforced by the application of the *DSM* and thus codified these so-called differences in ways that set the scene for generations of diagnostic practice. It is not so much that *DSM* created race, but rather it laid bare the internal racism of psychiatry right at the moment when science should have negated it, and which psychiatric science continues to repeat. The way these diagnostic ideas translated into treatment practices is the subject of the final section of this chapter.

Because of the lack of consistency or similarity from one state to another, it is not possible to provide a comprehensive comparison across the states, so the data presented here provides some snapshots into various aspects of the institutional practices, some more in depth than others. This is also the case when it comes to reporting actual treatment methods and their application. The third section of this chapter looks at prevailing ideas about and approaches to treatment in the mid-1950s, considering how available treatment modalities were operationalized differently for racial groups. The data here is not extensive; sometimes each of these states reported treatment data, sometimes they did not, and to find it required scouring hundreds of pages of annual reports, where it would be buried in a single paragraph. But there is enough to indicate that the science of psychiatry at the time enabled its own performance of the Jim Crow routine. This section of the chapter explores the way that the internal racism of psychiatry manifested in the different types of therapeutic programs that each facility developed and considers some of the implications of these discrepancies. But analyzing data requires an understanding of the very particular context of diagnostic practices in the mid-1950s, when American psychiatry was still largely concerned with the *origins* of disorders as the criteria for diagnosis.

Understanding the Diagnostic Context:
DSM-1 and Dynamic Psychiatry

By the mid-1950s, all three states under study here were clearly using the *DSM*. The *DSM* was first developed in 1952, born of an uneasy marriage between the remnants of military practice and institutional psychiatry. The need to collect data about types of mental illness had risen in the wake of World War II with unprecedented levels of what was then called "combat fatigue" or "war neurosis" and related nervous breakdown among soldiers despite the best efforts of the psychiatrists in the Surgeon General's office to weed out perceived weaknesses through its extensive Selective Service program.

Concerns about the stability of returning soldiers, as well as the society they were returning to, gave rise to the psy-science expert, who was now seen to hold the key to many social problems, ranging from juvenile delinquency to marital problems to serious and persistent mental illness. The willingness (or necessity) of families and communities to commit family members to institutions also rose after World War II. By 1953, the total number of people institutionalized in the United States for mental illness–related diagnoses reached an all-time high of more than 577,000 people.[5] Some method of consistent diagnostic classification was required to at least account for the vast numbers of people being committed and to track where possible what types of illnesses were prevalent.

However, the issue of naming and defining types of illnesses was in itself a fraught exercise. Several scholars have demonstrated the conflicting ideological and scientific positions inherent to American psychiatry in the postwar era.[6] Scientifically, the development of the *DSM* demonstrates the strong influence of Freudian psychoanalysis and psychodynamic psychiatry *and* an adherence to the more "disease process" method of classification and diagnosis exemplified by Emil Kraepelin. This is significant for the understanding of the use of the *DSM*, because the underlying method of creating those diagnostic categories was actually based on the supposed cause of illness rather than on a description of the symptoms.[7]

Using something like perceived cause as a diagnostic tool is exactly what allowed social, political, or cultural norms to pervade the science of psychiatry at the time. This is not to deny the importance of environment or trauma, but it is undoubtedly the case that cause was read differently according to race and gender by the majority of white male physicians doing the diagnosing. For some, the very fact of Blackness meant mental deficiency in the same way that the fact of femaleness meant hysteria. The psychiatric literature of the 1950s was steeped in both racialized and gendered assumptions about cause and symptomology, and this inevitably played out in the way that patients were diagnosed and then treated. The *DSM* remained unaltered until 1968.

Analyzing Diagnostic Patterns

Comparing diagnoses across the three states is complicated by a lack of consistency in reporting styles. Mississippi's biannual reports are particularly frustrating because they do not report diagnostic or treatment data by race at all, only gender; it is very possible the hospital at Whitfield did not bother to keep detailed records about the nature of Black illness and that only cursory attempts at diagnosis of Black patients were made. It may also be the case that the physicians at Whitfield were less obsessed with the alleged racial differences in psychiatry that seemed to prevail elsewhere. The fact that diagnostic categories at Whitfield were broken down by sex and age might indicate that gender was a more important mediator than race when it came to actual diagnosis.

The lack of diagnostic transparency could have also been a consequence of the lack of psychiatric expertise at Whitfield at the time, but this erasure may also indicate a kind of deliberate obfuscation. If the performance of Jim Crow in Mississippi was predicated on a logic of benevolent paternalism, then there was no need to record exact diagnoses along racial lines. The state could claim it treated all its disabled people with the same level of care. In the absence of detailed personal records, or even hospital policy records regarding diagnostic procedures, it is almost impossible to say anything about racial diagnosis at Whitfield.

But there are still some interesting things to note about what is available from Whitfield. In the biennial report ending June 30, 1955, the director, Dr. William Jaquith, reported 744 first admissions for women and 1,048 for men. Of these, the largest diagnostic category for women was "schizophrenic reactions," under which 257 cases were recorded. The next two highest categories were ones in which women had no clear diagnosis—that is, 122 were listed as undiagnosed and 71 listed as having no disorder at all.

Combined, these three categories accounted for 59.8 percent of all diagnoses.

The pattern for men admitted to Whitfield in the year 1955 was quite different. Of the 1,048 total first admissions, schizophrenia was attributed to 184 male patients, exactly half the rate as for women; 105 were listed as undiagnosed and 99 were listed without a mental disorder, which is close to 20 percent of all male patients. However, the categories "Undiagnosed" and "No mental disorder" constituted nearly 26 percent of all female diagnoses. These gendered differences, and the high rate of people being held without diagnoses, reflect the way that hospitals like Whitfield often worked as dumping grounds for broader social or domestic problems, to which women were particularly vulnerable. Without access to individual patient records, we cannot know if a person's symptoms simply defied easy categorization, or whether these people were then discharged or furloughed, but this kind of data raises questions about the way that admission and diagnostic procedures were implemented, and why people with no obvious mental illness were being held at Whitfield.

In Alabama, the link between public welfare and segregation was reinforced by and clearly represented in the annual reports, which were separated into two sections: one containing data for Bryce Hospital (white patients), and the other, data for Searcy Hospital (Black patients). In 1956, the Bryce section of the report covered the first 115 pages; the Searcy report ran for a mere 41 pages. The diagnostic data was presented in complex tables that reported diagnosis at first admission under the main categories of the *DSM*, and the Searcy section only listed those diagnoses with one or more patient. For 1956, the Bryce section recorded first-admission diagnostic data for 568 white men and 519 white women. For Searcy, first-admission data was recorded for 236 Black men and 258 Black women.

In 1956, Central State Hospital in Milledgeville, Georgia, recorded first admissions of 1,046 white men, 907 white women, 356 Black men, and 372 Black women. In the Georgia reports, the diagnostic statistics appeared all together in the same section but were separated into tables labeled "White Male," "White Female," "Colored Male," and "Colored Female." In the following pages, I compare select data points to try to identify diagnostic patterns in the two hospitals, and to hypothesize about what those patterns might signify.

One of the most contested diagnoses in the history of psychiatry is schizophrenia. In the 1950s, it was not precisely the same as we consider it today, nor was it a direct correlation to the earlier category of dementia

TABLE 3.1 Psychotic disorders diagnosed on first admission, 1956

Diagnostic data by race, gender, and state		Involutional psychotic reactions		Schizophrenic reactions		Affective reactions		Percent of total Dx
		#	%	#	%	#	%	
White men	Alabama	53	9.3	144	25.3	4	0.7	35.3
	Georgia	2	0.19	91	8.6	141	13.4	22.19
White women	Alabama	81	15.06	216	42.6	0	0	57.66
	Georgia	122	13	217	23.9	74	8.1	45.0
Black men	Alabama	0	0	57	24.1	16	6.7	30.8
	Georgia	0	0	83	23	51	14.3	37.3
Black women	Alabama	0	0	111	43.02	40	15.5	58.52
	Georgia	0	0	73	19.6	35	9.4	29.0

Sources: Table 2, pp. 38–41, *Annual Report of the Milledgeville State Hospital*, 1956, https://dlg.galileo.usg.edu/data/dlg/ggpd/pdfs/dlg_ggpd_y-ga-be450-pm5-ba1-b1955-h60.pdf; Table 6 (Bryce Hospital), p. 36, and Table 6 (Searcy Hospital), pp. 121–22, *Report of the Trustees of the Alabama State Hospitals*, 1956, https://digitalcommons.library.uab.edu/arash/.

praecox.[8] As historian of psychiatry Allan Horwitz has explained, the *DSM-1* represents a kind of transitional document, linking knowledge gained in the military with broader understandings of the impact of environment and stress on mental health.[9]

Illnesses that were not obviously linked to some kind of organic brain tissue damage were considered "psychogenic," exemplified by the use of the word "reactions." These reactions were generally considered the result of "interactions between vulnerable personalities and stressful life events, with Freudian psychodynamics emphasizing unresolved, unconscious conflicts that arise in early childhood. . . . Therefore, the manual used the term 'reaction' to characterize all of these types of disorders."[10]

The data from Alabama and Georgia in table 3.1 show shifts in patterns of diagnoses, which reveal a category in the making, subject to changes in both scientific understandings of cause and expression of mental illness but also highly influenced by social and cultural norms. Both states reported "schizophrenic reactions" as one of three main disorders: involutional psychotic reactions, schizophrenic reactions, and affective reactions. The *DSM* itself was vague on what constituted the difference between involutional, schizophrenic, and affective reactions, and also listed nine subtypes of schizophrenic reactions, making specific diagnostics difficult even at the time, let alone for those of us trying to understand them seventy years later.

Both schizophrenic and affective reactions were listed together in the *DSM-1* under the sentence "Disorders of psychogenic origin or without clearly defined tangible cause or structural change," while "involutional psychotic reactions" were listed separately as "disorders due to disturbance of metabolism, growth, nutrition, or endocrine function," which was generally read as shorthand for "melancholia" related to middle age (or menopause for women).[11]

Some interesting patterns emerge when comparing these diagnoses both within categories and across the states.[12] In Alabama, when represented as a percentage of diagnoses at first admission, gender was the decisive factor in the attribution of psychotic disorders, but racial patterns were still obvious. For example, Black women were diagnosed with affective reactions at twice the rate of anyone else—and not a single white woman was diagnosed in this way—whereas no Black patients were diagnosed with involutional psychotic reactions. This is significant in that these types of disorders were related to metabolic changes as part of the aging process and should therefore have transcended subjective opinions based on race. Affective reactions were judgments based on the behavior of the patient toward the clinician and were therefore subject to both race and gender biases and stereotypes.

Schizophrenic reactions was the most widely diagnosed for all women admitted in Alabama, accounting for 42.6 percent of white women's total diagnoses and just over 43 percent of all Black women's. Combined with the other psychotic disorders, this category accounted for nearly 57.7 percent of all white women's diagnosis and just over 58.5 percent of all Black women's.

This pattern was different in Georgia, where women were more likely to be given diagnoses from a broader spectrum across all categories, although almost half of the total diagnoses for white women came from these three psychotic disorders categories alone (45 percent). For Black and white women and Black men, schizophrenic reactions accounted for between 19 and 24 percent of all diagnoses, while it was attributed to only 8.6 percent of white men (compared to just over 25 percent in Alabama).

The most striking difference is the rate of diagnosis of schizophrenic reactions between the two states—it was twice as likely to be recorded in Alabama than it was in Georgia across all the race/sex groups except for Black men. These statistics indicate a lack of diagnostic complexity in Alabama and the tendency to over- or misdiagnose schizophrenia as a kind of blanket category. At this point in time, schizophrenia in Alabama was a female diagnosis, while this was not so much the case in Georgia, where white women and Black men were almost equally likely to be diagnosed with it.

But there is a striking similarity between the states, which is the complete non-diagnosis of involutional psychotic reactions for any Black patient anywhere. This category, which was considered related to the metabolic changes of middle age, was apparently not considered applicable to Black patients in either state. Without being able to cross-reference each of these diagnoses with the patient's age, it's difficult to explain this trend, but at the very least, it indicates a disregard for either the biological or the emotional complexity of Black life over the lifespan, as if those patients could not possibly experience the same metabolic processes as white people. In this pattern, the internal racism of psychiatry, based as it was on unscientific notions of biological difference, became particularly clear.

Racializing Alzheimer's Disease

The majority of other diagnoses seemed to fall into two main categories: "chronic brain syndrome" or "mental deficiency."[13] Understanding chronic brain syndrome is complicated because of the liminal space it inhabited between psychiatry and neuroscience and the emerging field of gerontology.[14] The picture is further complicated when trying to account for the presence of Alzheimer's disease (AD), recorded in the *DSM-1* under "Chronic Brain Syndrome associated with other disturbance of metabolism, growth or nutrition." This code included the word "presenile," which reflects the Kraepelian influence on the *DSM*, which differentiated Alzheimer's disease from regular dementia associated with aging because it had been recorded in people younger than sixty-five.[15] Given these patterns, it is impossible to say anything definitive about either the existence of Alzheimer's disease as a separate category or the process by which it was diagnosed.[16]

Senile brain disease is an interesting category, however, in that it was considered a mental illness because the *DSM* was still heavily influenced by psychodynamic approaches to diagnosis. As historian Jesse Ballenger writes, "AD and senile dementia were regarded by most psychiatrists of this period not as cognitive disorders produced by biological processes within the brain, but as mental illnesses produced by psychodynamic processes occurring between an aging individual and society. So conceived, dementia was not a well-bounded disease entity."[17] This broad psychosocial conception of dementia is reflected in the comparative data from Alabama and

TABLE 3.2 Chronic brain syndromes diagnosed on first admission, 1956

Diagnostic data by race, gender, and state		Cerebral arteriosclerosis		Senile brain disease		Percent of total
		#	%	#	%	Dx
White men	Alabama	133	23.4	10	1.7	25.1
	Georgia	306	29	0	0	29.0
White women	Alabama	103	19.8	14	2.6	22.4
	Georgia	143	15.7	131	14.4	30.1
Black men	Alabama	9	3.8	39	16.5	20.3
	Georgia	89	25	14	3.9	28.9
Black women	Alabama	7	2.7	38	14.7	17.4
	Georgia	97	26	22	5.0	31.0

Sources: Table 2, pp. 38–41, *Annual Report of the Milledgeville State Hospital*, 1956, https://dlg.galileo.usg.edu/data/dlg/ggpd/pdfs/dlg_ggpd_y-ga-be450-pm5-ba1-b1955-h60.pdf; Table 6 (Bryce Hospital), p. 36, and Table 6 (Searcy Hospital), pp. 121–22, *Report of the Trustees of the Alabama State Hospitals*, 1956, https://digitalcommons.library.uab.edu/arash/.

Georgia, which also demonstrates a lack of clear consensus between physicians in these two states about who belonged in what category.

Table 3.2 sets out the comparative data of chronic brain syndromes related to either cerebral arteriosclerosis (CA) or senile brain disease (SBD), the two most frequently used diagnoses in this category in 1956.

In Alabama, there is a striking difference between white patients being diagnosed on first admittance with senile brain disease versus Black patients. The proportion of Black men being admitted with this diagnosis was almost seventeen times the amount than for white men, and almost six times the amount than for white women, while the reverse pattern was true for cerebral arteriosclerosis. White patients, who were being admitted to the Bryce Hospital in Tuscaloosa, were far more likely to be diagnosed with CA than those being admitted to Searcy Hospital in Mount Vernon.

This overall pattern is almost completely reversed in Georgia, with some notable anomalies. White men, for example, were *only* diagnosed with CA. White women were roughly equally likely to be diagnosed with either CA or SBD, while Black men and women were much more likely to be diagnosed with CA than SBD.

In the absence of clear diagnostic processes in either state, it is difficult to hypothesize what the cause of this difference might be, but Ballenger's work on the thinking about senility and arteriosclerosis in the 1950s is helpful.

He argues that the "traditional view that arteriosclerosis was somehow causative in all cases of dementia in old age continued to appear in the literature. Thus the diagnosis of arteriosclerosis seems to have been greatly overused through the 1960s."[18] This was certainly the case in Georgia, where physicians at CSH were much more likely to use this diagnosis for everyone except white women. The diagnosis of senile brain disease could also relate to the thinking about the cause of that disease—that it was in fact a psychosocial pathology as much as a natural consequence of old age. If, as Ballenger argues, SBD was often conceptualized as a condition related to resistance to social change, with symptoms over which the patient was believed to have some control, it makes some sense why the admitting physicians in Alabama were more likely to attribute this kind of thinking about causality to Black patients, especially where any kind of resistance to social oppression was expressed.[19]

Chronic brain syndrome as a category of diagnosis also needs to be considered within the overall context of care for the elderly in this decade before the advent of Medicare and Medicaid. The two categories of chronic brain syndrome accounted for around 30 percent of the first-admission diagnoses for all sex and race groups at CSH in Georgia. State hospitals in the 1950s were facing a crisis of care as they became dumping grounds for elderly relatives, especially in states with no safety-net services for the aged.[20] This was painfully evident in Georgia, which had very few public facilities for the care of the elderly before 1965, and it relied solely on this one large facility in Milledgeville before it began a regionalization process.[21]

While there is no racial difference evident in the *distribution* of the diagnostic categories related to old age at Central State, there is a clear race-based difference in the *numbers* of overall admissions in these categories. White men (306) accounted for the largest number of first admissions with chronic brain syndromes, and white women were close behind with 274 total admissions. In comparison, there were only 119 admissions of Black women, and 103 Black men, meaning white men were admitted at three times the rate of Black men in these categories.

In Alabama, a similarly marked discrepancy existed: state hospitals admitted 143 white men and 117 white women with chronic brain syndromes, but only 48 Black men and 45 Black women. Black families were possibly less likely to voluntarily use the state hospital system for elder care if they could avoid it. But there is also the very real possibility that the Black elderly are less represented in the state hospital systems in Georgia and Alabama because they did not live as long, and that Black men in particular may have experienced other forms of institutionalization through the criminal justice system.

Defining Mental Deficiency

The other major diagnostic category used in 1956 was "mental deficiency." Mental deficiency under the *DSM-1* was broken into two categories, and the distinction between them was related to perception of cause. That is, the first type (x) was described as "disorders due to unknown or uncertain cause with the functional reaction alone manifest; heredity and familial diseases of this nature: mental deficiency (familial or heredity)," and the second type (y) was described as "disorders due to undetermined cause: mental deficiency, idiopathic." Each type had three subtypes: mild, moderate, or severe.[22]

The distinction between heredity and spontaneous types of mental deficiency would have been grist to the eugenicist mill but seems to have been irrelevant at the actual point of diagnosis, as none of the reports from Alabama or Georgia distinguish between the two types, nor do they break down the diagnosis by subtype. Again, there are some interesting differences between the states and between race and sex groups.

In Alabama, there is a very clear discrepancy in the diagnosis of mental deficiency between the white patients at Bryce and the Black patients at Searcy. The raw numbers themselves are relatively low: 12 white men, 4 white women, 17 Black men, and 15 Black women were newly admitted with this diagnosis in 1956. It is immediately striking that more Black people were diagnosed this way.

In Georgia, the number of people admitted in this category was higher, reflecting the larger population at Central State overall, but the greatest proportion of diagnoses was reserved for Black women: 13.7 percent of first admissions for Black women were classified as "mentally deficient," 4 percent higher than those of Black men, roughly double the rate of white men, and 10 percent higher than the admissions for white women. In Alabama, the rates of the diagnosis of "mentally deficient" were higher for all patients and higher again for Black patients. There was a clear difference here in diagnostic practice, demonstrating the way that white physicians at Searcy and in Georgia were using different criteria for Black patients, criteria that likely reflected embedded and racist assumptions about the allegedly lower intelligence and rational capacity of the Black person.

An analysis of diagnostic data—of any data that appears to fall along so-called racial lines—needs to be treated very carefully. If race is a social construct, then using statistics—a tool of biomedical white supremacy—could be seen as giving scientific credibility where none is due. Taken out of context, statistics like these could serve to reify the very idea of racial difference, and indeed they have already set the groundwork for misdiagnosis today. What I am arguing here, however, is that these statistics, and the people who collected them, served to create racial difference as biology in the first place. Diagnostic practices were *not* race neutral but instead were highly social and politically constructed categories, which changed according to the opinions and beliefs of the diagnosing physician. These processes could be entirely different from one state (Georgia) to another (Alabama), and even between facilities in the same state (Alabama).

Yet the veneer of science lent, and has continued to lend, authority to diagnostic difference that maps alongside the socially constructed category of race, in ways that shaped and reflected both public and psychiatric ideas about psychological difference. Diagnostic categories were not simply biased at the level of the individual practitioner but reflected broader social and psychiatric thinking about the alleged inferiority of the Black psyche. When those differences were codified by statistics in the 1950s with the advent of the *DSM*, they became the foundation for future belief and practice, handed down over years often unquestioned or unaltered. Because of this, racial politics that created and normalized segregation in psychiatric spaces was supported by seemingly scientific categories. Together, this creation of difference was used to justify approaches to therapy and treatment, revealing the inherently racist assumptions of psychiatric theory and the way it was applied in the Jim Crow South.

"All Recognized Types of Therapy"

In his introduction to the 1956 annual report from Central State Hospital in Milledgeville, superintendent Thomas Peacock gave an overview of the approach to treatment at this large hospital, which held more than 11,000 patients: "Psychiatry, more than any other branch of medicine, is in a state of flux, because of its theoretical approach. Those of us who have devoted years of our lives to its study are often perplexed by its rapidly changing tides."[23] The true extent of Peacock's confusion would be revealed by a major Atlanta newspaper exposé a few years later, but it was already evident in the ad hoc approach to treatment and therapy at CSH. This was not in itself a problem unique to the South, but it reflected the way that large hospitals ended up being a kind of dumping ground for all kinds of mental disability, including epilepsy, learning disabilities, schizophrenia, and the dementia associated with old age. This was the case because the respective state governments were reluctant to spend money on any of the states' "defectives"— so long as there was somewhere to put them where they would be out of sight and out of mind.

Peacock himself was not unaware of these issues, or the way that the hospital was perceived by the public. If he was overwhelmed by the changing nature of approaches to psychiatric treatment, he was also defensive about their utilization at Central State, claiming that the hospital employed the latest cutting-edge technologies in order to make the hospital something other than custodial.

In the same report from 1956, Peacock appealed to Judge Kemper, the director of the Division of Public Welfare, to pay attention to the great work being done by Central State and the people who worked there. "Despite the fact that some of our self-appointed critics and well-meaning but misguided friends refer to the hospital as being custodial in nature only," he wrote, "living testimony in the form of numerous ex-patients who have been restored to their loved ones and their rightful places in the community refutes such claims. Records also bear out the fact that this hospital has for many years provided recreational and occupational activities for the patients; and that it has been among the leaders in state institutions in the use of insulin, metrazol, and electric shock therapy, tranquilizing drugs, and in fact all recognized types of therapy."[24] Peacock's comments about the different types of therapy show the way that hospitals were desperate to find and use any means at their disposal to manage the behavior of the people the state confined, and sometimes to return them to a state of well-being.

Insights into the ways these therapies were applied are contained in the medical and psychology department reports from Central State Hospital. The assistant superintendent and director of the medical program, Dr. R. W. Bradford, was responsible for reporting the somatic types of treatments that were administered. He did this in a descriptive summary, with no breakdown of treatments by race or gender; but even so, this summary shows the extent and types of interventions being used.

The most common treatment was electroshock therapy—what we now call electroconvulsive therapy (ECT). As at Tuskegee, electroshock was considered cutting-edge technology at the time. Originally introduced to American hospitals in the 1940s, it became a highly potent tool for managing patient symptoms.[25] Its use and intent, however, was not always therapeutic when it came to Black patients, but in this era, its ability to modify patient behavior made it particularly valuable. In 1956, Dr. Bradford wrote, "We continue to make extensive use of electric shock therapy with good results," reporting that "three thousand, nine hundred and thirty-four (3,934) patients were treated and thirty thousand, seven hundred and twenty-six (30,726) treatments were given."[26] He stated that "eight hundred and forty-nine (849) patients were reported as having been restored; two thousand, four hundred and twenty-three (2,423) were improved and six hundred and sixty-two (662) as unimproved."[27] There is no indication of what constituted "improved," but it is safe to assume that Bradford was looking for a modification of the symptoms associated with severe delusions, aggressive or extroverted behavior, or a more active affect in relation to depression. The implication here is that the mitigation of certain types of behaviors, which were heavily racially coded, and a more manageable patient were what constituted success.

Without detailed and individual reports, it is not possible to tell which groups of people were specifically being given ECT or for what behavior or diagnosis, but 3,934 patients equaled more than one-third of the total inpatient population of 11,701. It was also slightly less than the total number of all patients, not just first admissions, classified as schizophrenic (4,275). It is impossible to tell whether ECT was being used as a therapy specifically for the treatment of schizophrenia or rather for the behavioral symptoms that made people hard to manage regardless of their specific diagnosis.

The most striking part of this scenario, however, is the sheer volume of treatments. If 30,726 treatments were administered in the single year between July 1955 and the end of June 1956, then an average of 84 treatments occurred every single day (counting weekends). This equates to roughly 10.5 treatments per hour (assuming an eight-hour day). In real time, I am sure it was more than this. This is a significant number of treatments, suggesting a factory-like approach that would have allowed little time for proper sedation or aftercare. These practices raise many questions about the logistics of ECT administration, the safety of patients undergoing it, and the care of patients post-treatment. There is also no direct evidence, including photos, about the way ECT was administered to Black patients in this hospital.

Two other somatic therapies were in use at CSH in the mid-1950s: insulin coma therapy and Metrazol shock. Both methods were designed to mimic the aftereffects of an epileptic seizure, when the patient might experience a reprieve from delusions or heightened anxiety and appear relatively calm and lucid. Both Metrazol and electric shock were performed without sedation and resulted in broken bones and, as we now know, broken memories and affect.[28] Insulin coma therapy required the administration of excessive amounts of insulin to create a diabetic coma, and at CSH in 1956, it "was used on two hundred and thirty-nine (239) cases, receiving a total number of one thousand and seventeen (1,017) treatments."[29] Both insulin and Metrazol were discredited by the early 1960s as completely ineffective and dangerous.

Eventually Metrazol and insulin were supplanted by the arrival of psychotropic drugs like Thorazine and Serpasil, which were officially FDA approved in 1955 and quickly pushed into use along with other major tranquilizers, like lithium. The records around drug utilization are also frustrating. Exact names of drugs administered are not recorded in the CSH annual report, but Dr. Bradford's summary suggests they were extensively used as early as 1956. "We have used to good advantage the tranquilizing drugs," he wrote. "Three thousand, two hundred and eighty-two (3,282) patients were treated and we are well pleased with the results from their use. Of this number two hundred and thirteen (213) were reported as having been restored; two thousand, four hundred and seventy-four (2,474) were improved and five hundred and ninety-five (595) as unimproved."[30] Significantly, there is absolute silence on the racial or gender breakdown of the use of any drug, so it is impossible to tell their efficacy, let alone their use, among the Black patients at CSH.

There is one particularly telling piece of information that does say something about the highly racialized therapeutic environment at Central State Hospital in the 1950s. Apart from the medical department, CSH was home to a psychology department. It was new, only five years old at the time, and headed by John T. Rowell, chief clinical psychologist. Rowell was committed to implementing a psychotherapy program and reported that he and his small team had performed 919 psychological tests (including the Rorschach and Bender-Gestalt tests) and that they had 15 current patients in individual psychotherapy and 182 participating in group psychotherapy. Rowell also reported on a psychotherapy "activational program," the goal of which was to "create a therapeutic atmosphere in which more concentrated psychotherapy could be given," and it consisted of group activities, music therapy, and informal psychotherapy.[31] Rowell was quick to differentiate this from recreational or occupational therapy, explaining that "these activities were not designed for entertainment but directed toward therapeutic goals of group participation and have resulted in arresting the regressive process for most patients in those settings where used."[32]

Significantly, the settings in which this kind of activity were taking place at Central State Hospital were in the white sections only. Rowell reported the department had seen 210 white male patients and 315 white female patients over the past five years, and that the success of the psychoactive therapeutic program was "an accomplished fact on the White Female Service."[33] While they had hoped to make more progress on "the other services," at this point it seemed that the priority for psychotherapy was white women, revealing the racial and gendered assumptions inherent to the practice. Not only were Black patients apparently not considered suitable for or worth including in the program, it was also likely that the emphasis on white women reflected the prevailing idea that white women who were institutionalized were more likely to be suffering from environmentally related neuroses than organic or psychotic illnesses and thus were more likely to respond to "talking therapy."[34]

Some of these same assumptions and patterns are evident in Alabama during the same time, but there are some differences worth noting, including the heavily racialized use of ECT. Because Alabama ran two entirely separate facilities, one dedicated to white patients and one to Black, the racial comparison is much more overtly reported and strikingly obvious. Superintendent James Tarwater was quick to report all the cutting-edge technologies in use at Bryce, at the same time as he acknowledged that the system was overcrowded and underfunded.

Like Thomas Peacock in Georgia, Tarwater was defensive about the perception of his hospitals as purely custodial and spent a great deal of effort explaining to the governor and the board of trustees the need for additional money so that a more active therapeutic regimen could be implemented. "With money appropriated, together with receipts from other sources, farm and land sales," he wrote, "we have endeavored to improve the care, treatment and living conditions of patients in several ways, specifically by the addition of personnel who are active in the treatment and rehabilitation of patients."[35]

There was only a nascent psychology program at Bryce Hospital in Tuscaloosa, with one full-time psychologist (Waters C. Paul) and one part-time PhD-prepared clinical psychologist, Dr. D. A. R. Peyman, who was appointed full time in 1956. Two other part-time psychology assistants and an administrative assistant were also hired that year. In 1956, the department administered 6,227 psychological tests to both patients and potential staff, compared to 1,017 conducted in 1953, its first year of operation.

TABLE 3.3 Use of electroshock therapy in Alabama state hospitals, 1956

	Male patients	Female patients
Bryce Hospital population (white)	2,385	2,612
Number of patients treated	609 (25.53%)	548 (20.98%)
Number of treatments given	10,026	2,997
Average treatments per patient	16.5	5.5
Searcy Hospital population (Black)	1,390	1,649
Number of patients treated	321 (23.09%)	939 (56.94%)
Number of treatments given	3,210	5,348
Average treatments per patient	10	5.7

Sources: Overall population data from Table 1, *Report of the Trustees of the Alabama State Hospitals*, 1956, p. 13. Figures for ECT use are given in Table 23: Surgical Report (Bryce Hospital), p. 89, and Table 23: Surgical Report (Searcy Hospital), p. 150, https://digitalcommons.library.uab.edu/arash/13/.

The department's active therapy program was limited, however. Dr. Peyman reported, "There were several psychotherapeutic groups conducted this year. One group consisted of patients from the Ladies Receiving Building and another of older chronic schizophrenic patients, and both were carried on for seven or eight months. There has also been individual psychotherapy for patients referred to this department by their hospital physicians."[36] Peyman reported about his attempts at using group psychotherapy in a small group of thirty-two white women diagnosed with schizophrenia in the journal *Group Psychotherapy* in 1956. In this study, he measured IQ scores before and after treatment and found that the greatest improvement (of only two points) occurred in the group that underwent both electroshock and the group therapy program.[37] In the same way that Dr. Rowell had in Georgia, Dr. Peyman focused only on white women.

Section 2 of the 1956 annual report from Alabama, concerned with the running of the all-Black Searcy Hospital in Mount Vernon, is only 30 pages (compared to the 130-plus pages for Bryce Hospital). Here there was no psychology department at all, and no report on the use or distribution of drugs. If Tarwater was sending drugs down to Searcy, there is no record of it. The main "therapeutic" technology in use at Searcy was electroshock therapy. A comparison of the data about its use at Searcy with the same data from Bryce in Tuscaloosa is set out in table 3.3.

The annual report for Bryce Hospital in 1956 did not include a breakdown of all the patients in the hospital by diagnostic category, only for first or readmissions that year, so it is not possible to track the correlation between ECT use and the size of the total "schizophrenic" population. Nevertheless, some discrepancies are striking.

While use of ECT was reserved for only 25.5 percent of the white men at Bryce and 20.9 percent of the white women at Bryce, white men experienced the highest average treatments, with 10,026 treatments among 609 patients, equaling an average of 16.5 per person, which is much higher than that of any other patient group.

Most obviously problematic at Searcy, however, was the use of ECT for Black women. While the Black men were likely to be given more treatments each on average (10 compared to the women's average of 5.7), the percentage of men being subjected to electroshock was 23 percent, less than the rate for white men. But the use of ECT among Black women was more than twice the amount for white men. Nearly 57 percent of *all* the women at Searcy were subjected to ECT in the year ending September 1956, with an average of 5.7 treatments per person. This is a stark and telling difference, and it is hard to read or report it without a sense of outrage at the thought of the violence and terror this practice must have incurred among the Black women at Searcy.

The frequency of ECT administration in Alabama was much less than it was in Georgia: at Bryce, 13,023 total treatments were spread over 365 eight-hour days, which averaged to about 4.5 treatments per hour (compared to Georgia's 10.5 per hour). Apart from the population being much lower than in Georgia, I suspect this is also because the wards at Bryce were much closer together and there was less likely to be multiple machines and multiple operators. At Searcy, the rate of ECT was less; 8,558 total treatments administered over a year equates to about 23.45 treatments per day, 2.93 treatments per hour. This rate is in the context of a lower population (3,039 total), but it also likely reflects the reality of the staffing at Searcy, which consisted of only the superintendent, three assistant physicians, and a team of largely untrained attendants listed as "the nursing service," with no RN in charge. The lack of diagnostic complexity at Searcy translated to a direct lack of therapeutic complexity for Black women in Alabama. Searcy had no psychology department and no visiting or consultant psychologists, so no attempts at psychotherapy were reported there at all.

The brevity and scarcity of the biennial reports from Whitfield Hospital in Mississippi make it almost impossible to present a true picture of therapeutic practices there. In his summary at the beginning of the report for 1955–57, Dr. Jaquith summarized the impact of the new tranquilizing drugs and their cost for the hospital. "During the past biennium," he reported, "there has been a tremendous upsurge in the field of psychiatry and the use of new tranquilizing drugs. These drugs are a valuable implement in the treating of the mentally ill. We have used these drugs widely and as they are quite expensive this has caused us to dig deep into the General Fund to purchase drugs which will give the patients the benefit of every modern treatment."[38] Jaquith noted that "one of our neighboring states" had had an emergency legislative meeting to approve an increased state appropriation for psychiatric drugs, whereas Mississippi had not done so. This meant that Jaquith was paying for them from his own budget. Given how few paying patients the hospital had, this was a significant outlay, tripling his expenses for 1955 and 1956. He argued that the expense was necessary because not only did the hospital owe it to the patients to provide them with access to the latest technologies, but the drugs were also proving effective and enabled him to discharge patients at a faster rate.[39]

Most of the rest of Jaquith's summary from the 1957 report detailed the struggle he had retaining trained psychiatric staff in the absence of a larger psychiatric program in the state, reflected in the fact that the new University of Mississippi Medical Center in Jackson had no psychiatric beds, and students there rotated through Whitfield for twelve weeks at a time. Jaquith reported that Whitfield had been approved for a one-year residency program, and he hoped this would bring more trained staff to work at the hospital.[40] Jaquith frequently lamented the fact that "Mississippi suffers from an acute shortage of trained people to treat the ever-increasing number of mentally ill. There are very few psychiatrists practicing in the state of Mississippi at a private practice level. To serve more than 2,000,000 Mississippians, there are approximately thirty psychiatrists. Like all state mental hospitals, this hospital lacks many psychiatrists, psychiatric social workers, psychiatric nurses, and other top personnel. We have only been able to maintain a skeleton crew of trained people."[41]

In the 1957–59 report, Jaquith included a summary of "Methods of Treatment," which listed electroshock, hydrotherapy, group therapy, Antabuse therapy, drug withdrawal therapy as well as the widespread use of new drugs.[42] Antabuse was (is) a drug designed to treat alcoholism, a major problem for Whitfield. Interestingly, Jaquith noted that the use of insulin shock therapy had been discontinued at Whitfield and in most other places in 1956 (except for Milledgeville) and was no longer a credited form of therapy, not least because it was time and labor intensive.[43] Yet Jaquith did report on the occasional use of prefrontal lobotomies, which "from time to time . . . are performed by consulting neurosurgeons. These pre-frontal lobotomies are not done until every form of acceptable therapy has been tried and evaluated."⁴⁴ At no point in any of these official reporting documents (or anywhere else I have been able to find) does Whitfield list any cross-referencing data related to the administration, distribution, or expense of actual treatments.

At the same time, Whitfield struggled to develop and maintain a psychology department, which waxed and waned depending on the availability of staff. Some attempts at psychotherapy had been made, including a group therapy program run by a resident and a short-lived "exit group" on the receiving ward for white women, but these programs were difficult to sustain due to the time and personnel required.⁴⁵

It seems a given that these programs would apply only to the white patients, but there is evidence of therapeutic services for Black patients in other records. As was evident in the employment of Dr. Washington as the first Black physician in 1955, Jaquith demonstrated some slightly progressive tendencies when it came to recognizing the importance of racially concordant care, especially in his attempt to make Whitfield something other than a series of holding cells.

In the patient newsletter, *The Whit*, which ran for only a few years (1951 to about 1955), "the colored service" section reported on the presence of a young psychologist from Tougaloo College, Dr. Matthew Burks. Burks was at Whitfield for about a year (1951–52), during which he worked to institute a more rigorous psychological testing program and other activities that would "contribute in bringing the colored ward in line with the progressive ideas of Dr. Marshall, Dr. Jaquith and Dr. Daly."⁴⁶ (Marshall was the [white] superintendent of the Black patient service, and Daly was the [white] chief clinical psychologist for the whole hospital.)

Burks continued to report briefly in *The Whit*, writing in July 1951, "My activities at present include: testing patients, obtaining case histories, conducting individual and group therapy, and other forms of therapeutic activities."⁴⁷ Burks believed in the importance of an active program aimed at rehabilitation and recovery in which people could be returned to their communities, and he hoped that the work he was doing at Whitfield, which included public outreach, might go some way toward educating the Black public about the importance of mental health and reducing the stigma around mental illness.

That same year, Whitfield played host to its first series of student interns, also from Tougaloo College, as part of a class on psychopathology. This relationship between Tougaloo and Whitfield represented a genuine attempt to better educate Black students about mental health and psychiatry for the benefit of their communities. As student reporter Tommie Anderson wrote in *The Whit*, the students had learned that "mental illness is like physical illness. It has its diagnosis, prognosis, and treatments just as is found in physical illness." He reported that their time at Whitfield, and the emphasis on public mental health, had "inspired some who were interested in psychology, to help others of their race."[48] The program for training Black students and employing Black staff was evidence of some attempt at Whitfield to bring services for Black patients into better alignment with those for white, and for a short while this may have been partially successful. At the end of the first report from this class, an unnamed person wrote, "The colored hospital feels that its functions and services are a matter of personal pride and any observer will truthfully say that he can find no other hospital, white or colored, possessed of better administration or morale."[49]

Despite various issues with the official records, and the challenges of building comparisons across three states, the data demonstrates that these large hospitals struggled to function as anything more than custodial. Administrators and staff knew that better approaches were possible but were hampered by the refusal of conservative state legislatures to spend any more than was necessary on the states' most undesirable people. When this general apathy and neglect intersected with existing racial attitudes and structures like segregation, amplified by the already existing internal racism of psychiatric practices like diagnosis, the situation for Black patients became dire.

Superintendents tried to use any technology at their disposal to reduce their population size and control inpatient behavior (whether this actually cured people or not), and this meant that approaches to diagnosis and treatment were often ad hoc if not downright abusive. When these practices occurred in deeply racially divided spaces, then the opportunity and circumstances for dismissive, disrespectful, and neglectful care were rife.

Disparities in diagnostic practices were supported by prevailing psychiatric ideas that held that there was something intrinsically different, and therefore inferior, about the Black psyche. This led to a lack of diagnostic complexity for Black patients and an overreliance on the general, poorly understood category of "schizophrenia," especially for Black women.

In this moment, in this first application of the *DSM*, prevailing attitudes were codified into diagnostic practice that became scientific knowledge, handed down almost unaltered into the present. And where Black patients were more isolated, as in the case of Searcy Hospital in Alabama, the hostility and violence of white supremacy was unleashed against the Black patient through an overreliance on electroshock therapy, surely one of the most terrifying of medical technologies ever invented.

But electroshock and tranquilizing drugs were not the only ways of keeping patients quiet and under control. The most prevalent "therapeutic" technique in all these spaces was "occupational therapy," and for Black patients, this mostly took the form of intense, involuntary, and backbreaking manual labor. Explored in more detail in chapter 4, this patient labor constituted not just a performance of the Jim Crow routine but an active replication of plantation relations, which relied on the exploitation of Black bodies. But that exploitation did not go uncontested, and patients, families, and communities worked hard to remind hospital administrators that Black people were not simply free labor but human beings.

Part II **Performing Jim Crow in the Asylum**

4 Negotiating Daily Life

Milledgeville GA
May the 23 1952
State Hospital
The 3 Hall

Dear NAACP I would like to have a job with you all I am hear have been heare for 10 years working hard for 9 years and father has been dead for 6 years and I do not no nobody to sin me out this place I will stay with them and pay your time getting me out this place. . . . I will work Jacksonville Fla anywhere you is got a job for me I am willing to work for I do work hard and don't get anything for it at all at the hall Dr Smith and Dr T G Peacock the superintendent of the Milledgeville State Hospital I am out on the road working 5½ days a week [illegible]
yours truly
D. M.

Mr. M.'s letter is scratched out in pencil on two scraps of blue-lined notepaper, the only letter in the Milledgeville Branch file of the NAACP at the Library of Congress, stored in a slim acid-free folder dated 1943–1953.[1] The rest of the documents in this file are correspondence between the organizers of the local Milledgeville Branch and the NAACP head office about the difficulties of obtaining and sustaining members. In the mid-twentieth century, Baldwin County, of which Milledgeville was the seat, was home to 10,000–24,000 Black people, one of 16 other counties (out of Georgia's 150) with this small-to-medium-size Black population.[2] Most of the state's Black folks lived in Fulton County (Atlanta) or Chatham County (Savannah). Surrounded by other heavily agricultural counties, Baldwin's main claim to fame was that Milledgeville had once been the capital of the Confederacy. Perhaps unsurprisingly, by 1954 the branch had been forced to close due to a lack of members, and Mr. M.'s letter went unanswered.

Mr. M.'s letter is revealing in important ways that set the scene for this chapter. Its existence in the NAACP records indicates both the possibilities and the difficulties of resistance and agency for Black patients, and the scarcity of the records that document the lived experience of everyday life. The content of Mr. M.'s letter gives us a glimpse of that reality, highlighting the way that Black patients were seen as a biddable workforce rather than as a patient population requiring treatment. This positioning revealed a particular paradox in the history of institutionalization overlaid with the history of eugenics. If Black patients were considered disabled enough to be institutionalized, they were not considered disabled enough to avoid hard labor. This labor, and the way that Black patients were treated on a daily basis, replicated and reinforced the performance of Jim Crow relations. Mr. M. made those relations clear: They were relations of work, not therapy.

In Southern asylums, Black patients were positioned *beyond* therapy. Their everyday lives in the institution were shaped by the long history of slavery, the plantation, and sharecropping in the South, where the Black body and mind were considered suitable only for hard work that benefited white people. This long history intersected with the internal racism of psychiatry to reinforce stereotypes about the nature of the Black psyche, stereotypes that had themselves been formed on the plantation. These ways of thinking also shaped social and labor relations beyond the asylum, but they were particularly insidious inside institutional walls because they struck at the heart of Black subjectivity itself and framed the way that vulnerable people saw themselves and their opportunity for resistance. Mr. M.'s letter demonstrated this firsthand: He spoke only of his life at Milledgeville as a worker, not as a patient. He knew he had rights and a course of appeal, he knew to write to the NAACP, but his appeal for release was based on how he saw himself as a good worker, not that he was cured of whatever had led him to be committed.

In this chapter, I explore the ways that Black patients were positioned in Southern asylums and argue that the resulting practices reflected the deliberate tactics of the Jim Crow routine, aimed at the control and oppression of the Black body and mind in many of the same ways that had sustained slavery. While the psychiatric hospital was not exactly a plantation, and people were patients, not exactly enslaved, letters like those from Mr. M. challenge the narrative of benevolent paternalism that administrators told themselves and the public, and they belie the idea that daily life for Black patients was in any way therapeutic. Beyond the existence of hard labor, differences in the recreational and occupational therapy programs for white versus Black patients demonstrate the racism that pervaded psychiatric practice and the way that segregation allowed for the abuse and mistreatment of Black patients in particular.

At the same time, I attempt to explore the ways that Black patients themselves negotiated these practices and relations. Within a potentially totalizing regime, there are moments of resistance, glimpses of the lived experience and actions of patients like Mr. M as they fought to retain their humanity and identity as patients. If dehumanizing stereotypes about Black subjectivity shaped white physicians' and administrators' approaches to care, Black patients themselves rebelled against this construction when they could.

This chapter draws on a number of sources to try to unpack this dynamic, including state senate investigations, annual reports, and a rare patient newsletter. I begin the chapter with the patient newsletter in order to counter the undue weight given to "official" sources, and to center the patient voice where it exists. The newsletter provides a unique insight into the routines of everyday life while raising many of the key themes of this book regarding how Black patients were treated. It demonstrates how Black patients negotiated segregated psychiatric spaces and how these spaces reinforced broader Jim Crow social relations, how patients fought to maintain their humanity and identity as people with families and social connections, and how patients were put to work for the benefit of the institution.

The rest of the chapter supplements this patient view with an analysis of official sources regarding the idea of occupational therapy, highlighting the extractive value and significance of the work to which Black patients were subject. While it is the case that work of some kind was common for all patients in mid-century asylums, my analysis shows that the way the idea and practice of occupational therapy was rolled out in these three Southern states worked to reinforce and replicate the subjection of the Black body and mind, enabled by the preexisting racist ideology of psychiatry itself. More than that, I argue that the practice of forced work for Black patients drew on and reproduced long-running racial labor practices with their roots in the plantation.

How these practices were enacted and experienced can be hard to reproduce, and my attempts to do so here are partial and sometimes inconclusive. Official sources only tell us so much, and in some cases they are deliberately silent. These silences are themselves telling in that they demonstrate the way that Black patients were ignored or erased, considered not quite human. They are problematic silences because they obscure the reality of life inside the asylum, and they erase the ways that patients themselves experienced, performed, and pushed back against the violence of Jim Crow.

There are so few letters from Black patients in the official archives that I can count them on one hand (compared to the innumerable complaints from white families). Sadly, patient newsletters from inside the institutions are also hard to find or no longer extant. For example, Central State Hospital (CSH) in Georgia had two patient newsletters, *The Builder*, produced by the white patients, and *The Golden Star*, produced by the Black patients, but no copy of the latter has ever been found, and the remaining copies of *The Builder* seem to live in a private collection.[3] In Alabama, there appears to have been only a short-lived patient newsletter from the early twentieth century confined to Bryce Hospital (white patients only). I found no trace or mention of a similar paper for the Black patients at Searcy.

But for a few years in the early 1950s, Whitfield Hospital in Mississippi produced a patient newsletter that did document in quite intricate detail some of the rhythms and practices of everyday life, and this newsletter did contain material about and from Black patients. I first read about *The Whit* in Michael Murphy's PhD dissertation about the longer history of the Mississippi State Hospital.[4] Murphy used *The Whit* mostly to report on an attempted exposé from a white patient, which I will explore in more detail in chapter 4, but I wanted to read the newsletter for myself to see what else it might tell me. But finding a full set was in itself a challenge.[5] The Mississippi Department of Archives and History did have some scattered copies in the regular collection, but I found more editions in an unprocessed collection that belonged to Dr. William Jaquith himself. This collection was a gold mine of photos, newspaper clippings, and copies of *The Whit*, and it was from here that I was able to get a clearer sense of what everyday life was like inside Whitfield.

As significant and revealing as *The Whit* is, however, it still requires a careful "against the grain" reading in order to fully appreciate the challenges of life in a segregated psychiatric hospital, especially in the context of the emerging civil rights movement and the subsequent white backlash. That is, the tone and content of *The Whit* is often as telling and revealing in what is not said and reveals the way that Black patients needed to negotiate everyday life in a psychiatric hospital in a state dedicated to the potentially deadly performance of the Jim Crow routine in all settings.

Performing Jim Crow in *The Whit*

The Whit, established in 1950 as *The Whitfield Monthly Literary Chronicle*, emanated from the patient-led literary club and had an initial team of four patients as editor, assistant editor, and reporters, with three staff advisers, including Dr. Daly—the hospital's chief clinical psychologist.[6] Throughout October 1950, the literary club met several times to look at books brought in by Dr. Daly and to review the recreational activities and patient newsletters of other institutions, like the Owen Clinic Institute in West Virginia. By October 18, the club had twenty-nine members who had signed on to write stories for *The Whit*.

The first edition appeared in late October 1950 and consisted of four pages, all devoted to activities of the white patients. There is no mention of Black patients, but Willie H. posted a review of a book called *Where I Was Born and Raised* (1948) by David Cohn.[7] The book was described as a "discussion of life in the Mississippi delta," but Willie's review consists of six paragraphs concerning various so-called problems related to African American communities. In his review, Willie H. notes that the author argues that the problems of the Mississippi Delta are greater "because of a greater Negro population" and that many of these so-called problems are related to the apparent refusal of Black people to take advantage of local health services or to "feel an interest in his own race."[8] For Cohn, Willie H. summarized, this was a problem for white people not least because the Black female population in particular "nurses our babies, care[s] for the sick, handing [sic] our food, and comes in contact with us in many ways." Willie's concern here reflected the age-old hypocrisy of white efforts in public health, which mobilized in marginalized communities or borderlands largely for the protection of white health.[9] Willie H. finished his review by noting that while Cohn was often critical of the Black people of the Delta, "he also pictures Negroes as faithful and loyal to the white race."[10]

In this first volume of a patient-led newsletter in which no Black patients are themselves represented, the tone is set by a white patient, repeating the words of a white author. The themes that Willie H. identifies as important from Cohn's book give some indication of the broader environment that Black patients needed to negotiate at Whitfield, where "faithfulness" and "loyalty" also became markers of both good behavior and sanity itself. Relationships of paternalism and deference shaped the everyday life of Black patients at Whitfield, as well as the way that patients advocated for improved conditions and for their own release.

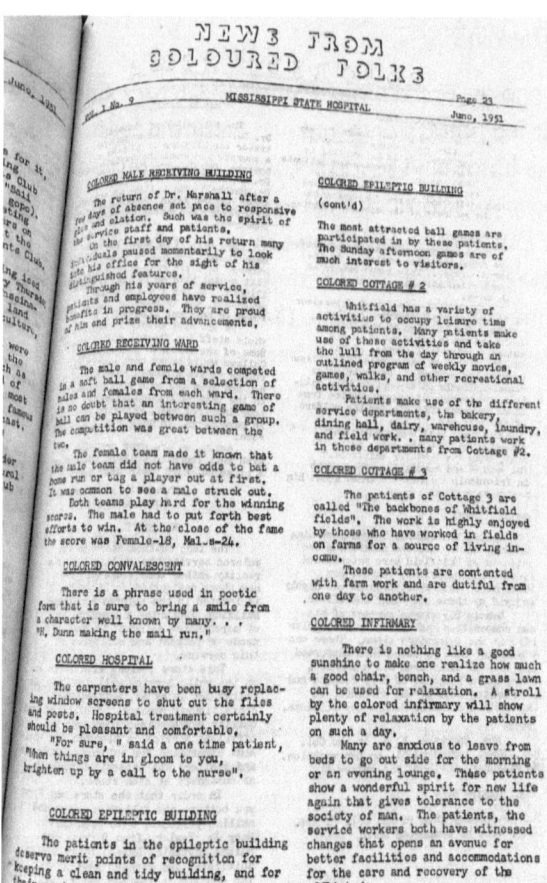

FIGURE 4.1 "News from Coloured Folks," *The Whit* 1, no. 9 (June 1951). Courtesy of the Archives and Records Services Division, Mississippi Department of Archives and History.

Writings by and about Black patients demonstrated the structures of segregation that discriminated against Black patients, but they also revealed the humanity, hope, and courage of Black patients as they sought to make sense of their confinement and to behave in ways that might have them considered "cured" enough to go home.

From its second volume, *The Whit* began to dedicate a page or two at the back to matters concerning Black patients. Variously called "Colored News," "Colored Section," "Colored Patients," or "News from Coloured Folks," (as in figure 4.1) this section gave an overview of activities happening in the segregated Black section of the hospital; tracked the movement of and relationships among patients, doctors, and attendants; and were used by patients themselves to seek help. The addition of this section of *The Whit* showed an attempt from management, especially Dr. Jaquith, to institute reforms in the wake of exposés and reports. At times the section indicated various kinds of treatment programs, but it also displayed several tensions in those attempts at treatment, revealing structural inequalities as well as the normalizing and disciplining purpose of both treatments and the patient newsletter itself.

In the next few sections of this chapter, I look at the ways that Black patients used *The Whit* to assert their humanity and identity as people with an illness who wanted to return home to their families and communities, and explore the relationships between patients and staff. I also use notes from *The Whit* to demonstrate the structural inequalities in relation to everyday life as a result of segregation, and the way that work was posed as a form of therapy.

The most striking element of the back section of *The Whit* is the determination of Black patients to assert their existence and identity as people with names and previous lives, who were not solely defined by their illness episode.[11] It also demonstrates the way that patients continually advocated for their right to go home. In September 1951, G.P.D.—a Black woman in the receiving ward—wrote, "Several of us are on the home list and we sure will be glad when someone comes to take us home," and C. M., a Black man, stated, "He likes his attendants and fellow patients very much, he gets along with everyone just fine, but he will be glad when he can go home."[12]

These types of sentiments became more frequent as more Black patients began to contribute to *The Whit*. In December 1951, C.H. from the male epileptic ward wrote, "I am doing just fine these days. I know we are going to have a big Christmas this year, but I won't be able to enjoy it too much if I am not at home. I wish I could go home and be with my family for Christmas, even if I have to come back. I believe if I could just spend Christmas at home it would be good for my mind, body and spirit."[13]

In April 1952, ten male patients from the disturbed ward made simple two-line entries that stated their desire to get well and go home. "I am very glad for a place to get well so I can go back home," wrote Eddie E., and Jimmie Lee J. added, "I just wait every day to hear my Doctor say I can go home." These sentiments were repeated by Tom F., Willie B., Richard R., John T., Benny P., Ollie S., Jeff W., and Cornell W.[14] And in a particularly powerful note in March 1952, one patient went to great lengths to remind readers of the humanity of patients like himself: "I, Clondike A, of Colored Male Epileptic . . . came to this hospital in July 1950 and this past month which was February 18, was my birthday and I am 41 years old. My home is in Cahoma County, Miss." He also pointed out that two of his fellow patients, Freeman

Negotiating Daily Life 97

and Walter P., "who are unable to write," also had birthdays in February, and that to Clondike, the patients in the Black male epileptic ward constituted "our family of one hundred."[15]

Comments like these not only demonstrate that patients were cognizant of and self-aware about their situation but also show that they came from a broad variety of backgrounds and had complex lives. For example, in March 1952, Willie J. wrote, "I have improved since I came here. Have been here for over a month. I will be glad when I can be at home so that I can provide for my wife and child and continue my medial course which was interrupted by my illness."[16] Willie J.'s comment demonstrates the way that he understood himself distinctly as a patient who had a life to return to.

Repeated postings across multiple volumes show the way that patients referred to themselves as sick, well, or improving, and demonstrate a clear expectation that they would be treated like patients, were there to recover, and expected to be able to go home. They also demonstrate the determination of Black patients to maintain social relationships that linked them to one another and to their communities of origin.

The pages of *The Whit* are full of notes and messages that mark the significance of relationships between patients and the ways that patients kept track of each other and their movements. For example, in July 1951, Cottage #2 reported that "W.M., better known as Pee-Wee, received a discharge for home. His absence is felt as he was humorous and brightened many faces with smiles among his cottage-mates." Similarly, "A.G. was happy to be returning to his family, and all his friends here wish him a happy future." That same month, Cottage #3 reported that "W.C. waved a happy and joyous good bye to friends in Cottage #3. He promised a visit back to see all his friends in Whitfield, after he spends some time at home."[17] In November 1951, an article from the Black male receiving ward paid close attention to the comings and goings of people: "We have had quite a few patients go home recently," the author wrote. "They were Willie H., Cleveland O., Curtis R., Ben T., Dave W., and Leon L. On the home list now are Quitman U. and Creed P. We shall miss them very much, but we are happy to see them go and wish them much success for the future."[18] This article also noted the importance of visitors for patient well-being, stating, "We have a lot of visitors Sunday from all over the State. Although the attendants have to work very hard on this day, it is a day of rejoicing for the patients. Many are made happy by the visits of their many relatives and friends."[19]

Statements like these demonstrate the ways that Black patients at Whitfield tried to retain their humanity through community and family connection, but they also indicate the loneliness of life at Whitfield and the lack of power some patients had over their own admission or discharge. The capriciousness of the admission and discharge process is evident in many of the short notes left by Black patients in *The Whit*. One short story demonstrates the way that patients could be admitted and easily forgotten. In August 1951, an unattributed note reported, "Will A. had been here twenty years and his people thought he was dead. But someone who knew him happened to come by and notified his people that he was still here. His people came and got him. Will is now on his way to Detroit, and very much 'alive.'"

Some patients who were discharged stayed in contact with their Whitfield family. In January 1952, O.L. (who might have been one of the attendants) wrote, "Walter S, who came to this institution two years ago, has gone home. A number of people have received letters from him since he left, saying that he was well and enjoyed being at home with his children. Walter was a lot of help around the hospital and everyone thought a lot of him. We were happy to see him go home, but we miss him very much."[20]

Patients also reported more than once on the death of a fellow patient. For example, in January 1952 "A Patient" noted that patients and staff alike "regret very much the death of Sam A. Sam was liked by everyone who knew him and he was known by a lot of people. He had been in and out of the institution for many years. . . . His sudden passing was shocking to everyone. Sam shall long be remembered at Whitfield by his many friends."[21] These snippets from patients, which clearly set out their complex social and family relationships, demonstrate an active resistance to the dehumanizing effects of life at Whitfield and the potential for social death. The process of alienation worked in two potential ways for the Black psychiatric patient: alienation from the self, which came with a category like mental illness; and natal alienation, as a result of long-term removal from the home and family. Patients were constantly reminding administrators reading *The Whit* that they were in fact part of a society, that they knew and cared about one another, and that they were missed and cared for beyond the asylum.

It is worth noting that in all these postings from patients, there is a repeated attitude of deference, which demonstrates the way that being considered well enough to go home was also a matter of how well a patient was able to perform and comply. To some extent, the postings by patients are themselves a performance of the Jim Crow routine, where the pleas to be returned home are framed within the broader context of Black deference to white authority as demanded in Mississippi at the time. Vulnerable patients knew they were vulnerable—in the context of broader unrest and violence, the lynch mob, and the Klan, patients approached their white caretakers with caution and extreme politeness.

One common mode of performance was the constant expression of gratitude, which worked to demonstrate a patient's competence and obedience, thus making them ready to be released. For example, in April 1952, Oscar M. wrote, "We have plenty of good wholesome food to eat and the water is so good, until it looks like I can't get enough of it. I hope to be going home soon and feel like I am well enough to go now." Early May A. wrote, "I am glad to be here and try to obey the doctors and attendants. I get plenty to eat and enjoy the shows and dances. Please pray for me so that I can soon go home." Annie Bell S. wrote, "I am thanking the good Lord, the doctors, and attendants at Whitfield have been good and nice to me. I obey the doctors, nurses and attendants. We have a good place to sleep. I enjoy the shows and dances. I want you to pray for me." Irene W. J. summed up the feelings of most patients when she wrote simply, "I have a good place here and I am enjoying myself. I like the good shows and dances. The nurse is good to me but I do want to go home soon."[22]

Sometimes expressions of gratitude were wrapped around concerns so as to soften any appearance of complaints that patients might have been making. In this way, patients demonstrated their agency and at times activism, but they did so in ways that kept them safe. And while patients were grateful for the food or the place to sleep or the recreation program, their comments also revealed deficiencies in these programs.

In October 1952, Jane B. commented, "I like Sunday best of all. I enjoyed all that good fried chicken and green peas and cake and Irish potatoes. I wish every day was Sunday so I could have plenty chicken to eat." Sundays were visiting days at Whitfield, and this comment suggests that the food may have been better on these days to impress visitors, and possibly deficient the rest of the time.

That same month, patient I. S. pointed out, "I would like a little more exercise than I get, but I guess after a while we can have a little more. I hope so. I sort of envy the guys on [sic] the cottages because they have more freedom than we do, but that's ok. I hope I can go home soon."[23]

Patients also noticed when their recreation program was altered. In April 1952, multiple patients commented on the cessation of the movie program. Willie E. wrote, "The shows aren't coming to us now for a long while. We don't know what the trouble is, but whatever it may be we hope it can soon be adjusted and our shows will be coming back again." Bob W. also noted the absence, writing, "The picture show has been discontinued for some reason I know not why but I hope it will come back soon."[24] These comments indicate that sometimes things were less that idyllic at Whitfield, but that it was difficult for Black patients to express their concerns as open complaints. They used *The Whit* to make comments that alerted people to their situation but needed to do so in a way that conveyed calm logic and gratitude, as these were attributes that signaled psychological improvement and behavioral control. These expectations of behavior as measures of cure were further tempered for the Black patient by the need to also meet the expectations and norms of the Jim Crow routine, which limited their ability to speak freely about how they were being treated at Whitfield.

The pages of *The Whit* are particularly informing about the activities available for Black patients and the ways that these were a particular performance of Jim Crow relations. A focus on activities was central to the idea that Whitfield was a decent place, and the first single page dedicated to "colored news," which appeared in November 1950, highlighted these aspects of daily life. It focused on two major patient activities, the glee club and the sewing room. The glee club consisted of both male and female Black patients who "sing Spirituals and are making preparations to sing Plantation Melodies and Semi-classics." It was noted, "We find it has been most beneficial to our patients."[25] The mention of spirituals and plantation melodies is notable. The glee club was run by two women, Lela Mannery and Olivia Hill—later in *The Whit* it is reported that Ms. Hill was the "Colored Recreation Director," but it is not clear if she is herself Black. Did she choose the spirituals and plantation melodies or did the patients make those selections themselves? If Hill was Black and the patients chose the songs, this activity might be interpreted as a kind of reclamation of identity and resistance and a recognition of the healing and racial uplift aspects of these types of song. But if she was white, this interpretation might need revisiting, as it raises questions about the politics and dynamics of having a white woman suggest plantation songs. This lack of clarity about racial concordance between employees and patients makes it difficult at times to unpack the intersection of psychiatric and racial power at Whitfield.

At any rate, the recreation program was an important part of life at Whitfield and was highly valued by patients and staff alike. During 1950–51, the program was assisted by two young women, LaPearl Younger and Lillian Parker, who were most definitely Black, having attended Tougaloo College to train in physical education. When they left at the end of August 1951 to return to their studies, their impact was duly noted: "Filled with energy and vitality these young ladies came to the hospital with an unselfish desire to make life brighter for the patients." Working with the director of the recreation program, Mr. Cottle, the students had established a program of light exercise, ball games, regular parties at each cottage, rotating movie shows, and a series of dances where patients from different cottages could meet one another and enjoy surprise "refreshments."

The "colored news" sections of *The Whit* are full of reports from staff and patients alike about how much these regular activities were appreciated. The summer months in particular were enjoyable for patients who were able to move outside, fall asleep under trees, and have picnics. In July 1951, Vera M. J. reported, "We had a wonderful time at the 4th of July picnic where a large number of patients gathered for a grand time with good music, plenty of dancing and refreshments."[26]

These outdoor activities also brought men and women together, which added "more enthusiasm to games, music and dancing."[27] The men and women also mixed to play games on Sunday afternoons. In June 1951, patients reported a spirited game of softball in which "the female team made it known that the male team did not have odds to bat a home run or tag a player out at first. It was common to see a male struck out. Both teams play hard for the winning scores. The male had to put forth best efforts to win."[28] It was noted that these afternoon ball games were also well attended by visitors, suggesting the importance of continuing regular activities that kept patients in touch with the rituals of everyday life and the communities and families they came from.

The sense of camaraderie among patients is particularly strong in a story from July 1951, where it was reported that in the male epileptic building, "watermelons are often seen among the patients. They purchase them themselves, after which they form groups and have a merry time eating, laughing and telling jokes. When the watermelon session is over, horse-shoe pitching usually climaxes the day's activities until the darkness forces the players to a reluctant finish."[29] Here is a sense of the possibility of autonomy and self-determination for patients, even while confined, and the importance of a quotidian ritual that marked a long hot Southern summer.

Sometimes patients got to enjoy off-campus events or excursions. The Colored State Fair was a regular highlight of life at Whitfield for Black patients. The October 1952 volume of *The Whit* was subtitled "State Fair Edition" and demonstrated the way that race relations inside Whitfield replicated broader Mississippi norms. White patients would attend the fair, which was held first, and a few days later Black patients would attend the Colored State Fair, which took place on the same site. These totally separate events meant that there was no chance of Black and white Mississippians socializing or having fun together, a situation that was never questioned or challenged by anyone, least of all patients.

For the majority, the opportunity to get out of Whitfield for the day and have some fun was something to look forward to. L.B. reported, "We are looking forward to a big day at the State Fair. Our wishes are that every patient here at the institution could be able to go along and help make it a big day for us." From Female Cottage A, E.E.M wrote, "We are now getting ready for the fair," and Nancy F. wrote, "We will be so glad when time comes for the Colored State Fair. I like to go to the fair and ride the hob horses and go all over the fair grounds and see lots of things." Henry C. summed up the anticipation when he wrote,

> We patients at the Colored Male Infirmary enjoy going to the Fair each year. We're looking forward to that day. We get our transportation free, and we don't have any expenses at the Fair. Everything is free for all, and we are very thankful. The greatest of all—each one is given some cash (money) to spend and of course we spent it eating and drinking and there couldn't be anything nicer. So we thank God for the very fine leadership of the members of the staff of the Mississippi State Hospital . . . We are thankful for our very fine attendants that are nice to see us thro' the Fair and other festivities that we enjoy so much.[30]

Yet there is some evidence that the fair was not an unalloyed joy for everyone. Of more than 2,000 patients in 1952, only 320 would be attending the fair. Nanie B. from Colored Female Cottage #4 wrote, "This is October and we are all looking forward to the Fair. Hope we won't get disappointed," indicating that even a regular event like the fair was not open to all.

The second edition of *The Whit* also reported on the recent Colored State Fair, at which the hospital had a booth exhibiting "crocheted bedspreads, quilts, embroidered sheets, towels and pillow slips. There were many beautiful crocheted vanity sets and doilies. Other patients made artificial flowers and there were a number of dresses on display. . . . The Mississippi State Hospital Booth was given first prize: a blue ribbon. A crocheted bedspread made by one of the patients was awarded a second prize." The article mentioned that the items for the exhibit were made "in the sewing room, under the supervision of Mrs. Jones and Mrs. Whittington."[31]

The sewing room featured regularly on the pages of *The Whit*, and I unpack its function as both a workplace and a therapeutic space later in this chapter, but this description paints a picture of lively, creative activity, drawing on long-running traditions of craft and quilt making as care work, and suggests that patient rooms and living spaces may have been brightened by these handmade items, assuming they were allowed to keep them.

Indeed, in the July 1951 edition, it was noted that in the Black TB hospital, "in the female ward, there is an interesting patient who enjoys an attractive room. The room contains the regular patient bed, a picture puzzle completely worked, and a tale of books and magazines. Not far away sits a bowl of delicious fruit, a small table radio furnishes soft music, and the daily programs that give a most home like and relaxing atmosphere." The patient, identified as E.C., reported, "I have been made to feel at ease by the visits of my friends, and their considerate thoughts for making my stay in the hospital a pleasant one."[32] E.C. saw herself clearly as a patient, temporarily dislocated but determined to hold on to her sense of self and her real life beyond the hospital confines, connected to her kin and community.

In the same way, M.D.—a patient in the Male Disturbed Building—kept up his "hobby" of creating delicious dishes—which he shared with other patients—using "various kinds of foods he is able to obtain," including rabbits and birds, which it appears he may have hunted himself.[33] These activities were important not only because they broke up the monotony of the day and kept people busy and stimulated but also because they reminded patients that they were in fact people with full lives beyond the hospital walls. These activities helped people maintain a sense of themselves connected to their previous lives, and helped people form bonds and connections with one another while they were hospitalized.

Religion also played a part in everyday life for Black patients, and Dr. Jaquith made sure that the Black patients had their own church and chaplain. In the April 1951 edition, a whole page was dedicated to the "Coloured Pastor," Reverend Hightower, who wrote a thoughtful meditation on "How People Get Lost" and appealed to Christian principles of compassion and empathy for patients, who were simply people who "have lost themselves, through their own foolishness, while others have been lost through somebody else's carelessness."[34] Reverend Hightower was replaced by Reverend Davis in August 1951. Davis had undertaken special training in mental health work, and so, as noted in the edition, he "understands the needs of the patients and is willing to minister to those needs."[35]

The church was a place of both religious and pastoral care, as well as an important space for community building, but it was not without challenges. In a snippet published in *The Whit* in November 1951, there is evidence of the way that church services sometimes took second place to other imperatives for patients. The new chaplain, Reverend Davis, had seen immediately that he would need to make some changes to his program if he hoped to meet patients' needs; he moved services from 3 P.M. to 9 A.M. on Sundays "because it was more convenient for a larger number of people. It allows us to complete our service on Sunday before visitors begin coming in. The patients then have the remainder of the day to see their visitors."[36]

Burks, the psychology extern, also wrote about improvements to the religious program, including the purchase of a new piano and more hymnals, and he hoped that this would facilitate the expansion of the choir. He praised "the ladies, for being so faithful in helping to support our efforts," but hoped that more men might attend services and participate in the choir in the future.[37] The involvement of Burks in the religious program demonstrated the way that church and spiritual life was considered a central part of a therapeutic atmosphere and provided space for patients to continue to retain their religious practices as part of their identity and humanity.[38]

A careful analysis of *The Whit* demonstrates several other structural issues at Whitfield, such as differences in the types of recreational programs and the level of attention that white versus Black patients received. These discrepancies indicate the way that segregation permeated all aspects of life at Whitfield. Seemingly innocuous things like Christmas celebration agendas and the recording of birthdays in *The Whit* show the way that daily life for white patients was far more complex and well managed than it was for Black patients.

The section of *The Whit* reserved for Black patient news was always the last four-to-five pages, never more than that, in a twenty-six-to-twenty-eight-page document. The rest of the pages were lengthy details of other programs held for white patients, including listings of film showings by cottage and club meetings, like the garden club or the literary club, from which Black patients were excluded. White patients had access to a library and a recreation hall, and there were often long listings of birthdays by patient name. Black patient birthdays were never recorded in *The Whit*. And at Christmas, events for the white patients and their families took precedence, with the chapel and dining hall dedicated to white patients on Christmas Day and Black patients having a much more limited schedule of activities.

For example, the November 1951 edition of *The Whit* includes a "Calendar of Events for the Coming Holiday Season," with a long list of activities for white patients, including multiple pre-Christmas parties, a Christmas Eve pageant with delivery of Christmas stockings to patients, then a mass

Negotiating Daily Life 105

and a tea dance on Christmas Day. The Black patients' calendar of events was much shorter. There was a Christmas Eve pageant scheduled for 2 P.M. on Christmas Eve and then stockings delivered Christmas morning. There were no religious services at all, and the Black patients had to wait until January 2 for a New Year's dance. It was also the case that gift drives did not always extend to Black patients, who noted the lack of gifts by "hoping there might be enough for them this year."[39]

If these discrepancies were reported and published in *The Whit*, which was then distributed back to patients, there is no reason to assume that Black patients did not also see and notice these patterns and feel them keenly. The polite comments being made by Black patients expressing their gratitude and obedience stand in stark contrast to the ways that they were actually being treated when compared to white patients and demonstrate that they knew exactly where they stood in the hierarchy of things at Whitfield. The blatant discrepancies and the measurement of conditions at Whitfield by what was acceptable for white patients were designed to make clear to the public where their tax dollars were being spent and to reinforce to the public that services provided to Black patients met the standard for benevolent paternalism only, a standard for which Black patients were always expected to be grateful.

In this way, *The Whit* demonstrates that Black patients in Mississippi, people who were at their most vulnerable, knew very well what sort of behavior was expected of them, where they stood in the hierarchy of state spending and public sympathy, and what role they were required to perform in order to be considered sane and secure their release. The Jim Crow routine demanded polite deference and subservience from Black patients, even while mentally ill, and thus the possibility of sanity was indelibly linked to a subjectivity considered acceptable by and to white people, defined by them, and designed for their comfort. For Black patients, the demand from white people to perform the routine deliberately replicated plantation relations and worked to reinforce white supremacy in the daily life of the hospital.

Beyond the details of everyday life, *The Whit* tells us very little about the therapeutic regimen employed at Whitfield for Black patients. Activities and a recreational program, in and of themselves, are not actually therapy. *The Whit* demonstrates some brief attempts from Jaquith to try to bring more formal approaches to therapy to the hospital, even for Black patients. For short-term psychology extern Burks, creating an active daily schedule that fostered human connection and put smiles on people's faces was in itself "vital and important as part of the treatment so necessary for the recovery of mental patients. Happiness, which is the key-word to good mental health, is found in activity."[40] In his short reports for *The Whit*, Burks talked mainly about the therapeutic value of the recreational program at Whitfield and differentiated it from other forms of activity, such as work.

For example, in January 1952 he wrote, "Many of us feel that when we come to Whitfield we are going to a place where there is all work and no play. But that is not true."[41] Burks was not entirely correct, however. There is an abundance of evidence in *The Whit* that many patients spent the majority of their time occupied by some form of manual labor that served to maintain the institution as much as it did to serve an ostensibly therapeutic purpose. In the next section, I look at the way occupational therapy was interpreted and used, how it was rationalized and operationalized, and what it signified for Black patients in the shadow of the plantation.

"They Call It Occupational Therapy"

The issue of labor in asylums is as old as the issue of the asylum itself and has been discussed extensively by historians of psychiatry, disability, and incarceration. Existing scholarship demonstrates how normal and widespread a practice it was, and how it was linked to broader social, political, and economic rationales.[42] Administrators, superintendents, and psychiatrists themselves barely needed to justify it because they relied on a long tradition of the idea of "work as therapy," which originated in the idea of "moral treatment."[43] Often credited to Philippe Pinel in Paris, moral treatment was "moral" in that it was argued to bring a more humane approach to treatment, but it was also moral because it acted on patient behavior rather than being a "medical" approach.[44] Reformers like Pinel, Samuel Tuke, and the Quakers in Pennsylvania all argued that restraint, chains, and physical violence were not conducive to the treatment of mental illness; rather, kindness, compassion and a supportive, family-like environment based in productive occupation were what was needed.

The most influential proponent of this method of institutional organization in the United States was Samuel Tuke, who also had thoughts on the idea of occupational therapy before it became a distinct specialty. In 1815, he wrote to the new superintendent of New York's Bloomingdale Asylum that "the introduction of employment amongst the patients . . . is of the utmost importance in the moral treatment of insanity." He did not mean employment in terms of work in exchange for pay; he meant employment in terms of "having something to do," explaining that "the employment of insane persons should, as much as possible, be adapted to their previous habits, inclinations and capacities, and, though horticultural pursuits may be the most desirable, the greatest benefit will, I believe, to be found to result from the person being engaged in that employment in which he can most easily excel."[45]

During the boom period of psychiatric institutions in the mid-nineteenth century, new designs like those developed by Thomas Kirkbride were established on large tracts of land outside urban centers, ostensibly to remove disturbed people from their stressful original environment and to act as a kind of "retreat."[46] Rural locations that lent themselves naturally to "horticultural pursuits" seem at one level benign but were part of a very deliberate approach to population management. As historian David Rothman has argued, institutional superintendents "designed and implemented an orderly and disciplined routine, a fixed, almost rigid calendar, and put daily labor at the heart of it."[47]

Work was seen as one way of keeping people healthy (through activity in the open air) and also a constructive way of "passing the time"—noble pursuits to be sure. But it was also a disciplining and normative technique: "steady labor would train inmates to proper habits, bringing regularity to disordered lives."[48] Historian Heather Murray has suggested that being occupied, even when the labor might be considered a form of social control subject to exploitation, was better than the "automaton" patient who spent their days staring out the window, and avoiding this stereotype was certainly one motivation of superintendents and administrators.[49]

To some extent, approaches to care and treatment had always been shaped by prevailing social attitudes toward the mentally ill as much as they were by scientific advancement.[50] Despite several attempts at reform of the institutional care system, the psychiatric patient was still seen as a financial and social burden, an attitude tempered by scattered attempts at empathy or bursts of public exposure and reform. Public empathy itself was tempered by the demands of industrial capitalism for a productive workforce, which permeated all aspects of American life so that even the disabled had "no right to be idle."[51]

Throughout the nineteenth and twentieth centuries, moral treatment and occupational therapy evolved to reflect these underlying ideologies more clearly. Even the early theorists of occupational therapy as a profession argued for its significance in not just keeping people "occupied" while in institutions but in training or retraining them for productive wage-earning work outside the institution. This is all well and good if the patients themselves wanted to work or would benefit from such a program on their release. But when it was forced labor from which the patient gained no benefit, then a more critical analysis is required. In American asylums, the inescapable "political economy" element to the use of patient labor undercut the discourse about its use as therapy.[52] In the South, this political economy was shaped by the Jim Crow routine, where racial capitalism reflected both the legacy of the plantation and the new forms of labor relations that were designed to benefit white society and keep Black communities down.

But there were some cracks in the discourse and use of patient labor and occupational therapy that show not everyone believed they were the same thing. Differences in approaches along both gender and race lines show the ways that work as therapy was a deeply problematic practice in Southern asylums. And there was a tension at the heart of patient labor that administrators themselves were not unaware of. For example, when he arrived at Whitfield in the late 1940s, Dr. William Jaquith expressed his concern about the extent of the farmwork there. As he recalled to a reporter at his retirement in 1979, "In 1950, I told them I'd never been a farmer. We closed the farm and the dairy herd. If a patient was well enough to work here, he was well enough to be at home."[53] This is a particularly telling statement from the only physician employed at Whitfield at the time—that there was no medical or psychiatric justification for the use of hard labor for patients.

But other evidence suggests the farm did not immediately close. It continued to appear in the biannual reports and in the Board of Trustees minutes, although it is never made clear in these sources whether patients were working the farms. However, there are many and frequent references to the ways that patients contributed to the running of the institution in the patient newsletter. These references provide an unusual glimpse into the meaning and significance of work within the hospital and even how it was experienced by patients themselves.

The way that work and occupational therapy in Mississippi were constantly conflated is obvious from one of the earliest posts in the Black section of *The Whit*. In June 1951, a staff person representing "Colored Cottage #2" wrote, "Whitfield has a variety of activities to occupy leisure time among patients. . . . Patients make use of the different service departments, the bakery, dining hall, dairy, warehouse, laundry, and field work. Many patients work in these departments from Cottage #2."[54] There is a clear elision here between the idea of "making use" of the service departments and working in them—do they exist for the patient or for the smooth running of the hospital? And in this same edition, a representative from "Colored Cottage #3" wrote, "The patients of Cottage 3 are called 'The backbones of Whitfield fields.' The work is highly enjoyed by those who have worked in fields on farms for a source of living income. These patients are contented with farm work and are dutiful from one day to another."[55]

There is a lot to unpack in these few short sentences. These comments, written by someone who was not a patient, are a performance of the Jim Crow routine in many ways: They normalize the expectation that the Black person would be content and comfortable with hard labor, a convenient fiction within the hospital that reflected broader social relations. In reality, the patients were "the backbones of [the] fields," of the hospital even, because without them there would be no food for the rest of the hospital. The ability of the hospital to function, to feed its staff and patients, came at the expense of the backbreaking labor of Black patients, whose experience was erased through the assumption of what they were content with and what they enjoyed.

The word "dutiful" is particularly telling because it speaks to the paternalism of the Jim Crow routine, the expectation that the Black person would be kept at the lowest rung of social and productive life and be happy to be so. It muted the possibility of agency or resistance, and suggested that the good patient was a compliant, obliging, deferential one. It also reflected a sense of obligation to the hospital from patients, an expectation that they should be grateful to be there, for whatever happened to them there, and that their labor was simply expected as what they owed to the institution that was supposedly caring for them. These expectations and assumptions were jumbled up with the justification for work as therapeutic, which makes it harder to parse out the abuse and exploitation inherent to this labor, especially in the absence of patient voices.

For example, in August 1951, a staff person wrote in some detail about the nature of work in the main kitchen located in the Colored Male Receiving Ward. These comments are worth repeating in full:

> W. H., R. A., and J. W. are very good helpers in the Receiving Ward kitchen. Their work makes it possible for organized group work in setting up the tables with meals for the patients and cleaning of the dining room and kitchen after each meal. All kitchen helpers work to fulfill an accepted responsibility. Because of their abilities in such group work, supervision of the kitchen routine is less dictatorial. These patients get pride and a feeling of normal usefulness in doing

their work satisfactorily. After the routine of kitchen duties are done, there are periods of rest and relaxation. Since everyone believes in the slogan "all work and no play makes Jack a dull boy," the schedule carries with it an outlet for recreation.[56]

In these comments, the writer demonstrated the conflation of forced labor and work as therapy. It may well be that patients took pride in their work, and that it kept them occupied in an otherwise dull place, but it is impossible to tell if that was truly how the work was experienced by the patients themselves.

The fact that kitchen work was valued because it was "less dictatorial" indicated that other forms of work were potentially more problematic, and the justification for the therapeutic nature of the work was undermined by the emphasis on equal time for rest and relaxation, suggesting it was therapeutic only because it was exhausting. The idea that work was a normal and "accepted responsibility" of patients does not negate the fact that the work was forced and exploitative, at the same time that it might have been something to break up the monotony of the hospital routine. It also does not negate the fact that the three men named in this commentary were also in fact patients, yet they are positioned as "helpers," providing care labor for other patients. Historian Wendy Gonaver has demonstrated the way that care labor of Black and enslaved patients was central to the running of the Eastern Lunatic Asylum in Virginia 100 years earlier.[57] The same patterns were repeated at Whitfield in the 1950s, long after slavery and peonage were abolished and fair labor standard laws were passed.[58]

Work at Whitfield was also highly gendered and reflected broader expectations and norms for Black women in Mississippi. There were two main places of work (usually not even couched as therapy) for Black women: the sewing room and the kitchen. The efforts of the women in the sewing room make frequent appearances on the pages of *The Whit*, from the creation of quilts for the fair to the production of clothing for the hospital. A short report in August 1951 gave some indication of the extent of the work undertaken by women in the sewing room. "If you really want to see some stitches made," the report stated, "visit the colored sewing room. They have a standing order of garments to turn out each month. They not only turn out their order, but do many things beside. In one month alone 1605 pieces were issued from the sewing room."[59]

The writer reported that about twenty-five patients were usually employed in the sewing room, and they were supervised by Mrs. Jones and

Mrs. Crosby (it is not clear if they were Black or white women). In September 1951, the writer of the report commented that the women were looking forward to the state fair, where their quilts and crochet pieces would be displayed, but they were also making dresses to wear from "a large supply of new cloth." The reporter noted that "because of their faithfulness to their duty, and the joy and pleasure they display in doing their work, these ladies deserve an opportunity for such an outlet which affords even more pleasure and recreation."[60] Again, the slippage between work as therapy/recreation and duty to the hospital was evident, and the assumption that the women enjoyed the work and took pride in it was used as justification. I do not doubt that the women did get a great deal of satisfaction out of sewing—especially quilting, given its significance as a form of homemaking, crafting, and activism within the African American community. But that still does not make it therapy, in and of itself.

There is little that can be considered therapeutic about the sheer scale of production from the sewing room: on average, each woman was making sixty-four items of clothing per month, or two per day. There are rare glimpses into how the patients themselves felt about their work in the sewing room. In one such example in January 1952, a patient remarked, "We already have a large order of new clothes ready to be shipped out to different buildings. We hope the patients will enjoy wearing them as much as we enjoy making them."[61] This work must have been laborious and difficult—some of it by machine, some of it by hand, but all of it essential to the running of the hospital, saving the administration many thousands of dollars a year, and not just on clothes.

In a report from February 1952, it was noted, "We are working on our big order for the first of the month. Straight-jackets, coffee strainers, clothing for the patients, cold frame clothes for the florist department are among the many articles made at the colored sewing room."[62] Mrs. Jones, one of the supervisors, also brought a visitor to see the work being done. This was not sewing as occupational therapy; it was domestic labor produced on a small factory-like scale, requiring a high level of organization and supervision. And not only were the patients making clothes, but they were also making the very things (straitjackets) that could be used against them if they disobeyed or were less dutiful.

If work was fashioned as therapeutic, as a way to relieve the boredom of daily life in the hospital, then perhaps it was so in the regulated routine of mass production, the whirring of machines, the rhythmic back and forth of a needle and thread through cloth. But it is also possible that a different kind of boredom may have prevailed in the repetitive motions of mechanical work, the timed and regulated discipline, the lack of rest or relaxation.

There is one small note here that hints at the conditions of work: "We have refreshments every Wednesday," the reporter wrote. "Patients enjoy it very much and look forward to Wednesday coming."[63] Not only were there not refreshments *every* day, but the existence of them once a week worked as a kind of lure and reward and served to break up the monotony as a respite from working long hours, especially in the hot summer months. I have little doubt that these conditions were not considered problematic by the people who administered them but were seen as a sign of goodwill from white to Black, couched in a rhetoric of self-congratulation and paternalistic generosity, the flip side to white supremacy being white saviorism, of course.

The significance of food preparation as care work was particularly pertinent at Whitfield, and there is strong evidence that Black women performed much of this labor. The most striking example of the way that Black women cared for other patients through food preparation, and the way this work was exploited by white administrators, was demonstrated in a photograph I encountered in two forms in Dr. Jaquith's scrapbooks.[64] The first image I encountered was a large black-and-white photograph, unlabeled, that showed two Black women standing behind a white woman seated at a kitchen table. The Black women were dressed all in white and held plates of food: one looked sideways at the camera and the other, a shy smile on her face, gazed downward. The woman seated looked down at her plate of food, a smile on her face. I had no idea what the photograph signified.

In a different scrapbook was taped an undated and uncredited newspaper clipping with a different version of the photo attached to a story. In this photo, the woman at the table is named as Mrs. Jaquith. The story is titled "Guest Cook of the Week" and refers to the women behind Mrs. Jaquith as "inmates of the hospital."[65] The story goes on to detail the way that Mrs. Jaquith, born and bred in New Orleans, was a terrible cook when she first married Dr. Jaquith, who insisted that she learn lest they starve. According to the story, she rapidly learned to cook via phone calls to her mother, using her grandmother's recipes. The reporter noted the sparkling-clean kitchen she was working in and asked how she kept it so tidy, and Mrs. Jaquith explained that she cleaned as she went and did not go to bed until every dish was washed. Then, the reporter added, "She has help part of the day from 'two of her girls,' as she calls them." The Jaquiths lived on-site at

Whitfield, and from this story, it became obvious that they availed themselves of patient labor for their own domestic purposes.

It is significant that Mrs. Jaquith did not have white women working for her in this way. Rather, the use of Black women was deliberately designed to reinforce the position of the Jaquiths at the top of the Whitfield hierarchy, replicating broader social relations and reminding the public and patients that the place of the Black person, as a patient or a civilian, was in the field or the kitchen. In this way, not only were patients performing labor essential to the efficient running of the hospital within which they were confined (in fact, without that labor, the hospital would have become unviable), but the exploitation of their labor in very particular ways was a performance of the Jim Crow routine. If the entire economy in the history of Mississippi had been built on the back of the unfree Black person, then Whitfield was no exception. In this broader social, political, and economic context, the mundane, punitive, and coercive use of Black patient labor made a lie of the idea of work as occupational therapy.

The dissonance between the theoretical justifications for patient labor and the way it worked in practice were particularly evident in Alabama. In September 1948, state senator Albert L. Patterson visited both Bryce and Searcy Hospitals, and the archives contain a typed transcript of conversations had with various staff and patients, as well as private conversations between the senator and his two committee members, Mr. J. P. Shelton and Mrs. Rose Emmett (and whoever was taking notes).[66] These minutes reveal a great deal not only about everyday conditions and practices but also about the attitudes that underpinned them.

One particularly telling comment came at the end of the visit, when the committee members met with various institutional administrators. The senator summarized his inspections by saying, "You are getting a lot of work out of the patients and are to be commended for that," to which assistant physician Billy Partlow said, "I think they call that occupational therapy." The senator noted, "They must be given something to do," and superintendent Tarwater responded, "That is true."[67] But "given something to do" was different for Black patients than it was for white patients, having a much more extractive nature and intent. This extractive labor also occurred in the context of significantly worse conditions and overall hostile attitudes toward Black patients.

When he visited Searcy—the Black-only hospital in Mount Vernon—Senator Patterson encountered some of these issues firsthand but failed to see them as problematic. He noted the way that Black patients were forced to wait outside in all weather for their meals, the lack of recreation facilities, the lack of personal liberty, and differences in the way that people were confined. "How is it kept so quiet?" he asked. Miss Clue, assistant to superintendent Dr. Harry Rowe, replied, "The patients are on good behavior, the doctors are going through on their daily checkup now." Patterson asked if any of the patients were dangerous, and Miss Clue replied, "Yes sir, we have a good many dangerous ones," and when asked how they managed those patients, she reported, "We have rooms in which they are confined."[68] In the same conversation, Mr. Shelton asked, "Do you have any padded cells," to which he was told no; when he then asked, "You have crazy folks here?" Miss Clue replied, "Yes sir, plenty, and they are mean and dangerous."[69]

This question from Shelton is particularly interesting, because it raises the question of who else was he expecting to encounter at a hospital for the mentally ill? Leaving aside the pejorative use of "crazy," Shelton's comment suggests that not everyone at Searcy was in fact mentally ill, and that the incarceration of the non-mentally ill Black person was standard practice. It also indicates that they were seen first as workers, not as patients. Miss Clue's response about "mean and dangerous" folks also spoke to an attitude of contempt, disgust, and fear that was not evident in comments about white patients. It is a disturbing and dehumanizing comment coming from a staff person and indicates a distinct lack of empathy, which would have created a hostile environment for patients. Later, Dr. Rowe explained to the visiting team that epileptics required close supervision because "they bite and fight each other."[70] These attitudes were not expressed in any of the comments about white patients, who were more likely to be left unsupervised and had access to personal effects, church services, and musical instruments.

The underlying belief in the danger posed by Black patients meant that there was no free space in which they could move around or exercise. Some patients simply sat on their beds all day, or on various ward porches. Further comments from Dr. Rowe, however, indicated the use of more forceful types of confinement. "These rooms on the side are used with patients who are restless and bother the others," explained Dr. Rowe, to no response.

The committee then went to the second floor of the men's ward, where "confinement rooms for worse patients" were located. Here, Senator Patterson said, "You don't have any beds up here," and Dr. Rowe explained that they placed mattresses on the concrete floor for the patients at night. The senator questioned the lack of bars on the windows, and Dr. Rowe explained that "it [already] looks too much like a jail." There are no images linked to

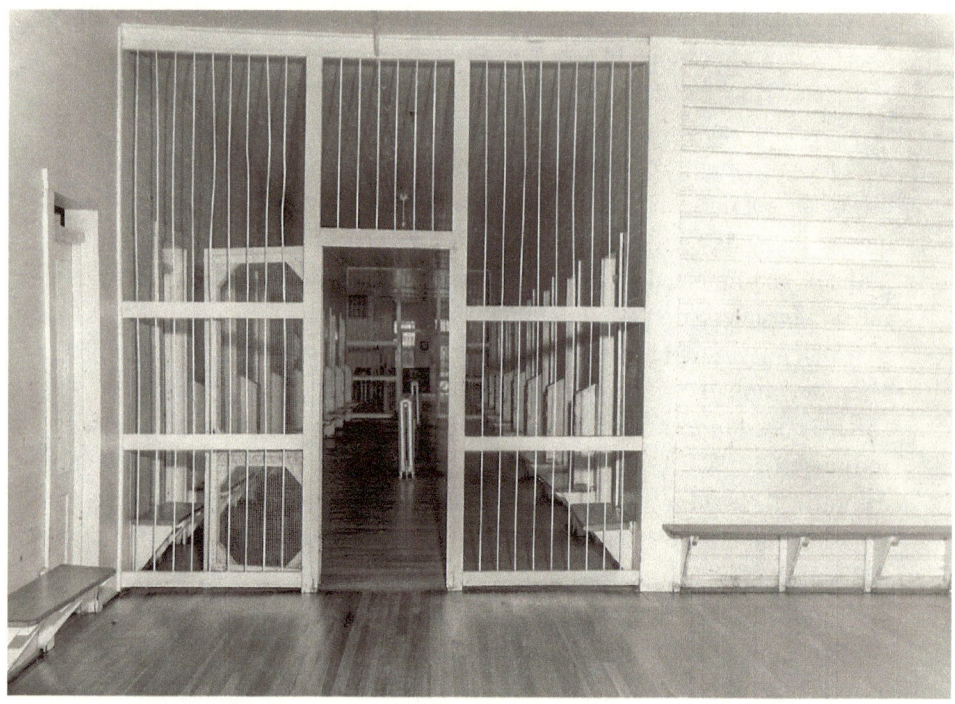

FIGURE 4.2 Patient dayroom, Searcy Hospital, 1949. Alabama Building Commission Photos, ADAH.

this particular report. However, in an image from the building commission (see figure 4.2), which visited Searcy a year later to repair walls, ceilings, and porches that had not been touched in forty years, small cubicles are visible along the walls of a long hallway.

Down the middle of the hallway are some oil heaters, and the line of cubicles is closed off from the main room by a metal cage-like door. If you look closely, there are little metal loops above each tiny bench, suggesting that patients, at one time or another, could have been tied up.[71] There is no note on this photo, so I cannot be sure that it is the same room that the senator visited, but regardless, there were indeed rooms at Searcy that looked very much like a jail.

The jail-like atmosphere was reinforced, intentionally or not, by the actual physical construction of Searcy, which existed solely inside the original Civil War fort walls. It was not and had never been designed as a hospital, and the inner space of a mere forty-two acres housed multiple wards, administration and facility buildings, and a small farm. The committee focused a great deal on the farming enterprises and the use of work, and articulated both as necessary for patient and staff upkeep and for amusement or occupation.

An administrative assistant pointed out that all the patients who were able were moved out to "farms and to the dairy," meaning the larger property beyond the main wall. When Patterson asked whether the patients were forced to work, he was told, "No sir, it is voluntary," but if patients wanted to work, they were given the opportunity to do so.[72] In the post-inspection chatter, Patterson noted, "They need more recreation, more exercise and entertainment, the institution is weak on that point," and then followed this comment with, "They should have more of the inmates working at Mt. Vernon. They do not have enough work."[73]

Mrs. Emmett summarily conflated work and recreation when she responded, "And that comes back to the recommendation that they need more recreation and exercise." The senator agreed, finishing their inspection of Searcy with the comment, "They need the right kind of director that could teach them to work etc. I believe this would cut down their number of inmates. So many of them were sitting around, and that is enough to run anyone crazy."[74] The senator was no psychiatrist, so it might be unreasonable to expect him to know that there are therapeutic options for the treatment of patients. However, his comments reflect the custodial nature and purpose of Searcy, and the common belief that work was all that was required. But they also reveal that the people who should know about therapeutic options were either ignorant or simply not using them.

The focus on farming in this report demonstrates the easy acceptance of the custodial function of a place like Searcy and its link to broader extractive labor practices in Alabama. As part of the inspection tour, the senator's committee also visited the State Farm Colony for Negroes at the Jemison Center, where he talked to Mr. H. G. Barr, the superintendent. The Jemison Center, as I set out in chapter 2, was actually located about eight miles north of the main Bryce Hospital campus in Tuscaloosa, across the Black Warrior River near Northport, Alabama. Mr. Shelton from the senate committee seemed already clear on the way that the Jemison Center, or the State Colony Farm, as it was also called, worked.

Before Mr. Barr could say a word, Shelton explained to the senator: "This place takes them at any age. They all go first to Mt. Vernon and the best workers are transferred here."[75] After Shelton confirmed the practice with Barr, the discussion turned to the type of farming and the crops produced: 200 bales of cotton, 3,000 bushels of corn, 5,000 bushels of sweet potatoes, 73 hogs, 78 chickens, 400 turkeys, 98 white-faced beef cattle, 210 guernseys

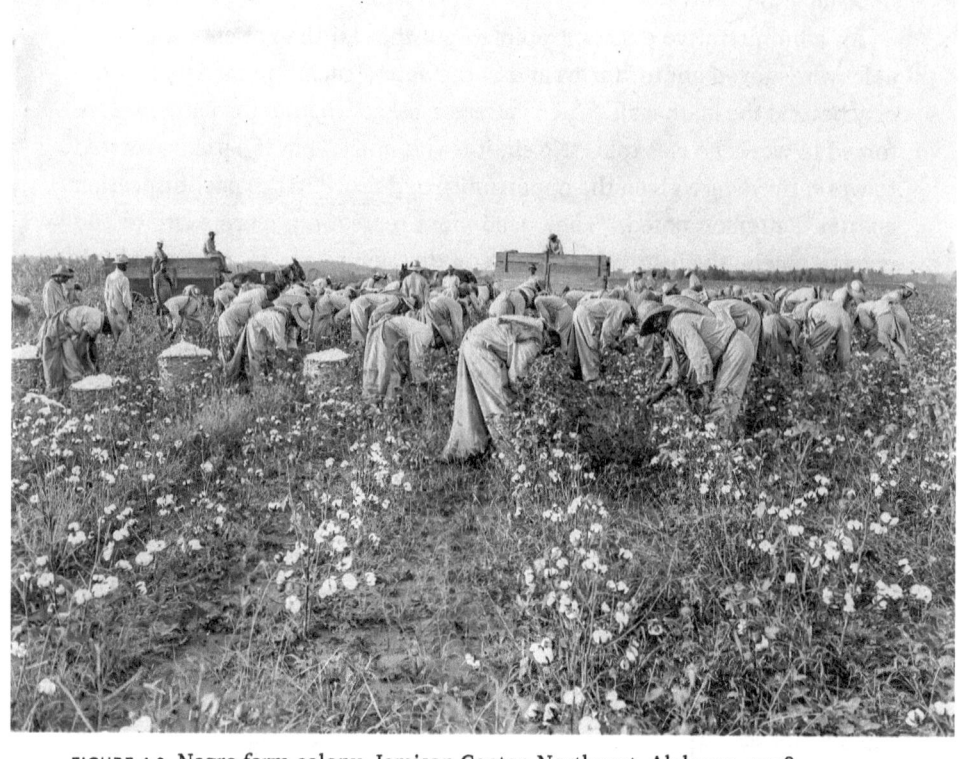

FIGURE 4.3 Negro farm colony, Jemison Center, Northport, Alabama, 1948. University of Alabama Libraries Special Collections.

for milking (200 gallons of milk sent straight to Bryce). The excess turkeys sold for about fifty cents per pound, and that money went into the general fund for running Bryce Hospital. The acreage of these farms was extensive: 240 for cotton, 930 for corn alone, with a total of 1,500 acres being worked by about fifty-five Black patients, who all slept in the same wooden building together. This farm was run by Mr. Causey, who also hired four local workers, who were paid between $90 and $105 a month.[76]

I found some photos of these farm colonies in the Hoole Special Collection library at the University of Alabama in Tuscaloosa, which now occupies the same land that was once Bryce Hospital. Figure 4.3 depicts a scene that could very well be a Southern plantation but has the words "Negro Colony Farm" scribbled on the back in pencil. It shows a group of Black men bent over picking cotton by hand, while other men watch from horse-drawn carts. One man at the front has his face turned to the camera. The field is vast, stretching into the distance, blurred around the edges with heat and dust. The fact that this photo was taken at the Jemison Center, now a hospital, once a plantation, viscerally demonstrates the continuities in labor practices in Alabama which permeated even the so-called hospital setting.

Despite the high level of productivity, the conditions for patients working at the Jemison Center were less than ideal. The committee noted the leaking walls and ceiling, the fact that patients did all the productive farmwork as well as all their own laundry and dishwashing, and that they did not seem to have enough to eat: steamed beef, light bread, rice or grits only.[77] Mrs. Emmett noted, "Their storage room was bare. They do not have much to eat," and the senator agreed: "I was certainly not impressed with what they had," he stated, and Mr. Shelton reiterated the point: "I do not believe they have enough to eat."[78]

The committee also noted that the "inmates," as they called them, had little time for recreation, had no access to church services, and were allowed only the bare minimum of personal effects—for example, a radio to share. In all these elements, the "colony farm" model for patients was indistinguishable from prison farms operating in these states at the same time.[79] Extractive labor was the sole purpose of the Jemison Center, justified by the same rhetoric that had been used to justify slavery.

One exchange is particularly telling in this regard. In addition to superintendent Barr, the committee members spoke to an unidentified Mr. Robertson—he seemed to be the farm manager. Mrs. Emmett asked Robertson if "these people work good," to which he replied, "Yes mam. They are better satisfied when they are working. They are not so well satisfied when it is raining or cold weather, and they cannot get out. We try to let them get out to the barn at least on bad days, for an hour or two."[80] Senator Patterson asked if the doors were locked (yes) and whether they ever whipped any patients (no). Mr. Robertson also noted that sometimes people ran away, and so they needed to be closely supervised. That supervision often took the form of a white man on a horse (see figure 4.4).

At the Jemison Center, or the State Colony Farm, the rhetoric of "it was good for them" was used to justify both custodial conditions and relentless work, in the same way confinement and hard labor were justified on the plantation and the prison farm. This framing reflected a particular performance of the Jim Crow routine in relation to the prevailing norms and expectations regarding Black and white labor relations in postwar Alabama.[81] That is, it reflected Alabama's reliance on extractive labor for

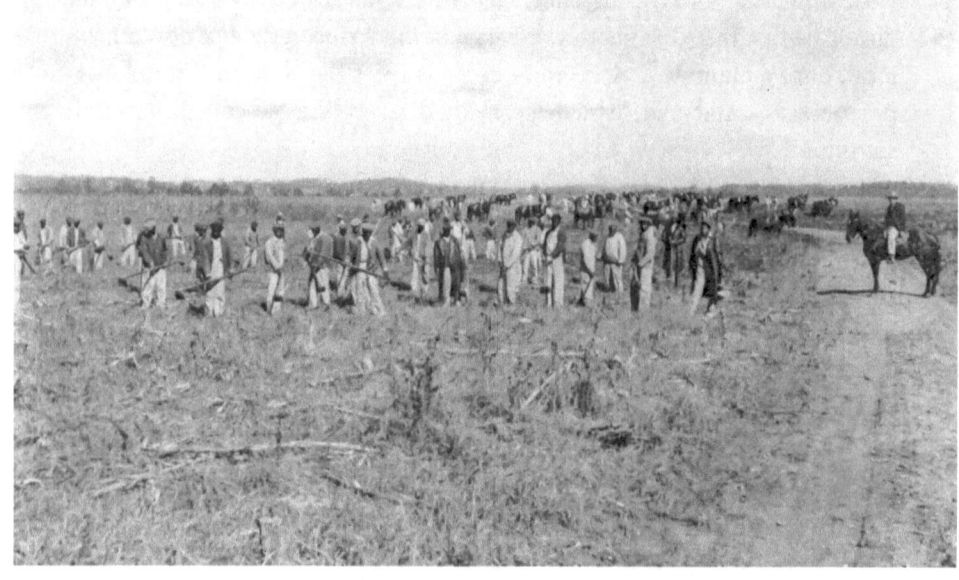

FIGURE 4.4 State Farm Colony for Negroes, Report of the Trustees of the Alabama State Hospitals, 1946. Courtesy of the Reynolds-Finley Historical Library, the University of Alabama at Birmingham.

agricultural production and its continued belief in the suitability of the Black body for that work, even at the intersection with illness or disability. At the same time, the emphasis on "occupational therapy" reflected the limited treatment programs in place in these so-called hospitals, especially for Black patients. It is particularly telling that the senator (who was not, obviously, a psychiatrist) asked no questions about actual psychiatric therapies, and neither was he told anything.

Throughout the 1950s, occupational therapy (OT) as distinct from farmwork became more prevalent in the official reports from Central State Hospital in Georgia, reflecting the rise of OT as a distinct profession with its own training and accreditation.[82] In 1956, occupational therapy was a relatively new program at CSH, which, the superintendent believed, separated that hospital from purely custodial institutions (as if Central State was not one). "The occupational therapy and recreation departments are likewise expanding to the wards," superintendent Thomas Peacock wrote:

> In addition to the benefits directly derived from keeping the patients occupied, the program has also stimulated the attendants and heightened their interest in improving conditions on their wards. A wholesome rivalry has sprung up among them, each group vying

with the other in efforts to make its surroundings more attractive and in improving the morale and comforts of its patients. Dr. Yarbrough has for many years given supervision to the occupational therapy activities in the white male department, most of it being centered in the Boland Building and at the "Log Cabin," where patients engage in woodwork and growing roses, chrysanthemums, and other flowers of show type caliber.[83]

In extolling the virtues of the program, and the improvements in conditions and morale it encouraged, Peacock admitted that there had been severe deficiencies in these areas previously.

Major discrepancies based on race prevailed, however. For example, while extolling Dr. Yarbrough's work with the white men, the superintendent made no mention of any similar activities for Black men. A garden club with multiple groups existed only for white patients.[84] And in 1956, Mrs. Maude Boone, the supervisor of the OT aides, made it clear that occupational therapy as we might think of it today was still new and developing for white patients at CSH, while being almost nonexistent for Black patients.

Boone wrote that three new OT aides (two white and one Black) had been hired for occupational therapy in the Rivers Building, which housed both Black and white patients, separated by floors, for the treatment of tuberculosis. She requested more space and supplies for workshops in the Howell and Boland Buildings (both housing white patients only) and noted that "the Occupational Therapy Shop in the Washington Building is badly in need of more space[,] and more equipment could be used in that shop."[85] The Washington Building was one of the largest buildings on the campus and located the farthest away from all the others—it was where most of the Black male patients lived. Mrs. Boone noted that Dr. Bailey had recently "returned" to his position as director of the clinical service for Black patients and had "shown great interest in occupational therapy," which made her hopeful at least that OT for the Black patients might become more prevalent than it currently was.[86]

Sewing and handicrafts, presumably for women, were also part of the OT program at Central State Hospital; Boone reported that "the Occupational Therapy Department had a very nice exhibit at the fairs in Macon and Atlanta last year, where the work of the [white?] patients was displayed. They had first prizes in quilts and embroidery which were displayed on television[,] and the patients enjoyed seeing the work. This year we hope to have more space for displaying their work and a larger quantity of articles to display."[87] Boone also mentioned the production of the patient newsletter, *The Builder*, as part of the OT program, separating *The Builder* from the *Golden Star*, the Black patient newspaper, which she does not name: "A paper is being printed weekly for the colored department," she wrote, "and many patients are interested in writing for the paper. They do all their editing and reporting. This has created a lot of interest in the colored department." The fact that no copies of *The Builder* or the *Golden Star* seem to have survived for public view is a terrible loss, given how much insight into patients' lives and experiences was possible through an analysis of *The Whit* from Mississippi State Hospital.[88]

Tellingly, the recreation department report for CSH was barely a page long and demonstrated the lack of real amusement for Black patients here. In the 1956 report, the program director, Bruce Posser, wrote, "This past year also saw the establishment of a Colored Recreation Center. One of the pavilions was turned over to this department and is used by the Colored Department for the majority of events. The patients come to the Center to play cards, games, ball, and dance. This has enabled the Colored Department to expand its program. In addition to the above, we have had our annual barbecues for the white and colored departments, as well as picnics and wiener roasts."[89]

Other recreational activities were supplied by local church groups and bundled in with the other activities and services provided by the social services department, which did not clearly differentiate between services for Black or white patients, but it is not clear that Black churches or volunteer groups were included. The United Church Women were particularly active in arranging funding for new televisions, donating books and magazines, and providing a whole new set of furniture for dayrooms in various wards, but there is no mention of any of these services being provided specifically for Black patients.[90] For Black or white patients, recreation was the bare minimum that a hospital like CSH should have provided, and it was no substitute for actual therapy. It was merely a panacea, a way to pass the time because actual therapy was expensive or impractical; and for Black patients, work as therapy was, as Mr. M.'s letter had made clear, a simple fact of life.

Since its origins, work at CSH had followed clearly demarcated race and gender lines.[91] As Mab Segrest notes, "White men were gardeners. . . . Black men lived and worked on a "colony farm." . . . White women were seamstresses and colored women worked the laundry."[92] The annual report for

1956 includes a category called "Industrial Therapy," which detailed the costs of supplies and equipment for a sewing room, shoe repair shop, mattress factory, and broom shop.[93] In the same report, it was suggested that the horticulturalist be allowed to plant an orchard and a vineyard to offset the cost of buying jams, preserves, and jellies, noting that the hospital had a "sufficient labor force to man such a project, which can provide useful occupational therapy for patients at the Institution."[94] These kinds of gardening activities however, were reserved for white patients. Black patients in Georgia, like their counterparts in Alabama, were much more likely to find themselves picking cotton.

CSH ran two large colony farms, and they were run very much like the Jemison Center farm in Alabama in that they were situated away from the main hospital campus and patients lived on-site in dormitories. There was no therapy on the colony farms other than work. The best description of the work they performed, and the conditions for patients who worked on them, is included in the reports of the business administrator and the Farm and Dairy Division.

In his report, Mr. Joe Boone, the institutional business administrator, requested financial support from the state for a number of substandard buildings, most of them housing Black patients. He called attention to the state of Colony No. 2 (also known as the State Farm for Colored Males), which housed 110 patients (the report by the Farm and Dairy Division noted that the dairy operation from Colony No. 1 had been moved to Colony No. 2).[95] Operations at Central State Hospital included an abattoir for hogs, raised on-site; dairies; and broiler and egg "projects," as well as a cannery and a bakery. These "productive units," as they were called, operated at least in part on patient labor and produced "$1,956,614.24 worth of farm and dairy products at a net cost of $1,250,012.81, showing a net profit of $706,601.43."[96] The level of production here was intense, highly mechanized, and large scale. Central State Hospital created its own ecosystem for the town of Milledgeville and surrounding Baldwin County, employing local laborers, contractors, supervisors, and assistants. Yet it managed a substantial profit because of the use of patient labor. Matters were also complicated by proximity to the prison system. The approach to work for patients developed in parallel with the labor camp and convict leasing system so rampant in Georgia at the time, and at times the prison and hospital farms were literally adjacent to each other.[97] It was easy for patients and prison inmates to be swapped between institutions, and common for prisoners to work in the hospital kitchen.

Negotiating Daily Life 123

There is, of course, no questioning the use of patient labor in any of these enterprises, and even though meticulous income and expenditure tallies are kept for every aspect of their operation, there is never a clear accounting for the number or type of patients used, or a reckoning of exactly how much their labor saved the hospital, and therefore the state. It is only through cross-referencing with other records or sections of the report that I can find out anything about the existence of Black patients here at all. Unlike Searcy in Alabama or even Whitfield in Mississippi, the fact of segregation existed unquestioningly and was noted in the use of the term "colored service," but there was no separate report from or about that service. The information about Black patients is bundled in with the detail about the hospital overall, and if that is not deliberate, it is at least obfuscatory. The performance of the Jim Crow routine took a different tenor in Georgia, where the records made it look like Black and white patients were treated the same, indicating at least a tacit knowledge that they *should* be. The reality, of course, would turn out to be something else.

To some extent, the reliance on work as therapy across all institutions deep into the twentieth century was exacerbated by the science of psychiatric treatment itself, which before 1950 was based largely on the management of behavior, especially the behavior of large populations in remote places. This meant that cure and recovery were tenuous possibilities for anyone, let alone the Black patient who was already marginalized. While it might be tempting to argue that labor for psychiatric patients was a universal aspect of inpatient care and came from the good intentions of moral treatment and occupational therapy, the evidence itself suggests that this was not entirely the case. In all circumstances, North or South, work was work, not therapy. There is evidence that patients enjoyed it at times, if only to relieve the otherwise relentless boredom of institutionalization, and for some patients, it did provide basic skills that could be used on release.

But for Black patients in Southern asylums, its therapeutic benefits were overshadowed by the obviously extractive and forced nature of the work. Administrators justified the work through a rhetoric of therapy, but other evidence clearly revealed the hypocrisy of that framing and is belied by the obvious reality that the institutions would not have functioned without the forced labor of Black patients, the literal "backbones" of the hospital to which they had been admitted in the hope of cure, recovery, and return home. The hard labor of long days in the field are difficult to characterize as anything other than plantation practices, reinforced by racist ideas about the lack of complexity of the Black psyche and the imperviousness of the Black body to pain, even when technically disabled.

The use of work specifically in a hospital setting for patients, who were not actually inmates even though they were often called that, signals the simultaneous impossibility and immutability of Black disability. That is, Black patients were fit to work in the field because they were always already beyond therapy, beyond psychiatry, and beyond recovery. At the same time as they were disabled enough to require eugenic confinement, they were paradoxically not disabled enough to avoid hard work. The lie of occupational therapy was exposed in the nature of the work undertaken by Black patients (and the justifications for it), which merely served to reinforce and replicate white supremacy and Jim Crow law and custom within and beyond the hospital walls.

These conditions and practices were not necessarily new to anyone paying attention. Alternative sources of information about the daily experiences of patients in the nation's psychiatric hospitals had come under scrutiny from the media at various times in the postwar period. These reports and exposés, the subject of chapter 5, provide more information about life for Black patients and the work that people were doing outside the system to try to raise awareness. But there were limitations to this kind of activism, and it sometimes had unintended consequences.

5   Exposing Southern Snake Pits

Jackson, Miss.
259 Oferrell Ave
Dec. 5, 1947

Dear Sirs,
I have been Cheif of Patol at the State Hospital for the insane people at Whitfield Miss for several months and they are making slaves out of the colord patient out there they work them from before day to after dark one of the Big Shots by the name of Stagg shot one of the patient eyes out and the Day Superin by the name of Smith carry a gun all the time I am torning my resisnation in and quiting please do not mention my name if you want to see me contact Dr S D Redmond and he know how to get in touch with me.
Your truly
/s/ Hull Watkins

I found Mr. Watkins's letter in the papers of the NAACP Legal Defense Fund at the Library of Congress, in a file called Hospitals, Miscellaneous Cases.[1] It signifies a lot in a few short sentences. First, it is safe to assume that Mr. Watkins was white, because no Black man was the chief of anything run by the state of Mississippi in 1947. Mr. Watkins knew enough to write to the head office of the NAACP Legal Defense Fund in New York City, and that act speaks to the role that white moderates and liberals played in Mississippi's civil rights battles yet to come. But Mr. Watkins knew enough to not make himself known—he hid behind a request for anonymity and resigned rather than confront directly the situation at Whitfield. Even so, Mr. Watkins's letter is significant because it is direct evidence of the reality of that system and demonstrates the many ways that Jim Crow was performed in the Southern asylum on a daily basis. The letter speaks to the level of violence and the overt practices of white supremacy that made daily life in these institutions so dangerous and traumatizing for Black patients, and it makes a clear connection between the history of slavery and the so-called therapeutic practices being used in asylums, exposing the gendered and racialized use of farmwork. The letter is significant because it is so unique, one of very few concerned with conditions for Black patients, yet I could find no evidence of it having an immediate impact.[2]

The timing of Mr. Watkins's letter, however, is highly significant. The period immediately after World War II was in many ways transformational in American psychiatry. Concerns about the state of mind of returning veterans, as well as the ability of the nation to adjust to postwar life in the shadow of fascism and communism, spurred a rapid expansion of the psy-sciences into all aspects of American life.[3] At the same time, a great deal of attention began to be paid to conditions in the nation's psychiatric hospitals largely because of the role of conscientious objectors (COs), who had been sent to work in psychiatric hospitals during the war to replace the nurses active in the war effort.[4]

COs effectively became whistleblowers and contributed to a growing public concern about horrific conditions that the media compared to the POW and Nazi death camp images they had been subjected to only a year or two before. America's claim to greatness and democracy were surely undermined by the hypocrisy of its treatment of the mentally ill and disabled, which had been so violently exposed and opposed in the fight against the Nazi regime. These concerns were bolstered by major stories like Albert Maisel's "Bedlam 1946," published by *Life* magazine in May 1946, and Albert Deutsch's *The Shame of the States*, published in 1948. Public imagination was also stirred by Mary Jane Ward's 1946 book *The Snake Pit*, about her experience at New York's Bellevue Hospital, which was made into a movie starring Olivia de Havilland in 1948.[5]

Mr. Watkins's letter hinted at the impact of these public concerns even in the Deep South. If top-down policy and legislation like the Mental Health Act and the creation of the National Institute of Mental Health were designed to address structural problems, it was popular culture and media coverage that stood the best chance of shifting public attitudes. The flip side to the official state records, like senate studies, APA inspections, hospital annual reports, and even patient newsletters, which I used in other chapters, are the public writings of journalists. In this chapter, I look at the way newspapers or other public writings in the period after World War II and before 1960 sometimes inadvertently, sometimes deliberately, sought to inform the public and improve conditions, and in so doing revealed information about the Black patient experience.

At the same time, these exposés and sources are also important for what they do not say and for their limitations in effecting fundamental change. In pursuing a "reform" agenda, newspaper exposés and popular writings often ironically served to *expand* the reach of large, centralized hospitals, which remained indelibly segregated, especially in the South, and therefore acted as a kind of nonreform reform.[6] And the majority of exposés focused on conditions for white patients, but they were often supported by hospital administrators themselves as a way of raising public sympathy and therefore hopefully government funding.

Dr. Jaquith at Whitfield used the pages of the patient newsletter *The Whit* to reproduce letters that had been written by a white patient in the late 1940s and smuggled out to the *Delta Democrat-Times*. These letters had provoked a major US Senate investigation and sparked a long-running interest on the part of editor Hodding Carter about the state of Whitfield—and of mental health in Mississippi more broadly. At the same time, journalist Albert Deutsch turned his attention to Milledgeville in Georgia, and his concerns were then taken up by Black publications like *Ebony*, by local doctor Peter Cranford, and eventually by the Pulitzer Prize–winning reporter Jack Nelson in the *Atlanta Constitution*. In the rest of this chapter I use these published writings to analyze the ways that the patient experience was represented, looking specifically for information about Black patients and teasing out the gaps and silences around their experience. The way that Black patients are or are not represented, in form as well as content, reveals a great deal about the way Jim Crow at the intersection with mental illness was performed in the popular media and press, and reveals deeply embedded ideas about the nature of the Black personality, the overlay with eugenics and criminality, and the limitations of even progressive journalists when it came to matters of race.

Hodding Carter, Hayden Campbell, and the *Delta Democrat-Times*

From about 1946, a white patient at Whitfield, Fred Chaney, had been smuggling letters out to friends, relatives, and politicians, including the governor, about the conditions at Whitfield.[7] He also sent letters to newspaper editors, including Hodding Carter at Greenville's *Delta Democrat-Times*, who began extensive coverage of conditions and debates about Whitfield from early 1947.[8] This coverage was not specific to conditions for Black patients of course—while Carter himself was a supporter of civil rights, he was also a known conservative about Black–white relationships and a proponent of slow change in Mississippi until later in his life.[9] For Carter, though, it likely made strategic sense to focus on conditions for white patients, because he was writing for a white audience with limited sympathy for Black people in Mississippi, let alone those confined in a mental hospital. This was a frequent tactic—the white patient as the face of abject neglect and abuse in campaigns to raise awareness and funding for the institution as a whole. And behind every story about those conditions for white patients is the unspoken reality of the exponentially worse conditions for Black patients.

Carter was well aware that Black patients existed, of course. When he began his coverage of Whitfield, before Dr. Jaquith arrived, the hospital was under the stewardship of Dr. Charles B. Mitchell, who argued in the *Delta Democrat-Times* (*DDT*) that "mental disease shows no respect for color or creed."[10] Mitchell's main complaint about the problems faced by Whitfield were related to the lack of a state expenditure for the facility, which meant that he was feeding patients on $0.78 per day when the US Public Health Service recommended that the minimum spent should be $2.50 per day. Mitchell also argued that it was impossible to run an institution the size of Whitfield when the medical superintendent (himself) had his decisions and requests undercut by a business manager who was a direct appointee of the governor. There was no other oversight of Whitfield at this time.

Mitchell's complaints were supported by an inspection from state senator Fred Jones, who visited Whitfield in January 1947. His inspection was covered extensively in the *DDT*, which reported on Jones's determination that "conditions there [were] as bad as they were in concentration camps in Europe." He cited a lack of nutritious food, leaking pipes, no heating, and overcrowding so bad that there were no beds, just mattresses on the floor that "could be piled in the corner during the day time in order to give the inmates space in which to move around."[11] Jones then went on to chair a joint legislative committee, which "termed the conditions at Whitfield intolerable" and supported a bill sponsored by the State Medical Association calling for the administration of Whitfield and the state's other mental institutions—like the white-only hospital in Meridian and the state school at Ellisville—to be placed under the control of a five-member board. Governor Wright agreed to support the bill if both Dr. Mitchell and Mr. Dyer (the business manager) resigned from Whitfield, which they did.[12] The board was instituted, and Dr. William Shackleford became the superintendent, with sole oversight.

This was not the end of problems, however, and continued investigations and complaints revealed that Shackleford was highly problematic. In an article from December 1948, the *DDT* stated that an official report on conditions at Whitfield known as the Boswell Report should have been made public and presented to the investigating legislative committee, but apparently it was tabled at the time.[13] The same article reported that another politician, Senator Hayden Campbell, had taken up the Whitfield cause and undertaken his own investigation. Apparently Campbell's efforts were not being taken seriously—other politicians seemed to think that Senator Jones's earlier investigation and the pending Boswell Report would be enough, or that the testimony of patients was not something to be taken seriously. But Campbell's investigation was based on his own repeated visits to Whitfield and firsthand discussions with a number of ex and current employees and patients.

Carter referenced this investigation in an editorial on January 16, 1949, titled "Mississippi's Snake Pit," making a direct link to the popular book and film. In his editorial, Carter wrote that even if there had been minor improvements, "Representative Campbell has secured a lot of evidence, and we see no reason to doubt the grim story he tells." Carter summarized Campbell's reports as a "testimony of brutality, lack of sufficient equipment, mismanagement, possible side tracking of funds and improper medical care."[14] He also referenced Chaney's letters as evidence of how much work was still to be done at Whitfield, publishing another editorial five days later in which he summarized Chaney's letters as recommendations.

In April 1949, Carter published the results of Senator Campbell's investigation in a series of four articles in one week. In these articles, written by Senator Campbell himself, details about the level of violence were presented, with numerous stories about the role of attendants in these practices. One story spelled out the existence of a "goon squad": a group of patients who were used by attendants to attack other patients, often leaving people to die from their injuries. Attendants themselves were accused of whipping patients, "male and female, and on the colored service too," Campbell's anonymous source reported.[15] There was no mention of any shootings of colored patients, however.

Therapy itself seemed nonexistent, while physical violence as a form of behavior control was rampant. Treatments like "tight packs"—wrapping a patient in wet blankets attached to a wooden board or iron bed—were used as punishment for alleged transgressions, often leading to kidney and other organ damage, if not death.[16] Another frequent punishment was to move patients who had transgressed in some way into the "disturbed ward," where they would be left to fend for themselves.[17]

In an article titled "Filth and Neglect Are Rule at Hospital," Campbell reported on his own observations of various buildings and the infirmary, where patients lay on concrete floors, or five women to a mattress, or on beds with no sheets, surrounded by excrement. He reported his conversations with ex-patients and ex-attendants about the lack of medical oversight, the lack of actual treatment, no clean sheets, food with no variety and no fresh fruit or vegetables, and the firing and rehiring of substandard staff.[18] For Campbell, the only answer was a change of leadership, requiring the replacement of Dr. Shackleford. Campbell made the point that an actual psychiatric graduate was required to establish some kind of therapeutic regimen at the hospital.[19] Carter agreed, and in his editorial the following day, he wrote, "Mostly, the folks we have talked with believe that the basic concept of management there is wrong. Mostly, these people think that rehabilitation of the mentally sick should be the first task of any such hospital. Occasionally there is one who believes that the hospital should be maintained just as a place of confinement for the criminally insane but even those people don't want mistreatment in the place of confinement. . . . So we'd better demand a new method of treatment to make certain that the old system doesn't remain in usage."[20]

However, none of these articles specifically mention conditions for Black people beyond the single mention of attendants whipping patients in "the colored service." For the most part, the "default patient" is white, with Black patients existing only in the margins or between the lines. There is no mention of a Black patient being shot—all of the people who were injured by beatings that are named are white people. But in correspondence between Senator Campbell and Hodding Carter, there is more detailed information about the impact of the abuse, violence, and corruption that prevailed and its implications for Black patients.[21] And it was in these papers that I finally found a link to Mr. Watkins's letter.

Senator Campbell's investigation involved unannounced visits to Whitfield during which he demanded to be taken to various buildings and was then able to talk to individual staff or patients. He also had people contact him after his visits, or he was given names of people to talk to later and went to visit them at home, or they would come talk to him at his office. He kept a list of these people with notes about what they might be able to tell him, and whether they would be willing to testify to the legislative committee, and then he compiled the results of his observations and conversations into a final report.[22] The report contained greater and more graphic detail about the nature of the corruption and the leadership problems than the *Delta Democrat-Times* had published, and Campbell used names to call out the people he thought were to blame. He started at the top with Dr. Shackleford, who had not even visited many of the buildings since taking over as superintendent in 1947 and who did little to improve things. Campbell and Carter both blamed him for the willful ignoring of abuse and complaints.[23]

Campbell found that corruption was rife at all levels of the institution and that the men named in Hull Watkins's letter were the prime suspects. Campbell learned from Mr. Godbold, who was in charge of the commissary at Whitfield, that large amounts of sugar, tobacco, and other foodstuffs were being ordered but not making their way to patients. For example, "The negro kitchen was using more sugar per week than all the other kitchens at Whitfield combined" and in one week had ordered 500 pounds over the usual 200 pound allocation. This order was approved by none other than Mr. J. O. Stagg, the business manager of the institution. The business manager was technically the second-in-command of the institution, answerable only to the superintendent himself. The fact that Stagg went about his business with a gun in hand, ready to shoot Black patients, was not mentioned. When Godbold asked Stagg what to tell the investigator about the excess sugar and where it was going, "Stagg told him to tell the investigator to go to hell, it was none of his damn business." The same was true of an excess tobacco order, which Godbold believed was being sold or traded. Godbold told Campbell, "More than enough food was coming to Whitfield to feed the patients. Yet the patients are not getting enough food."[24] Stagg was also responsible for watering down milk and not serving the fruit that was ordered, as well as overstocking the cold storage so that the meat went bad but was fed to patients anyway.

But it was Fred Smith who Campbell particularly disliked. Watkins's letter named him as the day superintendent, and Campbell's notes reveal that Smith was in fact the "Supervisor of the Colored Service and Deputy Sheriff at Whitfield." The use of the title "Sheriff" is telling, as it demonstrated the already existing carceral atmosphere at what was supposed to be a hospital and signified that his duties were conceived in a carceral vein rather than medical or therapeutic. Campbell and others, called Smith "the Bootlegger of Whitfield" and set out in great detail his propensity for whiskey, the supply and drinking of it (remembering that Mississippi was technically a dry state at the time, yet Whitfield was home to many alcoholics). Smith involved "his negro attendants" in his bootlegging operation and was frequently found drunk at work. Campbell also named Smith as one of the employees guilty of using state cars and state gasoline for private purposes.

Yet even with all this activity, these were the only references to "the Colored Service" that Campbell made in his investigation. He mentioned many of the wards that he visited in his notes, and not one of them was in the Black section of the campus. He mentioned "negro attendants," but he did not list any in his notes of people he interviewed. And it is unlikely that any would have come forward to talk to him voluntarily. If the two people in charge of the hiring and firing of attendants, like Stagg and Smith, were not above shooting a patient, they would not have been above treating untrained Black staff with violence and intimidation.

Campbell never set out the details of how Black staff interacted with Black patients, but I assume that involvement in a bootlegging operation run by their gun-wielding supervisor may not have been entirely voluntary. And if it was, this can be hardly surprising, given the low wages and poor working conditions for Black staff. In the context of these reports and investigations, it is notable that Senator Campbell never mentioned the shooting of a Black patient or the working of patients like slaves on farms, and that the general conditions for Black patients did not rate a single mention. Here in real time is evidence of the way that certain stories are deemed worth repeating and reporting on, while others disappear into the ether.

There are, however, two stories not related to Campbell's investigation that Carter published during this time that reveal the intersection between Whitfield and other forms of institutional confinement for Black people in Mississippi. The fact that these stories exist show that someone was thinking about the existence of Black patients in the maelstrom of Whitfield. Hodding Carter himself wrote an editorial on January 26, 1947, regarding "the story behind the headlines." The story dealt with the committal of "Charles Ferguson, a 13-year-old Negro boy who slew two Negroes during a robbery." Carter praised the judge, jury, and social worker who conducted an investigation into the boy's background and found "a tragic picture of a mentally defective child, not responsible for his act and handicapped in background, care and health."[25] Carter was pleased by the "enlightened" decision to send the child to Whitfield Hospital rather than give him "a sentence of death or commitment to Parchman" (the notorious prison farm) and quoted the testimony of the assessing psychiatrist, Dr. Estelle Magiera, as the saving grace, because Charles was diagnosed as "a middle grade mental defective with epileptic equivalent states." But the rest of Dr. Magiera's assessment states, "We further recommend that Charles Ferguson never be allowed to return to the community where he would be a danger and a menace." Of course, what else is to be done with a child who did actually kill people, even if in self-defense? Of course, it is better that he be at a psychiatric hospital rather than an adult prison as bad as Parchman.

What the article did not say is that Charles could have been referred to Ellisville State School, where other "mentally defective" children were located. But in the same way as it had for Thomas Hurston twenty years later, the psychiatric hospital acted as a de facto prison, even for children. It is also the case that Charles's crime was killing two Black men who had been breaking into his house. There can be little doubt that the Blackness of the perpetrators was considered something of a mitigating factor—if Charles had murdered two white intruders, his case would not have made it past "the hanging bridge."[26] But it is also the exceptional nature of the way Charles Ferguson was treated that is an alert to the fate of other Black children caught up in this system. At the end of the article, Carter tellingly wrote that the "handling of Charles Ferguson's case is a far cry from the inattentiveness to the case histories of juvenile and adult wrong doers that too largely marks their day in court."[27] In other words, people with mental and intellectual disability, especially Black people, did *not* usually have their backgrounds and medical histories considered before being consigned to death or Parchman. Charles Ferguson's story acts as a kind of symbolic marker for all the stories like his that were not told and represents thousands of others killed and confined because of a disability.

Then, on September 4, 1949, a story ran on page one titled "Whitfield Board Will Ask for Raise in Funds" (see figure 5.1).[28] This story demonstrated the effects of two years of exposés and investigations, as a five-member board was now instituted to oversee all three of the state's mental hospitals. The article reported that Dr. Shackleford had resigned and that the board was seeking a graduate psychiatrist to take over and install a therapeutic program. The board recognized that only a significant increase in funds—which would allow for the hiring of more and better qualified staff as well as increased wages—would address the systemic problems at Whitfield. The requested funding amount was for a total of $8,385,963 for the three hospitals (more than a $3 million increase over the existing budget), $1.5 million for the white-only hospital in Meridian, and $1.8 million for the white and Black children's hospital in Ellisville. The budget was also intended to provide for an occupational therapy program to be instituted.

Nested against this article was a story about a Black woman named Emma Wright. She had been admitted to Whitfield with bruises and other injuries

Whitfield Board Will Ask For Raise In Funds

Want An Extra Million Dollars For The Next Two Years To Improve Conditions

JACKSON, (UP) — The State Mental Institutions Board will recommend to the 1950 legislature that Whitfield Mental Hospital, which has been the object of several recent investigations, receive an appropriation of $5,656,101 for the 1950-52 fiscal biennium over $2,300,000 more than it received for the present two-year period.

The board also will ask that the appropriation for the East Mississippi Mental Hospital at Meridian be upped by $979,450 and that the Ellisville state school for the feeble-minded receive $556,061 more than the appropriation granted by the 1948 legislature.

The board will ask for $8,285,963 for the three mental hospitals, an increase of $3,423,824 over the 1948 appropriations. The board's recommended appropriation for the East Mississippi hospital is $1,543,820, and for Ellisville $1,086,039.

To Budget Group

The board's recommended appropriations will be turned over to the State Budget Commission which will study the suggested amounts requested and then make its recommendations to the legislature.

Board Chairman R. C. Stovall, of Columbus, said that "the proposed budgets embody what the state board considers is a necessary minimum for providing adequate medical and psychiatric treatment to the mental patients of our state. It is now up to the state legislature."

The additional money would be used to increase the medical and nursing staffs at the hospitals, to install an occupational therapy program for all patients able to benefit by it, and to increase pay for nurses and attendants.

The board will recommend that a graduate psychiatrist be named as director at Whitfield. The former head of the institution, Dr. W. Lawson Shackleford, resigned a few weeks ago.

Recall Charges

The hospital at Whitfield was the object during many months of constant attacks by Rep. Hayden Campbell of Hinds county who charged that patients were receiving "poor and inhuman treatment."

Campbell told the United Press today that conditions had improved considerably during the past few weeks, but added that "I am not through with Whitfield yet by a long shot."

Stovall said that with the additional funds asked for the hospital would be able to properly screen and train patients and estimated that once a proper program is set up the hospital will be able to discharge annually a third of the patients who enter each year.

"At the present time," he said, "Whitfield's services are more custodial than remedial. That's because we lack funds to provide an adequate staff of psychiatrists, nurses, attendants and proper equipment. We are going along almost in the dark ages because of lack of funds."

Whitfield Doctor Says Insane Woman Has Been Bruised

Several sources of information revealed Saturday that Emma Wright, whom prisoners say was beaten by the jailer in the Washington County jail, was admitted to the Whitfield institution on August 30, sustained at least one bruise on her thigh and complained of being beaten in the Greenville jail.

Sheriff Hugh Foote, however, told the Delta Democrat-Times Saturday afternoon that the woman might have received the bruise from a fight with "another Negro woman named Georgia" which occurred in the jail.

Emma Wright was imprisoned in May or June of this year after she admittedly murdered her baby with an axe, and remained there, one informant said, because she was "a good worker" and did washing for county employees.

Didn't Act Insane

She was not taken to Whitfield until August 30. Sheriff Foote explained Saturday that "she didn't act crazy when she first came to the jail," and that she had therefore not been sent off immediately.

Jailer J. W. McElwee told the Delta Democrat-Times Saturday afternoon that "for a long while the woman seemed to be doing fine and we put her in with the other women and let her do some washing and ironing."

He emphatically denied that the woman had received any bruises in the jail. "She certainly didn't have any bruises when she left here."

Dr. B. J. Marshall of Whitfield, who examined her Saturday morning, said she was "probably a maniac" and said he could not understand why she had not been brought immediately to Whitfield for examination after the murder.

He told the Delta Democrat-Times that the woman's father from Arcola had appeared at Whitfield Saturday morning to see her and expressed concern about her physical condition. Dr. Marshall said he then made a thorough physical examination of Emma Wright and found she had a bruise on her thigh. She told him she had been kicked in the side and on the legs by the jailer in Greenville.

The woman was admitted to the hospital on August 30, he said, but because of her "definite disturbed condition," he had not examined her physically immediately but that she had been sent to treatment wards.

Had Prison Psychosis

He could not say whether or not she had been mentally ill at the time of the murder but added that she had a "prison psychosis." "Why wasn't she brought here after the murder?" he asked.

Tom Moseley, Arcola Justice of the Peace, said Emma Wright was brought to his office in May

(Continued on page 2)

FIGURE 5.1 "Whitfield Doctor Says Insane Woman Has Been Bruised," *Delta Democrat-Times*, September 4, 1949. Image courtesy of Delta Democrat-Times.

after spending some months in the Washington County jail after allegedly killing her baby with an axe. She was first reported to a local Arcola police officer, who called the deputy sheriff and state investigator. They took her to the county jail in Greenville, where she appeared before Tom Mosely, a justice of the peace, who "decided as soon as we saw the woman that she was crazy." Mosely said that he turned the case over to the sheriff, expecting that the woman would be committed to Whitfield.[29]

Jail officials took a different view, however. The sheriff said that she did not seem crazy when she got to the jail, and jailer J. W. McElwee reported that "for a long while the woman seemed to be doing fine and we put her in with the other women and let her do some washing and ironing." An anonymous citizen raised concerns that she was being kept at the jail "because they liked her and she did washing for them." That person managed to get the attention of county attorneys, who had her seen by two Greenville doctors who suggested she be taken to Whitfield for examination. Once at Whitfield, she was seen by Dr. Marshall who was astonished that she had not been brought immediately to the hospital. Both Dr. Marshall and Ms. Wright's father were concerned about her condition and discovered bruises, which she claimed were the result of being beaten by the police. It was only when she was committed to Whitfield that she was able to reconnect with her father, who had been looking for her.[30]

In both the physical placement and in the contents of the story of Emma Wright, there is a glimpse of how these systems worked as a kind of parallel space for Black patients. Hodding Carter did not bury this story. He put it in full view on page one, right next to a story that talked about reforms at Whitfield. I have no idea what he was thinking in doing so, but it was a deliberate choice, as all editorial choices are. Emma Wright's story quite literally runs parallel to the "end" of a long-running investigation that focused entirely on white patients, demonstrating the way that even newspapers performed Jim Crow on a daily basis.

The remainder of the official reports and other newspaper stories contained nothing about the conditions or admission processes or treatment and care for Black patients at Whitfield. Not a single investigator thought to walk to that side of the campus; no one commented on the actual shooting of a Black patient. Black patients were relegated to the margins of an official investigation and to being a side note to a story about the outcomes. In fact, their entire existence was a footnote that never got written. Everyone knew they were there, but few people seemed to care. Everyone knew how bad things were for white patients, but who thought to document the conditions for Black patients?

It is also the case that Charles Ferguson and Emma Wright only made the newspapers because they were the objects of white benevolence, rescued from the prison system by "the good people" of Whitfield. And in that rescue, it was made obvious that the Black disabled were profoundly at the mercy of white men in positions of power. It did not matter that a Black woman was "probably a maniac."[31] She was capable of working for the county jail, and so that was where she stayed. In fact, it was argued that she "wanted" to be there, that the officers "let her" do laundry work for them. At no point was she the subject of the rule of law; there was no process available to her to appeal her condition or to find her family, who were looking for her. Emma Wright's story shows the ways that Black people could be transferred at will from one white man to another, put to work, jailed, and disappeared with no recourse and no formal commitment procedure.

Like the shot man referred to in Mr. Watkins's letter, an anonymous informer told her story, and then that informer slipped into the shadows again, fearful for their own safety in the face of such violence. Emma Wright's and Charles Ferguson's stories are used as evidence of the benevolent paternalism with which white Mississippi treated its Black citizens, single examples that showed the everyday performance of this particular Jim Crow routine.[32] And they are reminders, yet again, that for these two people we do know about, there are thousands of others who will remain unknown.

The last story that the *Delta Democrat-Times* ran about Whitfield for some time was published in December 1949.[33] The article reported on the ongoing activities of the investigating committee that had released a supplemental report that week. The report noted improvements and mentioned the appointment of Dr. William Jaquith, who was "credited by the committee with bringing about changes in personnel which the committee believes will be beneficial to a more harmonious operation of affairs at the institution." Jaquith, who went on to oversee Whitfield for the next thirty years, was not seen as a political appointment and was given full power to hire and fire as he saw fit. But the committee made the point that conditions could only continue to improve if significantly more funds were allocated to the institution.

Importantly, however, the committee called its report "final," arguing that their job was done, and that they found no evidence to back up Senator Campbell's claims of abuse and violence. So much energy and effort had been spent in the previous three years, from Fred Chaney, to Senators Jones and Campbell, to the work of Hodding Carter himself, and very little had changed. While the flurry of energy may have seen the firing of some staff, a rise in funds, and new leadership, it also came with the standard whitewashing of the Black existence. The ability of this type of exposé to reform anything fundamental about the way that a place like Whitfield worked was severely limited.

Albert Deutsch and *The Shame of the States*

The situation in Mississippi was not unique. Interesting parallels and comparisons can be drawn to Georgia and a series of investigations there. As the largest hospital in the country and the only public psychiatric facility in the state, Milledgeville was a source of repeated scandals and exposés in the mid-twentieth century, most of which were met with repeated political interference and defensiveness. Albert Deutsch covered this situation briefly in his book *The Shame of the States*, which was a compilation of his journalistic work for *PM*. Georgia was the only Southern state he visited, and even that was by accident. As he explained himself, his original plan had been

> to omit the states below the Mason and Dixon line. . . . I felt that the public conscience could be more readily aroused if I confined my reports to those Northern states representative of what was generally considered "the best" in institutional provision. The case for reform, it seemed to me, would be weakened if I went where some might say: "Well, anybody can come up with dirt if he digs deep enough into the South." Besides, people in the South, already skinned raw by Northern criticism, might get defensive and adopt a do-nothing attitude if subjected to yet another exposé by another Northerner. In terms of constructive reaction, the job could be done better by native surveyors.[34]

These comments by Deutsch are telling. They are evidence of the deliberate tactic of eliciting sympathy by appealing to the conscience of white people, for whom confinement, abuse, and bad conditions were unacceptable. They demonstrate the force of lingering attitudes about the "backwardness" of the South and the distrust and defensiveness this engendered, which would rear its head again in the move toward civil rights.

But the Atlanta Mental Hygiene Association encouraged Deutsch to intervene. At their insistence, he asked for but was initially denied access to

Milledgeville by the State Welfare Department, which oversaw the hospital at that time. This denial became a political tool for incoming conservative governor Eugene Talmadge, who took the chance to claim that current state leadership was "hid[ing] something," even though he had little real interest in how the state's mentally ill were being cared for.[35] But Milledgeville was already in the news because of beatings and murders that had taken place there, and the Atlanta Mental Hygiene Association believed that an exposé from someone like Deutsch was needed to bring awareness and change to the institution. Deutsch was finally taken to tour the facility in 1947 at the invitation of Governor Ellis, accompanied by Judge A. J. Hartley, the head of the State Welfare Department.

In his writing, Deutsch was quick to point out, "If I found shameful conditions at Milledgeville, they differed only in degree, not in kind, from those found in most American mental hospitals. The shame is not Georgia's alone, nor the South's, but the nation's." But in the rest of his short chapter, Deutsch was almost utterly damning of Milledgeville, which, he wrote, suffered from a lack of government spending on either patients or staff, including a state appropriation of 76 cents per patient per day, and merely fourteen physicians for nearly 9,000 patients. This meant one physician for every 633 patients, when the minimum official standard as recommended by the American Psychiatric Association was one for every 150. Some buildings had only one graduate nurse, others had no nurses at all, and there was only one social worker for the entire institution. The focus of recent spending was on a new $450,000 building for the criminally insane, where only eighteen such people would be housed, in line with the tendency of the Georgia state government to spend more money on prisons and policing than on health.[36]

Deutsch was also unusually clear about the impact of Jim Crow segregation. When he arrived at Milledgeville, he was shown around by the then superintendent Dr. Yarbrough, who had been in charge for forty years. Yarbrough was frank about the "'scandalous' conditions we encountered, especially in the colored sections." The disparity between white and Black accommodations was particularly stark to Deutsch, who noted that the only modern building was the Rivers Building for the treatment of tuberculosis. This building had separate wings for Black and white patients, which required the duplication of expensive equipment like X-ray machines, "illustrating the high cost of Jim Crow." Deutsch also pointed out that the TB building was the only building where Black patients received the same level of care as white patients, representing "the only part of Milledgeville where the hypocritical "separate-but-equal facilities" Jim Crow law of Georgia is observed."[37]

Significantly, Deutsch pointed out how segregation worked to make the Black patient invisible, pointing to the annual report written by the aforementioned Yarbrough. The default patient in these reports was always white. The Black patient only ever appeared when something new happened that revealed how bad the "old" was, or when a practice or policy was clearly marked as white, thus actively excluding the Black experience. For example, Deutsch remarked on the way that Yarbrough had reported on daily clinics held over a six-month period, in which white patients were interviewed to determine whether they had shown sufficient improvement to be released from the hospital. Deutsch remarked, "Nothing is said about interviews with the Negro patients for the same purpose," and I think it is safe to assume that this was because those interviews did not happen with Black patients.[38] In the face of appalling conditions and a complete lack of therapeutic programs, there was no reason for administrators to assume that Black patients might have improved—in fact, they already knew that they would not have, since that was never the goal. The thought that Black patients should be actively surveyed with a view to being released was unthinkable to politicians and administrators alike.

Deutsch also noted the way that segregation's impact was revealed at the moment of improvement or reform. New buildings or resources went first and foremost to white patients, leaving Black patients with leftovers. For example, a simple act of changing beds from wood to metal demonstrated that all white patients would now have the new beds, while only Black patients in "the new colored building" would enjoy this reform. Deutsch noted sharply that "colored patients in the old building still sleep in broken-down, vermin-infested wooden beds, when they don't have to lie on mattresses thrown on the bare floors."[39] These disparities were a symptom of the larger patterns of service provision at Milledgeville, which was reflected by its position in the national schema.

While Deutsch had started his assessment with the caveat that things were no worse at Milledgeville than anywhere else in the country, he then qualified that statement with the assertion that "physically, the best I saw at Milledgeville ranked with the best I've seen anywhere; the worst was the worst I had ever seen." There is no doubt that this worst was specifically applicable to the Black patients, especially in relation to treatment and care. Buildings were one thing, a therapeutic program quite another. In that regard, Deutsch was emphatic: "From the medical viewpoint the institution ranks with the lowest of the 190 state mental hospitals in the United States."[40]

Ebony and the Internal Racism of American Psychiatry

It would be impossible to cover here every other news story or exposé about Milledgeville State Hospital during the postwar period, but there are a few other key sources that reveal the nature of segregation within the hospital as well as the general invisibility of the Black patient in the journalistic and political scene.

A year after Deutsch published his short chapter about Milledgeville, the popular Chicago-based Black magazine, *Ebony*, ran a story about conditions for Black patients in the nation's psychiatric hospitals. *Ebony* frequently ran stories about disabled African Americans, especially when they could be positioned as having "overcome" a disability to succeed or achieve in some way, but this story about Black patients in the nation's psychiatric hospitals had no such silver lining.

The story ran in April 1949 and spanned multiple pages, starting with a direct reference to Mary Jane Ward's book and movie in the lead article, titled "Insanity: Mental Illness among Negroes Exceeds Whites, Overcrowds Already-Jammed 'Snake Pits.'"[41] This lead piece covered a range of issues related to the mental health of Black Americans, and painted a comprehensive picture of the many ways that the psychiatric system failed them. While it was not true that Black patients were "more insane" than white ones, the article made the point that "for two decades now U.S. Negroes have been going insane at a much higher rate than whites," signaling a growing rate of contact with the diagnostic and confinement system. While increased stress, anxiety, and neurosis were a reality of Black life, it was also the case that "in the last 40 years the number of Negroes in mental hospitals has multiplied by five times."[42]

The writer noted that there were only eight Black psychiatrists out of the nation's 4,432, and as noted in chapter 1, most of them worked at Tuskegee. And while the article went on to present photographs taken at Camarillo State Hospital in California (a racially mixed hospital), it did spend some time thinking about the difference between "northern" and "southern" approaches to psychiatry, in which segregation was the key variable. For example, it noted that "in the North all state hospitals have wiped out color lines among patients but most private institutions . . . refuse to admit

Negroes."⁴³ So while integration in Northern state hospitals might have been the new norm (the extent to which it really was is debatable), a de facto segregation existed due to a pricing barrier and the existing biases of psychiatrists themselves.

The journal took up this issue of bias over the page, but not before it made a very specific comment about Milledgeville Hospital. If lack of funding and overcrowding had led to institutions that were more like jails than hospitals for white patients, "then for Negroes the situation approaches Nazi concentration camp standards—especially in the South, where three out of every five colored insane are confined. Georgia's Milledgeville State Hospital has been cited by newspaperman Albert Deutsch as the worst in the nation and its Negro wards described as unbelievable 'this side of Dante's Inferno.'"⁴⁴ This reference to Dante does not appear in Deutsch's *The Shame of the States* as it was eventually published, but the reference made it clear that the editors and writers at *Ebony* were paying attention to these exposés and to the growing recognition of the importance of mental health work for Black people.

There are three related articles in this one April edition, covering issues from the bias of physicians to the creation of new clinics in Harlem. Importantly, the writers made clear that it was the racism built into the mental health system, especially in the South, that caused different conditions and outcomes for Black patients. In a second article in this April 1949 edition, the writer took issue with the idea that "a mania of persecution" was a form of neurosis in Black people. The issue was not that this fear was unwarranted but that it should be understood as an expression of the very real stress of living with everyday discrimination. The author quoted Dr. Orville Sheffield from Tuskegee, who argued that prejudice can be "a contributing factor" to what became classified as "neurosis," and that social circumstances like poverty, housing insecurity, and "all-round second class status forced upon the Negro by racial discrimination are keys to the mental sickness" allegedly finding prevalence in Black communities.⁴⁵

Racism in approaches to diagnosis and treatment were factors that kept Black patients from getting help even when they wanted it, so that in Southern hospitals in particular, they were actually underrepresented. In Illinois, for example, Black people were 6 percent of the population and 12 percent of the asylum intake, whereas in Georgia they accounted for 8.8 percent of the population and only 5.5 percent of the asylum population. The writer of this article argued that it was "lack of facilities as well as outright discrimination" that kept Black patients out of Southern hospitals and less well treated when they were admitted.[46]

Over the page, the writer picked up the theme of inequitable treatment to point out that "in Southern hospitals, for instance, white patients who get better treatment leave institutions at a much higher rate than Negroes."[47] The writer also noted the pernicious practice of using work as a form of treatment when it was really just free and forced labor, which kept Black patients tied to institutions and receiving less actual therapeutic treatment or opportunities for rehabilitation. For example, at a state hospital in South Carolina, Black patients—who made up 45 percent of the population—accounted for only 22 percent of the discharges. The writer argued that "one reason can be seen in the work assignments given Negroes. Some 50 colored patients worked as scrubwomen and 20 more got kitchen jobs while no whites were given such menial tasks."[48] While white administrators and clinicians were keen to call physical labor "occupational therapy," as discussed earlier, *Ebony* was not afraid to call out the practice for what it was—both inherently racist and therapeutically problematic.

For the writers in *Ebony*, racism and segregation were also seen to impact mental health because of the types of people employed as caretaking staff at hospitals. Segregation in ward staff was taken as a given because it was unthinkable that Black attendants should care for white patients or be placed in positions where they were not subservient to other white workers. The writer quoted a survey from the National Mental Health Foundation, which found that almost all the nation's segregated mental hospitals existed below the Mason-Dixon line, and more than half did not employ Black staff because "white patients would resent being directed and supervised by colored persons."[49]

The rationale of racial violence was also attributed to patients as a reason for segregation—that the patients themselves would not tolerate one another as much as they would not tolerate being cared for by people from a different race. But neither the writer of this article nor the author of the original *Snake Pit*, Mary Jane Ward, had much truck with this argument. *Ebony* reached out to Ward and found that "she and others who have studied U.S. mental institutions find little color bias among the insane themselves, but much among those who are supposed to cure the mentally unbalanced." Ward went so far as to say that she had seen "many examples of brotherhood in mental hospitals and I don't remember any instances of race prejudice. I think the average white patient regards the average Negro patient as a fellow sufferer. The employment of Negro doctors and nurses isn't likely to disturb the average white patient."[50]

Ebony finished its coverage of the mental health problem by arguing that in fact it was psychiatry itself that was biased against Black patients, even in the North, noting that "not only are Negroes denied hospitalization on an equal basis with whites but also simple psychiatric care. Few white psychiatrists will accept Negro patients for fear of losing their wealthy white clientele."[51] This fear and discrimination contributed to de facto forms of segregation beyond the state hospital and meant that Black New Yorkers who were not relegated to the snake pit at Bellevue were forced to seek help in the basement of a church in Harlem, at the only service operating for Black outpatients: the Lafargue Clinic.[52] The clinic director, Dr. Frederick Wertham, told *Ebony* that unless American psychiatry took a stand against its own internal racism, there was little hope for change. "As long as official psychiatry remains what it is today . . . we will have to continue working in a basement, in more ways than one." Wertham commented.[53] The Harlem doctor was right. These exposés by Deutsch and *Ebony* barely scraped the surface of the depth of the problem of racism and segregation in psychiatric practice, which even well-intentioned white doctors were unable to reform.

Dr. Cranford's Diary

One surprising source from this period that is neither an official report nor a newspaper exposé is a book from 1953 by a psychologist at Milledgeville. Dr. Peter Cranford's *But for the Grace of God* was an attempt by the psychologist to document the hospital's elusive early history, warts and all. It was not published at the time, but various editions have been publicly available since the 1980s: a 1981 edition through Great Pyramid Press in Augusta, a 1998 edition published by the Georgia Consumer Council, and a more widely available version published in 2008 by the Old Capital Press in Milledgeville.

The 2008 version is the one I am referencing here, and it includes two parts: part 1 consists of nine chapters covering the history of the hospital from 1834 to about 1952, and part 2 is called "The Inside Story of My Year at Milledgeville," which are excerpts from Cranford's diary. Cranford's work is useful because it follows quickly after Deutsch's visit and contains explicit information about conditions for Black patients. But Cranford's work was not known outside the hospital at the time. The 2008 edition includes a note from Cranford between the two parts in which he writes, "Thirty years have passed since the history was compiled. . . . In 1952 the original history was not acceptable to publishers since it was somewhat academic and because it might not sell outside Georgia. There was also a degree of political opposition."[54]

Cranford noted numerous times in his diary excerpts that his attempt to locate records and put the history of the institution on paper made administrators nervous. There was a lot for them to be nervous about. In the one year he spent at Milledgeville, Cranford documented a vast array of brutal practices and poor conditions, including for Black patients. In this section I will focus mostly on these comments rather than try to summarize the whole book, although it provides a good overview of the general chaos, corruption, and brutality that prevailed for all patients. The book is also notable for its attempt at humanizing patients, made possible through Cranford's close regular contact with them.

But Cranford himself found the history part hard to write, first because of the haphazard recordkeeping. In the preface to his book, he noted the effects of past floods and fires as well as the accidental burning of records by a patient who was cleaning out the superintendent's office. "To prevent a similar occurrence," Cranford ironically suggested, "it would be wise to preserve in some college library the large amount of crumbling yellow historical data now dumped in the abandoned old chapel on the fourth floor of the Center Building."[55] To get around this lack of records, Cranford spent a great deal of time talking to various personnel, including Joe Ingram, a Black attendant who had risen through the ranks in his sixty-year career at Milledgeville and eventually had a building named after him. Cranford thanked Mr. Ingram in the preface, noting that his "long memory was of invaluable assistance in locating records, describing personalities, and supplying the details of incidents about which the written facts were few."[56] Mr. Ingram showed Cranford where the records from the 1800s were piled like trash in the abandoned chapel, and Cranford's history of these early years is a good overview of the way that the hospital quickly became a dumping ground for most of Georgia's social problems—overcrowded, underfunded, and indelibly segregated.

The chapters in his history are organized by superintendents' tenure—the last chapter concerns Dr. Peacock's administration from 1948 until 1960, which is the period of interest for me, and documents a number of reports and studies that were made of the hospital in the late 1940s and early 1950s. These reports detailed the ease with which people could be admitted, that the average length of stay was twenty years, and that the primary form of "treatment" was electroshock therapy, used more as a form of patient control. In this chapter, Cranford documented the employment of refugee doctors from Europe, who he thought provided stability and empathy for patients.[57] Yet these doctors were largely attributed to "the colored service." In his diary, Cranford noted, "The colored patients are cared for by European refugee doctors who treat them kindly. The colored are lucky to be treated by those who have themselves greatly suffered."[58]

It is not clear from this comment whether Cranford meant that the European doctors were Jewish or were simply better than the white ones in terms of empathy. But there was an explicit link being made generally across psychiatry at this time about the hypocrisy of America's Jim Crow laws (and the nature of psychiatric hospitals) in the wake of revelations about Nazi atrocities. But Cranford was also hinting specifically at some of the same issues that had concerned the Black psychiatrists at Tuskegee—that the nature of African American history in the United States constituted a kind of collective trauma with obvious and measurable implications for Black mental health.

Cranford noted a few of the other ways that segregation worked at Milledgeville, such as the establishment of a new dental clinic where "the patients received good and sympathetic care but it was not generally available to the colored," and the fact that "the colored patients did not have adequate medical and surgical care or recreational facilities."[59] Part of Cranford's job was to teach psychological concepts to new staff, and in July 1951 he taught a class of thirty-five Black male and female attendants. He noted that during his lecture, "some strictly colored problems surfaced. There was much clamoring to be heard. When the hour was up I was taken aback by all rising, followed by a speech of appreciation from a male class member and much handshaking."[60] This interaction demonstrated the way that Black staff were interested in improving their knowledge and the way in which their training had been previously ignored. They also might have been speaking about patient issues. While Cranford does not specify what the "strictly colored problems" were, he noted later in his diary that his experience with both Black attendants and Black patients reassured him that "despite what is commonly believed about whites and blacks being different emotionally, there is no difference that I can detect."[61]

There are frequent mentions in Cranford's diary of his various discussions with Black attendants and the stories they would tell him about escaped patients and his attempts to help various patients through appeals to

Superintendent Peacock or to Governor Talmadge directly. But ultimately, Milledgeville proved too difficult for Dr. Cranford. His diary excerpts also detail his struggle to do any meaningful psychological work, the ongoing corruption and political infighting, and his battle of wills with Superintendent Peacock. Peacock grew nervous about Cranford's historical writing, and when Cranford resigned at the end of only one year, he demanded that he hand over the manuscript, claiming it was hospital property. Cranford refused, and that manuscript would eventually be published.

Before he left, Cranford made an interesting entry in his diary about the importance of public exposés for improving conditions for the mentally ill. On December 15, 1951, he wrote, "Historically, the best friends of the patients, and the most effective, have been the Atlanta papers. The people on the inside can't or won't talk. Those on the outside don't know or are powerless. The mentally ill are not protected against political forces which can undermine the work of the institution. . . . Alert newspaper reporting is necessary for the well-being of patients."[62] For the patients of Milledgeville, the most effective of those alert newspapers was the *Atlanta Constitution* and a reporter by the name of Jack Nelson.

Jack Nelson and the *Atlanta Constitution*

From March 1959, Jack Nelson began "what was probably the most memorable investigation of my career: the horrific conditions at Milledgeville State Hospital."[63] Nelson was well known in Atlanta for his reporting about government corruption, which he supported with meticulous evidence and witness affidavits as well as a clever libel department.[64] Concerns about corruption at Milledgeville from local (Baldwin County) state legislator Phillip Chandler set Nelson on the hunt for evidence about the hospital, where he found that "a purchasing scandal involving kickbacks to hospital and state officials created a situation in which the hospital's average expenditure per patient for housing, food, and health care was a paltry $2.52 a day."[65]

In his reporting, Nelson made overt reference to a number of previous reports and stories about problems at Milledgeville that dated back to 1916 and argued that too little had changed.[66] He set out the ways that approaches to the mentally ill went through cycles of short bursts of interest in reform and then long decades of neglect and apathy. He detailed the abject conditions, political interference and corruption, lax admission procedures, lack of therapeutic programs, understaffing, underfunding, violence, alcoholic administrators, experimental drug trials without consent, nurses performing surgery, lack of data keeping and record systems, theft of supplies and instruments, and the use of medical facilities meant for patients by families of staff.

In this one year alone, the *Atlanta Constitution* published at least sixty-three major articles about conditions, corruption, and neglect at the hospital.[67] Of these sixty-plus articles, six mentioned Black patients directly. We might wish for more, given the *Constitution*'s overall reputation as a moderate civil rights–supporting newspaper.[68] Indeed, in his autobiography, Nelson mentions that during his visit to Milledgeville, the superintendent, Dr. Peacock, interrupted their interview to take a call from Dr. Gibson, one of the hospital's surgeons. To Dr. Gibson Peacock yelled, "I've got that fella Jack Nelson from that lyin' Ralph McGill, communist-lovin', n___-lovin' *Atlanta Constitution*."[69]

But the situation at Milledgeville was not seen as a civil rights one, and the *Constitution*'s coverage indicated the taken-for-grantedness of segregation, especially in medical settings. The exposé is utterly scathing and ruthless in its condemnation of the hospital's administration and practices, as well as legislative and public apathy. But it did not explicitly condemn the practice of segregation. Even with the *Constitution*, some reading between the lines is necessary. As elsewhere, the default patient was usually white unless the qualifying word "Negro" (the *Constitution* deliberately and purposefully used the capital *N*) was used to specifically refer to Black patients.[70] Stories that did talk about Black patients did not shy away from the details but indicated the depth of despair and neglect hinted at by Dr. Cranford. Overall, there is a lot to learn from Nelson's exposé about the way that segregation worked to relegate Black patients to the margins of the institution in both reality and public discourse.

Nelson's writings relied largely on the testimony of various whistleblowers and sparked an immediate reaction—initially, of course, obfuscation and a violent defensiveness on the part of Dr. Peacock and the head of the State Welfare Department, Alan Kemper. But as Nelson remembered in his autobiography, "not all of the ensuing reaction . . . was negative. After the initial series and the interview with Peacock were published, the *Journal of the Medical Association of Georgia* reported that 'citizens throughout the state were shocked' and editorialized in favor of sweeping reforms. An embarrassed [Governor] Ernest Vandiver . . . asked the medical association to appoint a committee to investigate the allegations."[71]

This publicity also led to the establishment of a joint house and senate investigative committee and a mental health study committee. All the actors involved in the whistleblowing and investigation were white, of course. The legislative and study committees chaired by Baldwin County state representative Culver Kidd and an investigative committee of the Medical Association of Georgia (MAG) led by Dr. Bruce Schaefer were all white men. The problems at Milledgeville were documented by Dr. Joe Combs, who was listed as the clinical director of the white women's service. Combs was relentless and scathing in his critique of the administration of the hospital, which he saw as political, and of the running of programs, which he argued were custodial and not medical. The placement of the hospital under the auspices of the State Welfare Department had made the hospital a dumping ground for all sorts of problems and populations, including more than 4,000 elderly senile patients who had nowhere else to go, and far too many children and others labeled as "mental defectives."[72] Combs suggested that the hospital be moved under the administration of the state health department, and that the sister hospital for "feebleminded" children—Gracewood, in Augusta—also be moved to that department.[73]

Racial segregation was the ever present but barely spoken backdrop to all the discussion about reform and improvement. Combs's designation as the chief of the white women's service made that clear, as did his own suggestion that the clinical aspects of the hospital required three "chiefs": one for white women (his role), another for white men, and "one for all Negro patients."[74] This last suggestion would place more than 4,000 people under one director, and showed little concern for gender differences in the way that they were acknowledged when it came to white patients. This was the only suggestion that Combs himself had for Black patients specifically.

An unnamed whistleblower told Nelson that among other problems at the medical surgical unit (the Jones Building), the "Negro surgical patients have been—and still are—shuttled off to a clinic about a mile away immediately after operations because there are no facilities for them in the building housing the operating rooms."[75] This practice was particularly cruel and arbitrary, placing undue stress and risk on vulnerable patients simply because they could not be nursed in the same building. The unnamed clinic is also most likely to be in fact the Rivers Building, which Google Maps confirms was located "about a mile" from the Jones Building. The Rivers Building, as described in the Deutsch exposé and by Dr. Cranford, was the only other nursing care facility for Black patients on the campus, but it was for the treatment of tuberculosis. If this is where postoperative patients were transferred to, they were then rendered doubly vulnerable through exposure to TB infection. This movement of vulnerable patients demonstrated an unquestioned commitment to segregation, which both signaled and operationalized the belief that Black bodies at Milledgeville were worth less than even the minimum standard of care available to white ones.

The other way that Nelson's exposé made this clear was through a number of comments about the everyday living conditions of Black patients. These glimpses of everyday life came to Nelson via tours of the facility, which were undertaken from mid-1959 onward. In June, the joint legislative committee and mental health study group led by Culver Kidd visited Milledgeville and noted the way that elderly senile patients were packed in to run-down buildings alongside "mental defectives," and that there were still many wooden buildings considered fire traps holding white and Black patients alike.

But it was noted that "Negro patients have some of the poorest buildings at the institution. In one building of crumbling bricks there are some 700 Negro women. The ceiling, floors and stairways are wooden. The windows are barred. 'If this thing caught fire' a legislator said, 'you could never put it out. And the patients couldn't get out.'"[76] More details about these buildings and other conditions for Black patients emerged about a month later, when Governor Vandiver himself visited the hospital. In this visit to the hospital, the governor's party, which included investigative committee members and his wife, "made a painstaking inspection of two relatively small Negro wards."[77] The governor requested he be allowed inside these particular buildings, forsaking the planned "grand tour" of the entire campus. Both the governor and his wife were shocked and sickened by what they saw.

In the first building, they encountered 240 Black patients, and the description of their situation is worth repeating in full: "In the first ward Vandiver visited he saw 240 patients standing and sitting around doing nothing. Flies swarmed around the place and several patients batted at them with tattered straw hats. In the adjacent kitchen, flies had come through the window. There were no screens. The governor stopped to talk to several patients. One was a sixty-two-year-old man from Montgomery County. He had been in the institution since 1927. The man said he used to work on Dr. W. M. Moses' farm in Mt. Vernon."[78] Representative Underwood, himself from Montgomery County, also talked to the man, who had never had anyone visit him. He asked Mr. Underwood about people he remembered from Montgomery County and was sad to learn that many of them had long since died. Representative Underwood expressed his own sadness at the patient's lonely plight.

The tour continued to another building for Black men, but Mrs. Vandiver waited outside, saying that she did not "want to feel any worse than I already do." In the second building, which was a fifty-eight-year-old building once used as a prison, the governor again witnessed appalling conditions and a distinct lack of treatment and care. The building, Vandiver commented, "wasn't good enough for prisoners, much less sick people," and was marked by a lack of working toilets, only six for 120 patients, and two showers, only one of which was working. He noted that there were no lights in the bathrooms, and naked light bulbs hung from the ceiling in other parts of the building, which also had locked and inadequate exits, making the building a terrible fire trap. Vandiver was particularly appalled by the food, commenting, "I don't see how a dog could have eaten it."[79]

Also accompanying the governor was Dr. George Jackson from Kansas, where he was director of the then highly rated state hospitals (under Menninger supervision). During the tour of these Black patient buildings, Dr. Jackson spent some time talking to a few of the patients. The *Constitution* reported that one man Dr. Jackson spoke with had been in this one ward for more than twenty years and had never had anyone visit him either, apart from the "store keeper" in his hometown, who had also written a few times. In a particularly poignant moment, this patient's "eyes welled up when Dr. Jackson asked about his relatives. The man 'guessed' they had all died." Dr. Jackson called these men "forgotten people" and the conditions "sickening."[80] After the tour, Governor Vandiver expressed his shame and disgust, exclaiming that it was far worse than he had imagined and that improvements were needed on all fronts, and he exhorted the legislative committee to not delay in passing the required bills for needed reform.[81]

In both his autobiography and in the *Constitution*, Nelson recorded the success of his campaign and of the legislative committee's investigation. The MAG published its recommendations as the Schaefer Report, and in February 1960, the *Constitution* reported the unanimous legislative vote for a commitment to work toward a sweeping program of reform. Dr. Peacock and a slew of others were fired, and the internal departments of the hospital were restructured.

The *Constitution* reported, "Authority financing for a $12,210,000 building program was approved; a humane commitment bill was adopted; steps were taken to provide scholarships for study; . . . Gracewood and the alcoholism program were transferred to the Health department; a psychiatrist was added to the State Board of Health; mental patients who can afford to pay will be allowed to do so and the way was cleared for another interim mental health study committee."[82]

In his autobiography, Nelson reflected on this outcome, which he painted as a win all round: "All of the pressure from so many quarters," he wrote, "eventually brought more humane treatment and better health care for the patients. Many reforms were instituted, including a $12 million program to downsize Milledgeville and build regional mental health facilities around the state. I can't think of another story I covered that had such far-reaching consequences."[83] For Nelson also, it resulted in a Pulitzer Prize for Local Reporting and took his career in exciting new directions.

But it would be premature to think that these newspaper exposés would bring any meaningful improvements for Black patients. In Mississippi, for example, I was able to trace the continued employment of Mr. Stagg, including his promotion and pay raise.[84] And despite the millions of dollars for buildings at Milledgeville, the population there continued to expand, not decline. In fact, it could, and has been, argued that improvements and reforms actually expanded the capacity of these hospitals, providing fresh resources that did nothing to address the underlying ideologies of confinement or segregation.[85]

These practices would not seriously be challenged until the community mental health and civil rights movements of the 1960s, which, along with Medicare, provided both the impetus and the funding for a major overhaul of approaches to institutional—and segregated—psychiatry. At the same time, exposés like the ones at Milledgeville were themselves foundational to the continued pressure for alternatives to institutionalization. Newspapers were, as Dr. Cranford suggested, the best friend of the (white) patient because they were the main avenue through which psychiatric power could be actively and publicly resisted, and an important forum for the voice of the patient and family.

Access to public exposure was limited for the Black community, however. It was really only Black periodicals like *Ebony* that centered the Black patient and purposely attempted to report thoroughly and honestly about the internal racism of psychiatry itself. And the *Ebony* exposé itself was rare—psychiatric hospitals do not appear to be a subject for Southern Black periodicals more fully until later in the 1960s, and then it was in the context of the legal fight to end segregation.

This was especially the case in Alabama, where the major white newspapers made barely any mention of Searcy Hospital or conditions for Black patients at all. This does not mean that no one knew or cared what was happening to them. As the work at Tuskegee revealed, Black psychiatrists knew that the state hospital system was a problem, but they had no access to it as practitioners and were not in a position to advocate for patients there. That burden would fall on the shoulders of local families, communities, and legal activists, who relied on changes in federal legislation to bring an end to segregation in state psychiatric facilities.

Part III **Ending Jim Crow in the Asylum**

6 Planning Community Mental Health

June 24, 1946
Searcy Hospital
Mt. Vernon, Alabama

Now with reference to MJO being entirely well . . . I told you at that time that she was very peculiar and eccentric and she did entertain a good many wrong ideas about different things. Most of the time, she is able to be out on ward with other patients and gets along fairly well but at times she does give quite a bit of trouble and occasionally attempts to fight the other patients and the attendants. We do not believe she would be mentally capable of supporting herself if outside an institution and she would most probably in time become a public nuisance and might even become dangerous. We do not believe it would be advisable to release her from the institution here at the present time.
Harry S. Rowe. Assistant Superintendent

This letter from Dr. Rowe was written to Ms. O of Bessemer, Alabama, in 1946.[1] Ms. O. had been to visit her daughter at Searcy Hospital, some 193 miles southwest of Bessemer, and had not liked what she saw. Ms. O. wrote to the governor, whose office passed it on to Dr. Partlow, who was superintendent of the Alabama State Hospitals at the time, who passed it on to Dr. Rowe at Searcy. Dr. Rowe refuted Ms. O.'s claims that her daughter was being held against her will and being used as a secretary and a nurse, and refused her request to have her daughter released so she could bring her home.

The original letter from Ms. O. has been removed from the file, and there is no more correspondence recorded from her. There are many other letters like it in the State Institutions series at the Alabama Department of Archives and History, so many that I lost count. Twenty years of bulging files with letter after letter from people across Alabama appealing to the governor to have their family members released, letters from patients begging for their freedom, claiming they were the victim of family politics or would rather be in prison. They are usually written in pencil, attempts at cursive in a sometimes shaky script, looping handwriting sprawled across small pieces of lined notepaper, often indecipherable. Almost all of them were written about or by white people relative to their incarceration at Bryce Hospital in Tuscaloosa.

The response to Ms. O.'s letter is one of very few related to Searcy Hospital in Mount Vernon.[2] Written well before either the Community Mental Health Act or the Civil Rights Act, these letters indicate the ways that families and patients interacted with the state institution system, demonstrating their regard and concern for family and their desire to care for loved ones. Ms. O.'s letter represents several key tensions that run through this chapter: the need and desire for noninstitutional, community-based mental health services for affected loved ones; the absolute lack of quality services for people who needed them; and the political game-playing by state legislators, who also faced racist resistance to the potential integration or downsizing of state institutions. Exposés had gone some way to revealing the abject and racist conditions that prevailed in these institutions, but families and activists did not have significant power to intervene until the passing of several acts of legislation in the mid-1960s.

In this chapter, I explore the different ways that the states of Georgia, Mississippi, and Alabama approached the move to community mental health after the passing of Public Law 88–164, the Mental Retardation Facilities and Community Mental Health Centers Construction Act, more commonly referred to as the Community Mental Health Act (CMHA) of 1963. I am not interested here in the act's implementation, because that would take forever to try to document, and I know already that the CMHA was not actually implemented as intended. Rather, I am interested in understanding how planning for community mental health took place in the context of broader moves toward racial integration, and to what extent community mental health plans were shaped by or may have intervened in that process. The CMHA did not contain a nondiscrimination clause—that would come later—but it would be naive to assume that the Kennedy government did not know that community mental health would be affected by moves to create civil rights and nondiscrimination in federal facilities.

In the three sections that follow, I look at the way planning for community mental health was dealt with in Georgia, Mississippi, and Alabama, exploring the way that the process of planning exposed the negative impact of segregation in existing facilities, and considering to what extent the plans that were proposed might have contributed to ending or replicating de facto segregation outside institutions. The CMHA was passed on October 31, 1963, and the Civil Rights Act on July 2, 1964, but community mental health plans were not due to the federal government until 1965, after the passing of Medicare and Medicaid legislation. Both the Civil Rights Act and Medicare required integration of medical facilities in order to receive federal funding, a known fact that permeates every state's planning efforts, explicitly or not. The final section of the chapter explores the power and promise inherent in federal legislation, detailing the ways that administrators dealt with the complex connections between this succession of laws and their implications for mental health funding, which were frustrated at the state level.

As a bare minimum, community-based mental health services needed to be developed for all of a state's citizens equally, but there were ways that state legislators, consciously or not, replicated segregation specifically through a focus on geography. The dependence in all three states on a strategy of regionalization reinforced the reliance on existing institutional care and potentially replicated already existing structural problems that ran along racialized geographical lines. In this scenario, the Community Mental Health Act planning process threatened to do little more than move around the deck chairs on an already sinking ship, another example of a "nonreform reform."[3]

These problems were not wholly of the planner's making but were exacerbated by various states' responses and a lack of interest in mental health spending, especially where that intersected with racial tension. I try to unpack these tensions in this chapter to show the way that legislative and community activism were limited in reshaping the terrain of mental health service provision in the South in the 1960s. The argument here is that the so-called failure of the CMHA (as some have argued) was not so much a failure of funding or political will as it was a success of racism and white supremacy. The process of developing community mental health plans reflected a moment where fundamental change looked possible, but it also revealed the impact and the depth of the racism that would continue to act as powerful barriers.

Institutional Nonreform in Georgia

Georgia was the most proactive in planning for community mental health, not just because of public concern but because it had the most to lose financially. In Georgia's response to both community mental health (and later, civil rights), economic and political expediency prevailed over the need to maintain racial segregation, which demonstrated how flexible a social boundary that was in Georgia. This was not the case in Mississippi or Alabama, both of which had governors committed to maintaining segregation whatever the cost. That cost would prove to be significant for those states, but Georgia tried to adopt a more liberal position.

In early 1964, before the Department of Health, Education, and Welfare (HEW) had made clear its processes for community mental health planning or funding, the relatively new governor of Georgia, Carl Sanders, instituted a Commission for Efficiency and Improvement in Government. Sanders was a young governor, only thirty-seven when he took office, having "campaigned on a New South platform of economic expansion and racial moderation."[4] His attitude toward the implementation of civil rights was shaped by a desire not to be humiliated into compliance, to present a progressive image of Georgia, and to ensure continued funding. Sanders walked a middle line of conservative change and adherence to the law as the antics of extreme segregationists like Lester Maddox and Marvin Griffin fell increasingly out of favor, not least where federal money was on the line.[5]

In his approach to mental health, Sanders was supported by a long history of complaints, surveys, and liabilities related to the corruption, malpractice, and neglect occurring at Central State Hospital (CSH). Despite the efforts of previous investigations, like the Schaefer Report (discussed in chapter 5), not enough had changed at Milledgeville, and the advent of the CMHA gave the governor the impetus he needed to attempt wholesale reform.

In early 1964, he "requested the Surgeon General of the United States Public Health Service to make a report to the Governor's Commission for Efficiency and Improvement in Government."[6] The surgeon general passed the request on to the National Institute of Mental Health (NIMH), which put together a panel of consultants led by Dr. William G. Hollister, chief of the Community Research and Services branch of the NIMH. Hollister convened thirty-four people from within NIMH headquarters in Bethesda and from the local branch of the Public Health Service office in Atlanta. Consultants included psychiatric nurses; directors of various departments from well-known hospitals, including St. Elizabeths and the Menninger Clinic; professors of psychiatry, nursing, and aging from Duke, Harvard, and Michigan; and business administrators and statisticians from other state hospitals in California and Texas.[7]

The panel was given three months (June–August 1964) to survey the state of mental health services in Georgia, but with particular instruction to focus on the institutional care provided at Central State Hospital in Milledgeville and Gracewood State School outside Augusta. As the author of the report (who was not identified, although I assume it was Hollister or someone in his office) noted, there had been thirteen previous surveys of mental health services in Georgia between 1913 and 1959, and the recommendations of the latest, the Schaefer Report, had not been fully implemented. The panel also had no desire to duplicate work that was already happening as part of the comprehensive planning for community mental health.

Therefore, the survey had three distinct goals: "assistance to the state of Georgia in evaluating the institutional phases of its mental health and mental retardation programs," "examination of the alternatives for improvement of patient care in a large institution," and "provision of consultation resources to the State in the development of its mental health and mental retardation programs."[8] The panelists reviewed the previous reports about institutional conditions and undertook a series of visits to the institutions in question, speaking to key staff where they could. It was noted that because of the desire for a quick response, the report confined itself to major recommendations and was designed to serve as a blueprint to help with the comprehensive planning for community mental health funding.

Chapter 2 of the report summarized the main recommendations, and chapter 3 was a discussion of some of those recommendations in more detail. Because of my concern with the implications of both the Community Mental Health Act and the Civil Rights Act for Black patients at Central State Hospital in particular, I will focus on those recommendations pertinent to CSH rather than summarize the entire report (but it is worth reading in its entirety and can be located at the National Library of Medicine).

In the discussion section related to Central State Hospital (which they called Milledgeville State Hospital), it was immediately noted that "Georgia is the largest state east of the Mississippi River and is the only state in the United States that attempts to serve as large a population and geographical area with a single psychiatric mental hospital."[9] This meant that the hospital had become a dumping ground for nearly every kind of intellectual and developmental disability, alcoholism, elder care, mental illness, epilepsy, foster care, and sometimes simply just poverty, neglect, or homelessness. The physical arrangement of the hospital and its therapeutic practices reflected this dumping-ground mentality and was made worse by "an attitude of fear and apprehension about patients seldom seen among staff in other mental hospitals."[10] This attitude meant that "undue precautions are taken in allowing patients freedoms of the grounds, and they are not encouraged to shop, to attend recreational activities, or to participate in religious services in town because so many patients might overcrowd the small community."[11] This situation was made worse by the isolation of the hospital, its distance from other major centers of both resources and culture, and thus the difficulty of attracting and retaining properly trained staff. Therefore, the hospital, according to the NIMH, had become purely custodial and was out of touch with the latest thinking about patients' rights as well as with psychiatric theory and practice itself.

The main recommendation that the report made was that the state government itself would be required to step in and enforce changes at the state level that would begin a process of quality improvement and "decentralization" (not necessarily deinstitutionalization). The long-range goal was to make Central State Hospital into "a psychiatric treatment and rehabilitation facility for an assigned geographic region" rather than the single hospital for the whole state. In order for this to happen, several things needed to change.

First, conditions and practices at CSH needed to be streamlined and improved, which would mean "developing more therapeutic attitudes and climate, an individualized plan for each patient and use of local aftercare and rehabilitation." Second, the state needed to "reduce the diversity of the population," removing people who did not need to be there because they were not actually mentally ill. The report suggested that distinct units for the intellectually or developmentally disabled (I/DD), elderly people, alcoholics, and emotionally disturbed children be created within CSH so that their care could be specifically tailored, and that eventually separate facilities could be arranged elsewhere for these different types of patients. In fact, the report strongly recommended that the practice of admitting geriatric or I/DD patients who were not mentally ill be "immediately discontinued."[12] It also recommended that the "criminally insane, defective delinquent and the women prisoners now housed at Milledgeville" be brought more fully under the control of the Department of Corrections.[13]

Third, it recommended a radical reorganization of patients within CSH into "geographical units[,] each serving a primary region of the state." The report was, not surprisingly, overtly race neutral and made no direct reference to the passing or impact of the Civil Rights Act in its recommendations, yet the existence and consequences of segregation would have been evident to the report's writers. While all the recommendations were phrased within a broader framework of addressing inadequacies in both the hospital's facilities and the therapeutic nature of the program, if followed they would have forced if not integration, at least improvements in the situation for Black patients.

The most interesting of these strategies was the idea of moving patients into units based on geography, an idea that would have served multiple purposes. Primarily, this was articulated as a cure for "desocialization" and aimed to link patients with others from their home counties in order to facilitate connections and ultimately a smoother transition "home." It was also tied to the broader regionalization agenda of the report (and the NIMH), suggesting that once regional outpatient services existed, it would be easier to link patients to aftercare and employment services, returning them as "productive citizens" to their home counties. It was also argued that organizing patients by county would break down the habit of assigning patients on a behavioral basis, meaning the "elimination of security wards, disturbed wards, etc.," and would facilitate better staff-patient relationships, because mixing people with different types of illness should help to raise the standard of care and reduce the "dehumanization" of some patients over others.[14]

Yet the extent to which a geographical organization would have broken down racial segregation is debatable. It is true that if the units were organized along county lines, Black and white people would necessarily be placed in the same wards where those counties were themselves racially diverse. The flip side of this, of course, is that not all of Georgia's counties were actually racially diverse. Given factors like redlining and the urban-rural divide in Georgia, this could just as easily end up placing Black people with their Black neighbors, and white people with their white neighbors.

It could also have been a way to rearrange the pieces on the board to look like integration had been achieved in terms of the letter of the law, while replicating already occurring statewide geographical segregation. It was well known that some counties in Georgia had higher proportions of Black people than white, and a regional plan that lumped historically Black counties together would not have disturbed the status quo.

There were other ways that the report noted discrepancies in programs that hinted at an awareness of problems caused by segregation. Again, the language was very much about equity for all patients, as opposed to naming and calling for an end to segregation. But the greatest discrepancy, and therefore critique, was offered in relation to the industrial and vocational therapy programs.

Overall, the report's writers were extremely critical of the hospital's approach to so-called industrial therapy and argued that it was no longer acceptable for hospitals to rely on patient labor. The economic needs of the hospital could not be used to justify what the NIMH saw as exploitative and abusive conditions that dehumanized patients and used work as a substitute for genuine therapeutic approaches. The report pointed out that work assignments were "not related to the psychological needs of the patients" and did not "teach patients to adapt to job conditions they may encounter after discharge."

This argument is precisely the point that *Ebony* magazine had made in its critique of CSH twenty years earlier. For the NIMH, the rationale of work as therapy was completely undermined by the way that the "hospital's needs for labor have assumed much higher priority than therapeutic needs" and had led to working conditions that were "far from satisfactory" and demanded long hours. The report writers suggested a complete overhaul of the industrial therapy program "from both the economic and therapeutic standpoint" and recommended that "immediate plans should be made to launch a . . . program that would be therapeutically oriented and protective of the rights and dignity of working patients."[15]

In relation to vocational therapy, it was noted that the hospital had recently established a state-of-the-art facility on-site, which was staffed by personnel from the state's Department of Vocational Rehabilitation. But it was also carefully noted that it was failing to meet its potential because it was not available to all patients. By "all patients," it was clear who was affected: the report writers clearly called out the discrimination against Black patients when they wrote, "Vocational rehabilitation services have not been optimally implemented for many patients who could benefit from these services such as Negro patients, and certain groups of chronic patients."[16] In other words, no vocational rehabilitation services currently existed for Black patients. Therefore, the recommendation from the NIMH was to diversify the vocational rehabilitation program and to provide meaningful opportunities in communities that would help patients leave the hospital and engage in productive work in their home counties.

This particular recommendation is significant and telling in many ways. It clearly exposed the lie at the heart of the idea that patient work was therapeutic in any way. This report from the NIMH reflected growing community concerns about the dignity of patients and their right to be treated as patients—not just exploited as workers. The argument that "surely it was better they have something to do" is belied by this condemnation by the NIMH, which argued that the "something to do" was so inherently exploitative and dehumanizing that it was actually contradictory to any possibility of a therapeutic outcome. Therapy was not the goal of these activities; behavior control and economic imperatives were.

Growing community concerns about patients' rights and human dignity began the cycle of ending unpaid patient labor. And as Ben-Moshe has argued, the increasing inability of hospitals to justify the continuation of patient labor to underwrite their operations was a large contributing factor in the move toward deinstitutionalization.[17] If a hospital was no longer able to use free patient labor to maintain the hospital or feed other patients, then there was no more reason to continue the facade that it was therapeutic when everyone knew it was actually not. This was especially the case when it came to Black patients in Southern hospitals, who were always assigned to the hardest and most exhausting forms of physical labor that replicated Old South plantation life, and did not develop skills for an increasingly urbanizing and industrializing New South.

Following quickly on the heels of this report from the NIMH, the community mental health planning process served to expose the bad practices caused by custodial institutionalization. The extent of the problems at Central State Hospital were evident in the Comprehensive Community Mental Health Plan (CCMHP) that the state Department of Public Health submitted to the NIMH on December 21, 1965. Each state needed to submit one of these plans, as well as nominate a single state agency that would be responsible for the administration of community mental health funds.[18] Because each CCMHP needed to provide a survey of the current state of mental health services in each state, they are useful documents for providing a snapshot of service provision in the early 1960s.

The planning process itself took many years, but Georgia had a head start because of the NIMH survey and report. The Georgia CCMHP extended to nine chapters over ninety pages and included a set of 155 explicit recommendations covering all aspects of a statewide mental health, developmental disability, addiction, and vocational rehabilitation program, which it hoped would be "second to none" if realized.[19] The document included a map of Georgia's counties titled "Possible Locations of Comprehensive Community Mental Health Programs."[20] The map is telling in regard to plans for reorganization within CSH and the idea of regionalization itself. It clearly shows the suggested concentration of services in and around metro Atlanta: in DeKalb, Fulton, Cobb, and Clayton Counties, all majority white in 1960. Only Fulton County (the central Atlanta county and home to Grady Hospital), with its 34.7 percent nonwhite population, came close to providing services for Black patients.[21] Of the nineteen proposed regional programs, nine of them were designated for heavily white-majority counties in the northeast corner of the state, including Atlanta and above. Not a single service center was destined for a majority-Black county. Stewart County, on the border with Alabama, was home to a 70.5 percent Black population and had no service center designated there or in any neighboring county.[22]

The demography and location of these majority-Black counties track almost entirely with the historical location of the plantation Black Belt, and they remained counties dominated by sharecropping and poverty well into the twentieth century. Even if there were proposed centers in adjacent counties, accessing them relied on money and means for private transportation. The concentration of Georgia's Black population into these largely isolated and rural counties meant that any reorganization that used geography as the rationale would simply reinforce segregation in mental health services and would do nothing to disrupt the white population's access to treatment and care. This geographical and structural reality undercut prevailing ideas about the rates at which Black patients actively sought mental health care.

Under the heading "Scope of Mental Illness Today" in chapter 2, the plan contained a subsection titled "Utilization Rates," which the planners understood as important to future planning. Subsection D was titled "The Influence of Sex and Race on Utilization" and provided a breakdown of statistics regarding the use of services across the state (not just Central State Hospital). The plan noted that "in both races, males were found to utilize resources more than females," but the clearer discrepancy fell along racial lines. In 1963, white men utilized services at a rate of 14.68 per thousand, white women at 10.83 per thousand, Black men at 8.34 per thousand, and Black women at 6.64 per thousand. This rate for Black patients constituted only 19 percent of the total patient load, whereas they made up 29 percent of the total state population.[23]

Some reasons for this discrepancy were offered in the plan. In relation to gender, the planners hypothesized that perhaps the higher utilization rate among men was "explained by the position of the male in our society as the 'breadwinner.' When he fails to perform this function there is considerable social pressure to have him treated and rehabilitated as . . . fast as possible."[24] This is an interesting comment because it makes clear the link between mental health treatment and ideas about "productivity," which also explains for whom that treatment was more readily available and also more targeted as rehabilitative.

If the Black man was considered a "breadwinner," it was only in relation to his manual labor, and that idea shaped the available forms of "treatment," such as farmwork. It partially explains why the more sophisticated industrial and vocational therapy programs were available only to white men, and why the entire hospital system was weighted in his favor. There is a subsequent comment in the plan about why women overall might utilize services less, in which it is hypothesized that women "suffering from the same . . . emotional disorder may, in many instances, be retained in the home for a longer period because of child-caring responsibilities."[25] The not-so-subtle subtext here is that women's emotional distress was not seen as urgent, as serious, or as important to society to treat, and that her prime responsibility was not to her own health but to her role as a childcare provider.

But theses hypotheses shifted again when it came to the underutilization of services by Black patients, which the planners concluded was both a cultural and a socioeconomic issue. The socioeconomic effect was obvious to the extent that people in the lower socioeconomic class were less able "to secure or purchase psychiatric services," and this went some way to explaining lower utilization by Black patients, since there was "a much higher percent of nonwhites than whites in this class." This assessment was followed by the comment that people in this group "seem to have a higher tolerance level for pathological behavior."[26] There was a problematic conflation here between race and poverty—because the planners assume that most poor people were Black and most poor people tolerate pathological behavior, they assume that there was something intrinsic to Black culture or society that was pathological. Failing to separate these issues reinforced the idea that both poverty and Blackness were a form of pathology, but it also shielded the state from any self-awareness or accountability about its own assumptions or behavior toward Black communities.

These comments also failed to account for the history of segregation in mental health services, which the planners fully intended to replicate with the distribution of new services. Before 1963, Central State Hospital was almost the sole provider. Grady Memorial Hospital in Atlanta did not have a long-term-stay inpatient ward, so it transferred patients to Central State. Other regional hospitals did the same. Private practitioners who took Black patients (who could pay) were few and far between. And beyond these structural issues, there were very good reasons why Black patients might hesitate to commit themselves or a family member.

Not the least of these would have been the very public coverage in both the main Atlanta newspaper and various Black press outlets about the horrific conditions prevailing at Central State Hospital. An underutilization of

Georgia's public psychiatric services could also be read as active resistance to the psychiatric-carceral system, where Black families knew their loved ones were likely to be neglected, exploited, abused, or disappeared. In this sense, the "tolerance of pathology" may have been a greater sense of community care and compassion, and a decision to keep family and community members at home in order to keep them safe. This desire was certainly motivating Ms. O. in her letter to Dr. Rowe at Searcy in Alabama. But it does not account for those families who did want and need external help, like Mrs. Hurston in Mississippi.

Community Health and Massive Resistance in Mississippi

Mrs. Hurston's letter, written in January 1965, demonstrates the complex relationship between Black families and state institutions. When Mrs. Hurston sent her letter to the Department of Health, Education, and Welfare, both community mental health legislation and nondiscrimination legislation were in place, which the department well knew. But racism and segregation limited the services available to Black folks and resulted in an eleven-year-old boy being bounced in and out of jail for five years.

If the department thought that the promise of community mental health money might improve the prospects for Black patients in Mississippi, it was sorely mistaken. The Mississippi Comprehensive Community Mental Health Plan provided a clear overview of the problems besetting that state's mental health services in the 1960s but made no specific mention of issues facing Black families and communities specifically. The plan used a language of "improving services for all Mississippians" in order to completely avoid talking about the ways those services remained indelibly segregated—a standard tactic when it came to appeasing public concerns over impending integration. In the plan, the way that Mississippi in particular performed the Jim Crow routine was to resolutely refuse to admit it was performing anything other than the natural, divinely ordered, and universally sanctioned Southern way of life. However, the writers of the plan were open and honest about the limitations of the state's mental health program, and it is absolutely the case that any reorganization or increase in funding *would* have improved those services.

The major tactics that the planning committee suggested for improvement were interagency coordination and, as in Georgia, regionalization. Interagency coordination was a reference to the fact that like most of these states, the focus on single large institutions meant that those institutions were self-administering and autonomous. Interagency coordination in Mississippi would be facilitated by the creation of an interagency commission, which would be "established for ongoing planning, co-ordination, and multi-agency action in the implementation of planning recommendations."[27]

At the service provision level, the commission would also bring oversight to the entire state program, and foster links between agencies and institutions that should make it easier to move patients to the most appropriate facilities—that is, "services and facilities should be functionally related to provide ease of patient movement and continuity of care."[28] It was an extremely limited tactic, however, as it relied simply on improving links and programs between institutions rather than dismantling institutions entirely. Greater communication between agencies and institutions would actually work to widen the mental health net in Mississippi, which at first glance might seem like a good thing, because the more services there were, the more people should be able to access them. But if the underlying nature of those institutions and agencies remained unchallenged, especially in regard to racism, then it would bring no tangible benefit to Black families in particular. In this sense, it was a classic nonreform reform.

Regionalization was a potentially more powerful strategy because it explicitly sought to address the overreliance on the two state hospitals: Eastern Mississippi Hospital in Meridian, which was open to white patients only, and Whitfield Hospital, the only existing facility for Black patients. The CCMHP set out an idea for dividing the state into nine distinct regions, each serving multiple counties but "designed to make services available within a 50–60 mile radius of every Mississippi citizen."[29] Each region would be home to a Regional Service Complex, which would contain a mix of inpatient and outpatient services as well as specialized services for children, "multi-problem families," and alcoholics.[30] The suggested regions were based on the location of existing services and hospitals, large city and trade centers, and population numbers.

But as was the case in Georgia, regionalization also had the potential to reinforce racial segregation, because some regions, especially along the Delta and the southeast border, grouped together counties that might be considered more traditionally "Black," meaning they may have remained vulnerable to continued underfunding, reinforcing de facto segregation.

While the plan stressed the need for the development of more outpatient services, it did not break up the reliance on state hospitals. Rather, the plan argued that regional complexes should not include any facility with more than 100 beds for acute care, and if long-term care were needed, then patients would be transferred to the existing state hospitals in Whitfield or Meridian.[31] The plan also suggested that those state hospitals should be provided with the necessary resources to provide "more intensive" treatment to patients. The planners also argued that regional complexes should draw on existing resources and draw in more agencies that intersected with mental health needs—for example, "private medicine, general hospitals, welfare departments, health departments, schools, nursing homes, child care facilities, vocational rehabilitation services, courts and law enforcement agencies, any other facility or agency which possesses mental health service potential"—but should also "remain responsive to local planning and local conditions."[32]

There were both strengths and limitations to this plan. A regional complex, if fully funded, would indeed bring much-needed services to regions where none currently existed. The plan did clearly suggest that those services should not be for long-term care but should focus on outpatient services where possible. But in doing so, the plan also extended the web of agencies or services that intersected with mental health, and in a situation where those agencies were not adequately funded or where trained mental health providers were not available, the potential for involuntary incarceration increased, not lessened.

This is the greatest limitation of any such plan in a state like Mississippi that was hesitant at the best of times to commit more money to mental health services and was the worst in the nation in terms of numbers of practicing mental health professionals. As the plan clearly stated, there were only thirty-one psychiatrists in the entire state of Mississippi in 1965, and they were concentrated in six of the state's eighty-two counties—particularly Hinds and Rankin, which were home to the University of Mississippi Medical Center in Jackson and the state hospital at Whitfield, respectively.[33] Of these thirty-one psychiatrists, only thirteen were in private practice, demonstrating again the reliance on single institutions for trained professionals, especially for Black and poor folks who had no resources by which to access private care anyway. So long as these serious structural problems remained, the state would need to continue to rely on the large state hospitals, and as long as those also remained segregated and underfunded, the outcomes for Black communities would not be improved by the state's response to the community mental health planning process.

Other local conditions that could also have affected the development and success of outpatient services included the massive resistance to civil rights.

This resistance could easily have manifested into racial violence in those counties where Klan influence was strongest. As Jason Ward and others have argued, attempts at any racial reform, such as educational segregation or War on Poverty programs, faced outright violence from white supremacist groups, including the Klan.[34] In Mississippi, individual members of the State Sovereignty Commission and other white supremacist groups, like the Americans for the Preservation of the White Race (APWR), still had things to say about the possibility of integration that sheds some light on possible resistance to community-based mental health.

In January 1963, members of the APWR from Summit, Mississippi, wrote to the governor expressing concerns about a Black family in town.[35] Summit was a small town in Pike County in southern Mississippi. On the border with Louisiana, Pike County was home to more klaverns of the United Klans of America than any other county in Mississippi (eight in total).[36] In this letter, penned by W. Arsene Dick, the members of the APWR and the mayor of Summit complained about a Black family led by a pair of "drunken ne'er-do-wells," who "make no attempt whatsoever to provide even the barest necessities for their children."[37] After detailing the abject conditions in which the children were forced to live, including having to eat "meal and flour dry," the letter spoke to a situation in which "each act of theft committed by these children gets more bold. Private homes are robbed. Sunday evening they broke a window and entered a supermarket on the main street of Summit."

Rather than reflect on the fact that the children were starving and probably simply trying to feed themselves, Mr. Dick wrote that "the oldest is 17 years old and mentally retarded. He was sent back to Summit six weeks ago, having been in Whitfield for the last 18 months. He is plain mean. The next is a twelve-year-old and the leader of the group. In the last two years this boy has been picked up 28 times. He has been beyond the powers of the law as there has been no room in the State Reform School at Oakley." The townspeople were requesting that the governor force the superintendent of Oakley to take this twelve-year-old into custody for his repeated attempts to feed his siblings.

This appeal demonstrates the many ways that white people could and did try to use the state psychiatric and juvenile detention system as a solution for broader social problems, a situation in which children were often scapegoated for the failings of both their parents and the communities in which they lived. Rather than spend money on community-based solutions, the people of Summit deferred to state institutions, creating a situation in which poverty and disability were criminalized. I have no evidence that the APWR in Summit or elsewhere in Mississippi had thoughts about the impending move toward community mental health, but I have little doubt that the attitude displayed in this letter signaled a broader environment of fear of the mentally disabled and a "not in my backyard" mentality that would have made the establishment of outpatient and community-based services detailed in the CCMHP unpalatable if not impossible to realize.[38]

"The Crippling Preoccupation with Race" in Alabama

The atmosphere of distrust and paranoia about mental health services, and the eugenic basis of white supremacist rhetoric, also affected planning for better mental health services in Alabama. As early as 1959, the state legislature had attempted to develop a "mental health clinic bill," which would break up some of the reliance on the state hospital system and send more money to clinics like the one in Tuskegee. But the planning for the bill needed to be undertaken in secrecy.

A memo from John McKee, director of the Division of Mental Hygiene, was sent to all clinic directors on October 19, 1959, and explained why: "A number of legislators stated that they were told 'informally' by other legislators close to the Governor that he is 'going along with the KKK on this matter'. . . . The Mental Health Association has long been aware of the Klan's agitation about our clinics being 'brainwashing stations.'"[39] In this environment, moves to expand community mental health beyond the few mental hygiene clinics were stalled in Alabama until the passing of the Community Mental Health Act.

But even then, the atmosphere of racially charged politics and the backdrop of resistance to civil rights permeated the Alabama planning process. The author of the Alabama Comprehensive Community Mental Health Plan (Alabama CCMH Plan), newly hired state health officer Dr. Ira Myers, made a number of frank admissions. In the introduction, he wrote, "The antifederalism, the crippling preoccupation with race, the defensiveness inflamed by defeat, poverty and resentment of the efforts to change the people's value system have flared again."[40] In addition to the influence of what he called "anti-mental health extremists," Myers claimed that "these attitudes have not only slowed our state's progress in the quantity and quality of mental health services, training and research, but have cast a shadow over the planning process itself. Reluctance to accept federal funds and resistance to the concept of planning had to be overcome before the actual job of organizing to plan and study could begin."[41] Myers's comments indicate the way that racial politics and psychiatry were intrinsically linked and demonstrated the difficulty of planning in a state where the governor was busy yelling "segregation now, segregation forever" from the schoolhouse door.

Psychiatrists, administrators, and mental health associations in Alabama were well aware of the need to negotiate this heated environment in such a way as to appear race neutral, foregrounding "the needs of all the people of Alabama."[42] But the plan itself revealed the vast disparity in services that already existed for Black and white patients, especially in a state that already had nineteen full- or part-time mental health centers. The problem with these already existing centers was that they were "inadequate in the amount and kinds of services they can offer their communities. Primarily, the problem is one of manpower."[43]

The idea, therefore, was to use these existing centers as "the nucleus for the future development" of community-based services in a regional plan, but this rested on the ability to train and attract more staff to those regions. There were limitations to this idea in the same way that there would have been in Georgia—geographical segregation was a real issue, and proposed regions would have done little to improve that situation.[44] For example, Macon County, the site of the Tuskegee Clinic, was included in a region (M-15) with other poor, majority-Black counties—Russell, Bullock, Barbour, and Pike—rather than combining it with either Montgomery or Lee County, where bigger and better services and more white people already existed. In fact, in the same way as they did in Georgia, the proposed mental health regions track almost perfectly with the contours of the already existing Black Belt, Black not just because of soil but because of the majority-Black population.[45]

The planners were not overt about this fact, but they did come up with a complicated algorithm by which to determine the regional boundaries based on a "relative need" index.[46] A number of factors went into this determination: poverty, unemployment, crime, delinquency, population density, and access to existing industrial or medical centers. Region 15 (home to Tuskegee) was ranked sixth on the priority list, and surrounding Black Belt regions 17, 18, and 19 ranked twelfth, eleventh, and eighth, respectively.[47] Interestingly, Mobile County, home to Searcy Hospital, where 2,500 Black patients were already being treated, was ranked sixteenth on the list of priorities, signaling that there was less concern about areas that already had established services. This fact would have been of no assistance whatsoever to those 2,500 patients, who, as Dr. Rowe's letter to Ms. O. indicated, were not likely to be released into the community anytime soon.

As comprehensive as it was, the Alabama plan could not divest itself of the reliance on state institutions. The writers of the plan agreed with the prevailing literature that community-based programs were better because they could counter "the adverse effects of removing an individual from his natural environment" as well as "the disadvantages of long-term institutionalization as differentiated from the actual effects of mental illness," and they had the advantage of "involving families of patients in their treatment."[48] However, at the same time, the planners wrote of the need to improve the quality of care at existing institutions, adding, "Of primary concern is the need for having available a facility to which acutely disturbed patients can be immediately admitted. Currently these patients are often housed in the jail, posing a problem for the patient, as well as the police."[49]

Therefore, the planners agreed that the current state hospitals needed to be downsized, but they should be replaced by regional hospitals with only a 100-bed capacity, which would form a network with other outpatient services (almost the same idea as in Mississippi). While there is no doubt that inpatient facilities were (and still are) required for patients in acute distress, creating a system of regional hospitals was not deinstitutionalization so much as it was regionalization. And when those regions replicated patterns of geographic segregation, they left the underlying structural issues of underfunding and understaffing untouched.

The plan also included a detailed catalog of the existing problems in the state hospital system, including a whole section in a supplement document, dated March 1966. In this document, the planners actually argued for an expansion of the state hospital system, suggesting that two new 500-bed facilities be built, "one centrally located in the upper third of the state and a similar unit in the lower third."[50] This part of the plan suggested breaking up and making use of the existing facilities at Bryce in Tuscaloosa to include preventive and outpatient services, and then suggested new facilities in or near Montgomery and Tuscumbia or Sheffield.

This section of the plan lists six pages of repairs and improvements required at Bryce Hospital over the next ten to fifteen years worth more than $15 million, with another $2.3 million dedicated to expanding and improving operations at Treatment Center number two and the Jemison Center, the site of the massive farm operations. This was followed by two and a half pages of renovations and improvements recommended for Searcy Hospital in Mobile, valued at $10,239,000.[51] At no point did the Alabama planners mention the racial segregation that differentiated these institutions from one another, nor did they ever seriously contemplate getting rid of them.

The Alabama plan is unique in the context of these three states because of the level of detail and thoughtfulness—it contained ideas for every possible problem and population, from children to aged care, from prevention to alcoholism. Many of the ideas, if funded and operationalized, did have the potential to provide a diverse and dynamic approach to mental health and treatment, and speak to the level of awareness and commitment on the part of the state's mental health practitioners. But just like Mississippi, it was a plan that never sought to challenge racial segregation, and it was a plan never realized.[52] It was, as Dr. Myers had flagged, a plan that was hindered at every turn when it came to being actualized because of the state's obsession with maintaining racial segregation, which threatened federal funding. And mental health was just about at the bottom of the list of Governor Wallace's priorities in 1964, considering he was much more concerned about fighting the implementation of the Civil Rights Act and whining about the interference of "outside agitators." But it would be the Civil Rights Act, and then Medicare and Medicaid, that would finally force his hand.[53]

The Power and Promise of Federal Legislation

I have no evidence that the Kennedy administration had any formal *intention* for the Community Mental Health Act to act as any kind of leverage against racial segregation in psychiatric facilities, but this is not to say that they did not think that it might. Neither the CMHA nor the Civil Rights Act of 1964, not to mention the Medicare legislation of 1965, was born overnight. They were all formulated in a period of rising concern with human rights broadly conceived, and the rights of the patient as a person were also affected by the broader political, social, and cultural shift, which was concerned with the rights of the Black American as a person. Civil rights and patients' rights were not the same thing, but they were both manifestations of the ideas behind and moves toward social justice that prevailed during the 1960s.

While the Community Mental Health Act alone was not overtly designed to deal with segregation in psychiatric facilities, its planning and implementation is inextricably linked to the two acts of legislation that followed immediately after. But because Southern states like Mississippi and Alabama had applied for almost no federal funding for state psychiatric services and were not rushing to apply for community mental health money either, there was no real leverage with which to enforce change.

The Medicare and Medicaid Act—or the Social Security Amendments of 1965—is largely credited as the most significant policy for enforcing the integration of hospitals, as it promised large amounts of monetary support to states for indigent and elder care.[54] But psychiatric hospitals were excluded from Medicare and Medicaid funding because the federal government had no desire to reinforce those institutions, given it had just passed the CMHA, so funds were made available to poor individuals and for the creation of nursing homes to remove the elderly from psychiatric hospitals. These two measures gave states the means to move patients out of large hospitals and into smaller facilities or services, which Title VI of the Civil Rights Act now required to be racially integrated.[55]

The question of how Title VI regulations applied to community mental health funding, or to states that were deliberately not requesting funding, had already occurred to administrators and officials at HEW, who had been dealing with a barrage of correspondence from various states trying to understand the implications of Title VI for both existing Hill-Burton funding and new community mental health funding. At what point, for example, could a community mental health facility become subject to Hill-Burton funding if it had a certain number of inpatient beds, and would that then necessitate desegregation? And if no federal money was used to create new facilities, would the existing facilities still be subject to a nondiscrimination requirement?[56]

The legal technicalities were complex and taxing. On May 5, 1965, Edward J. Rourke, assistant general counsel at HEW, made a note that he had orally advised Robert Nash, the civil rights officer in the Public Health Service (PHS), that "if State mental health institutions receive no Federal or matching funds directly or indirectly under any continuing State program, the desegregation of such institutions would not be required, nor need be reported as an area of noncompliance by the State."[57] However, Rourke went on to add that if a state had any project, research, or staffing grant from the federal government, they would need to submit Form 441, demonstrating their adherence to nondiscrimination across all their services.[58]

Rourke made an important point over a small technicality that would go on to have major implications—that is, if any part of a state's mental health service was not in compliance with Title VI, then the whole system would be deemed not compliant and subject to investigation or withholding of funding. The means of securing Title VI compliance relied on filing Form 441, in which a state declared nondiscrimination in any research or project grants. That nondiscrimination was assumed to be current and active, not a hypothetical plan about what might happen in the future.

As far as the National Institute of Mental Health was concerned, this nondiscrimination should have also applied ipso facto to facilities built with federal community mental health money, especially because that money did not become available until all states had completed their comprehensive plans, submitted them and had them approved, and nominated a single state agency for the administration of service and funds.

The issue of the relationship between Title VI and its implications for community mental health construction and funding for staff was a pressing concern for Martin Kramer, the acting assistant chief of the Community Mental Health Facilities branch at the NIMH. In a discussion with NIMH and PHS officials in November 1965, he raised the issue of the need for nondiscrimination in staffing if community mental health was going to be successful or meaningful and not just because it was the law. A memo compiled by Donald Young noted that Dr. Kramer had stated "that in his opinion such a nondiscrimination regulation would be extremely important from a program standpoint."[59] Kramer made the important point that it would not be possible for any community-based service operating in an atmosphere of discrimination to adequately meet the needs of all its patients: "It is Dr. Kramer's judgment, for example, that many mentally disturbed Negro patients cannot be properly treated in a mental health center, the professional staff of which is by policy exclusively white. He indicated that it is often therapeutically desirable that such patients receive treatment at least in part at the hands of members of their own race."[60] Kramer was reiterating and reinforcing here many of the thoughts that had long been articulated by Black physicians themselves about the importance of racial concordance, an idea that had motivated the creation of the community-based clinic in Tuskegee. It also potentially provided a leverage against existing segregation in places like Searcy Hospital.

For Kramer, the move toward integration needed to be applied across the board to a state's entire mental health system, both in- and outpatient, and in staffing as well as construction funding. In his memo, Young also stated that he believed that Title VI did in fact apply to community mental health funding, especially at the level of requests for staffing grants. In fact, the NIMH was hoping to include an overt clause in its funding applications to that effect. In response, Rourke admitted that there was no official nondiscrimination clause in the CMHA but that if nondiscrimination could be argued to be therapeutically indicated, then the NIMH could reasonably make such a request of the applicant.[61]

The approach that a state took to develop community mental health plans was, therefore, necessarily linked to its broader approach to the implications of Title VI for nondiscrimination in medical services and its current funding status. Those actions were also shaped by broader social and political attitudes toward the concept of civil rights itself. If Georgia was more proactive in its response to community mental health, that was because the state's government officials wanted to be seen as forward thinking and progressive. They also knew how desperately they needed federal money, and with civil rights looming, they planned accordingly. In the same vein, Mississippi and Alabama, in terms of state politics, stayed true to type. Resistance to "federal interference" also meant resistance to federal money, and the political desire to be seen to be preserving states' rights drove politicians to play fast and loose with plans for government money, especially for the mentally ill, who were not desirable constituents anyway. Combined with the massive resistance to other forms of federal intervention aimed more explicitly at racial integration, community mental health plans were never likely to garner true popular support or state funding.

The extent and nature of the plans from both Alabama and Mississippi demonstrated that there were plenty of good ideas from the mental health professions themselves, along with a recognition that more money, more staff, and more local services were needed. But even the planners would not tackle the great big desegregation elephant in the room. That task fell on the shoulders of grassroots activists, who were concerned with integration not simply for upholding the law but as a means of improving the lived reality for Black patients in the South's hospitals.

7 Mobilizing Grassroots Activism

October 5, 1953
National Association for the Advancement of Colored People
Mobile Branch
PO Box 1091
Mobile, Alabama

We . . . respectfully ask your consideration of the matter of employing Negro doctors at the Searcy Hospital. We believe favorable action in this particular by you would win the approval of a vast majority of the citizens of Alabama. Likewise it would be a step in the direction of providing qualified Negroes with dignified employment in the state's public health service. We shall appreciate your taking such moves, as the governor of all the people of the commonwealth of Alabama, that would establish justice and fair play in the above mentioned instances.
Respectfully yours,
J. L. LeFlore, Secretary

On October 6, 1953, Governor Persons of Alabama received this letter from the then secretary of the Mobile branch of the NAACP, John LeFlore. LeFlore started his letter by expressing his concerns regarding rumors of tubercular patients not being separated from other patients at Searcy, which he posed as a commonsense public health problem. He then raised issues about pay and conditions of employees, including the salary differential between white and Black attendants, and pointed out that the living conditions for Black employees were considerably worse than those for white ones, though they were "paying the same board rate as the white employees. Another complaint indicates discrimination with regards to drinking fountains at the hospital."[1] LeFlore's final point to the governor, spelled out above, highlighted the need for more Black doctors to bring about some kind of racial parity in both the workforce and in approaches to patient care.

Most significant about this letter is the date. Prefacing both the *Brown v. Board of Education* decision and the formal medical civil rights movement, LeFlore's letter is an important indicator of the way that grassroots activists were extremely proactive in their fight against segregation, well before laws existed to support them.

In the same way as with community mental health, the medical civil rights movement did not start with the passing of Title VI of the Civil Rights Act in 1964, and it did not start with policymakers and legislators. As many historians have shown, the push for health rights for Black and minority Americans has as long a history as the active attempt to oppress them.[2] The process of establishing civil rights in psychiatric settings, however, was a fraught one, because it challenged deeply embedded and long-held stereotypes about the nature of the Black personality and the racist fears that justified segregation. Undoing this system required a combination of community pressure, grassroots activism, government intervention, and legal enforcement.

This chapter focuses on the work of grassroots activists linked with the civil rights movement and their concerns with mental health and psychiatry in the South. Beginning with LeFlore, I look at the way community-based activism inspired and informed legal moves toward psychiatric hospital integration. The NAACP Legal Defense Fund (LDF) relied on its networks of local lawyers and activists to help bring federal cases that would set necessary precedents, and with the judgment in *Simkins v. Cone Memorial Hospital* in North Carolina in 1963, activists like LeFlore in Alabama were able to press for similar action in other settings. This grassroots activism was also necessary to alert the Civil Rights Unit of the Department of Health, Education, and Welfare (HEW) about breaches of the Civil Rights Act, and LeFlore, other activists from the Medical Committee for Human Rights (MCHR), and student civil rights groups were central to this activity. But the move toward integration did not go unchallenged and was met with the same resistance from white supremacist groups as other attempts at integration did, setting the scene for a clash between state governors and federal enforcement.

LeFlore's Local Activism

John LeFlore (see figure 7.1) is an important figure in the history of civil rights, and Mobile an important site for workers' and voting rights.[3]

From his early days as a US Postal Service employee and secretary of the Mobile NAACP, LeFlore had been deeply concerned with the importance

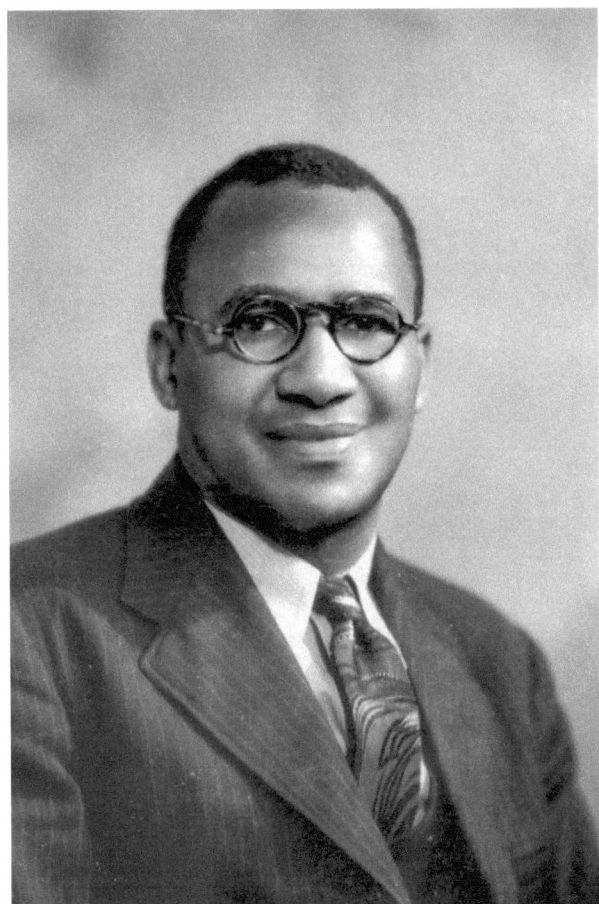

FIGURE 7.1 John LeFlore, c. 1942, Erik Overbey Collection, the Doy Leale McCall Rare Book and Manuscript Library, University of South Alabama.

of employment opportunity and equality under the law for voters and workers.[4]

His letter to Governor Persons received no official response that I can find, although it was marked up in various ways by the governor's office, indicating that they were paying attention (see figure 7.2).

LeFlore was in fact well known to the governor's office. When the state government banned the NAACP in Alabama in 1956, LeFlore had pivoted to help found the Non-Partisan Voter's League (NPVL) and became its director of casework in 1959. In this role, he was often the liaison between community groups and legal representation regarding all sorts of discrimination cases.[5]

From 1965, as part of his work as the chair of the Citizens Committee of the NPVL, LeFlore again took up the cause of the workers and patients at

**NATIONAL ASSOCIATION FOR THE ADVANCEMENT
OF COLORED PEOPLE**

MOBILE BRANCH

OFFICE OF THE

Post Office Box 1091
MOBILE 6, ALABAMA

Monday
October 5
1 9 5 3

RECEIVED
OCT 8 1953
GOVERNOR'S OFFICE

Hon. Gordon Persons
Governor, State of Alabama
State Capitol
Montgomery, Alabama

Dear Governor Persons:

 We respectfully call to your attention complaints reaching us that tubercular patients at the Searcy Hospital for the Insane, located at Mt. Vernon, Alabama, are permitted to roam indiscriminately among other inmates at the institution. This situation, if true, will certainly increase the likelihood of a spread of the disease among the persons confined at the hospital.

 We are quite certain that if this condition does prevail as reported to us, it is probably due to an oversight. However, the health danger involved would justify prompt action upon the part of proper authorities to correct the matter in question without further delay.

 In connection with another matter at the Searcy Hospital, we have been advised that salary differentials exist between white and Negro employees doing the same work. The prevailing policy, we were told, being to pay Negro workers considerably less than the sums received by their fellow workers of the white group for like jobs, education and training considered equal.

 Living conditions of the colored employees were described as poor, but with their paying the same board rate as charged white employees. Another complaint indicates discrimination with regard to drinking fountains at the hospital.

 We also respectfully ask your consideration of the matter of employing Negro doctors at the Searcy Hospital. We believe favorable action in this particular by you would win the approval of a vast majority of the citizens of Alabama. Likewise it would be a step in the direction of providing qualified Negroes with dignified employment in the state's public health service.

 We shall appreciate your taking such moves, as the governor of all the people of the commonwealth of Alabama, that would establish justice and fair play in the above mentioned instances.

Respectfully yours,

J. L. LeFlore
Secretary

cc:
Dr. D. G. Gill
State Health Officer

FIGURE 7.2 LeFlore to Persons, October 5, 1953. Governor Persons State Institutions Files, box SG12529, folder 4: FY1954, Alabama State Hospitals, ADAH.

Searcy Hospital. In June of that year, he wrote directly to Luther Terry, then surgeon general of the Public Health Service (PHS), complaining of continued "stubborn policies of racial segregation affecting both patients and employees" at Searcy.[6] LeFlore pointed out that not only were the hospitals racially segregated, but abhorrent practices were in place: "Patients from the Searcy Hospital are alleged to be compelled to go to Tuscaloosa by bus to work on a farm operated by the white hospital."[7]

He requested information from the surgeon general about the funding status of Bryce and Searcy, pointing out that their racial segregation put them in breach of the Civil Rights Act. Terry forwarded the letter to Robert Nash (civil rights officer for the PHS). Nash informed LeFlore that the PHS head office in DC did not keep that kind of information about individual hospitals, but he could find out from the regional office in Atlanta, to whom he was forwarding LeFlore's letter. "Incidentally," he added, "complaints have been recorded by others against these two hospitals and they will be investigated as soon as time permits."[8]

On July 22, 1965, LeFlore received an answer to his question from Carl Harper, the acting regional director of the PHS in Atlanta. Harper laid the groundwork for further action when he told LeFlore that Bryce was in receipt of federal funds. While Searcy was not, it could be seen as part of the same statewide mental health program operated by the board of trustees. "Since the Board has received Federal financial assistance for Bryce Hospital, it would appear that Title VI would be applicable to both," he wrote, a position reinforced by general counsel's comments to the National Institute of Mental Health (NIMH).[9]

Conditions for patients at both Bryce and Searcy were well documented in an investigation by law student Henry Stiles, who was working in Mobile with LeFlore as part of the Law Students Civil Rights Research Council. In July 1965, Stiles wrote to Ruth Adams at the LDF and told her that he had a series of complaint forms from workers and relatives of patients at Searcy, reporting that "the conditions there are appalling to us."[10] Stiles and LeFlore had been collecting information and signatures for a petition, which they then sent to a number of people, including James Quigley, the assistant secretary of HEW; Mr. Michael Meltsner, from the Legal Defense Fund; and Dr. Harry Rowe, the physician in charge of Searcy Hospital itself.[11]

In this petition, LeFlore and the signatories invoked their rights as both citizens and taxpayers to lay out four main demands: (a) the desegregation of all facilities and accommodations; (b) the elimination of discriminatory employment practices (including segregated work spaces and unequal conditions); (c) the employment "of properly qualified Negro doctors, nurses, technicians, clerks, receptionists, bookkeepers or other personnel"; and (d) "the indiscriminate admittance of patients to the Bryce Hospital and/or Searcy Hospital, without regard to race or color."[12]

The petitioners included a thorough listing of recent legal cases (such as *Simkins v. Cone* and two cases from Florida) that had addressed racial segregation in Southern hospitals, as well as reference to the Fourteenth Amendment and the relevant sections of the Civil Rights Act. The petitioners then demanded that Alabama's psychiatric hospitals "eliminate, within the next 60 days, all racial distinctions and discrimination which deny to any person or citizen equal services, rights and privileges at the said hospitals."[13] LeFlore knew precisely what the Constitution provided to Black Americans, and he intended to claim his community's full rights of citizenship.

In correspondence between LeFlore and the LDF, there was considerable focus on segregation's impact on the patient population. LeFlore's files contain handwritten notes detailing a kind of patient-leasing system in which "both Negro men and women are transferred to Bryce Hospital (Tuscaloosa) and Northport for farming. . . . Negroes stay on [the] farm at Northport, some of whom are transported by bus or truck to Bryce, then returned to Northport each night."[14] This site at Northport was the aforementioned Jemison Center. The notes also document that white employees were able to take Black patients home to work in their house and return them at the end of the day, a process similar to convict leasing. Reports from the relatives of patients detailed Black female patients at Searcy being forced to fill and cart wheelbarrows of coal from the pile to the kitchen, outgoing mail being censored or restricted, incoming mail being stolen, and patients being forced to leave their own wards and wait outdoors in all weather for the communal dining hall.

Stiles and LeFlore also received numerous reports of brutality and evidence of white supremacist violence within the psychiatric hospitals. In an affidavit, Mrs. Brown wrote that her son Joe Nathan Jr. "had been beaten by two white hospital employees, named Johnson and Newton. . . . My son took his father and me to one of the toilets and showed us welts and blisters on his left buttock which he said resulted from the two white men beating him up with a cut-off water hose. He explained that one of the men held him while the other one beat him after locking him up." While beatings and abuse were a common problem across all overcrowded and badly managed psychiatric institutions, Mrs. Brown was in no doubt about the racial implications of this attack, which she believed "was due to strong race prejudice in view of the fact that a number of white employees of this hospital are alleged to be members of the Ku Klux Klan." She linked this action to the broader environment of racial violence around Mount Vernon in which white employees of the hospital were in fact arrested only the previous week "after participating in a Klan rally at Mount Vernon and allegedly shooting into the house of a Negro woman and attempting to burn down her house."[15]

This report from Mrs. Brown was not mere anecdote; local newspapers carried the story as well. LeFlore often used his position on the editorial board of the local *Mobile Beacon* to raise awareness about issues related to discrimination at the hospital for both staff and patients. The *Beacon* covered the story about the Klan activity on August 6, 1966, in an article titled "Klan Terrorists Hit in Mobile County" and reported that John Henry Newton, a known member of the local Klan, was arrested for his role in the shooting and attempted burning. "Newton," the *Beacon* reported, "is said to be 18 years of age and to have recently had colored playmates, was released Monday on $2,000 bond; he is charged with arson and the destruction of private property."[16]

The charged atmosphere around Mount Vernon and Searcy continued; a week later, the *Mobile Beacon* ran another front-page story titled "Skirmish at Searcy Hosp. Causes Stir."[17] In this article, the *Beacon* reported that a Black employee, Willie Mays Jr., had been dismissed from Searcy because of an altercation with a white employee over the treatment of a patient. Mr. Mays, who worked in the kitchen at Searcy, reported that "it was 'feed-up' time and one of the male patients was seated at the table with his hat on. This white man said, 'what you doing with your hat on boy?' and judo chopped the patient as he snatched his hat. I called him where I was and said 'you shouldn't hit patients like that,' he said 'what you got to do with it' and slapped me across the face. My eye is still blood shot. Then I went into him." Both men were fired, and Dr. Rowe was "unavailable for comment," but the local community saw the incident as part of a larger series of racially charged incidents. A "number of area citizens converged on the hospital" in protest at Mr. May's firing and the violence against patients but were threatened with a call to the police chief. The article made a clear link between this incident and the Klan, stating at the end that "because of recent Klan activity in the area it is reported that most Negroes have armed themselves."[18]

This article, and the incident it records, speaks to the atmosphere of violence and fear in which both patients and staff at Searcy were forced to live, and the absolute lack of interest or protection that came from Dr. Rowe. For activists like LeFlore, the only solution was to integrate the hospital so that Black patients were not at the complete mercy of white staff and administrators. LeFlore could not have been surprised, however, that he received no other response to his letters and petitions than the reply of Searcy's Dr. Rowe, claiming it was the superintendent's decision about who was appointed to work in the hospitals.[19] The question of conditions for patients remained unaddressed. But LeFlore was not the only one raising such concerns. At the same time, the Medical Committee for Human Rights was providing care for civil rights workers in the South, and the issue of mental health was high on their agenda.

Psychiatry and the Medical Committee for Human Rights

During the Freedom Summer of 1964 in Mississippi, volunteers with the Medical Committee for Human Rights, led by Dr. Leslie Falk as the Mississippi field secretary, became increasingly cognizant of the significance of mental health in the civil rights struggle, and their work on the ground exposed both the inadequacies and the racism embedded in the state hospital systems. John Dittmer has written extensively about the history and work of the MCHR, and while I will not repeat that work here, my own research in the MCHR archives demonstrates the particular ways that the MCHR intervened at the intersection of psychiatry and civil rights.[20]

Beginning with a concern for the mental health of civil rights workers, MCHR volunteers were made aware of the nature and deficiencies of existing psychiatric facilities in Mississippi in particular. But MCHR work soon expanded beyond the health and welfare of civil rights workers to the communities in which they served (despite restrictions against practice), and at times MCHR clinicians were actively involved in negotiating mental health care for Black Mississippians. This work revealed not just the conditions of care and the impact of segregation but also the attitudes of communities and families themselves toward psychiatry.

In the years following Freedom Summer, the MCHR was actively involved in documenting civil rights abuses and lodging complaints with the Department of Health, Education, and Welfare, and in this activity they helped to hold HEW accountable for its own inaction and built evidence and support for Legal Defense Fund work. In addition, the MCHR was often led by psychiatrists. One of Dr. Falk's very first and most important contacts in Mississippi was Dr. Robert Smith. Smith had briefly been employed at Whitfield in the early 1960s, and Dr. Alvin Poussaint, who became the MCHR's Southern field director, was also a well-known psychiatrist.[21] Other white Northern psychiatrists acted as directors of local chapters of the MCHR in the North, and some of them went on to form the "radical caucus" of the American Psychiatric Association.[22]

In the first instance, however, the problem of mental health became a concern of the MCHR in relation to its own volunteers and local civil rights activists. It was obvious to volunteer psychologist Robert Coles that many of the civil rights activists were suffering from what he called "battle fatigue."[23] As Dittmer noted, "Providing psychiatric care and 'rest and recreation' for burnt-out civil rights workers became an important function for MCHR."[24] This care revealed the great toll of civil rights work in the context of white resistance, surveillance, and the constant threat of violence. A memo from Dr. Josephine Martin, based in New York, spelled out "the psychiatric problems that emerge from the civil rights movement" as "the youth of the participants, the separation from home (often for the first time), the close living, the constant stress and the real external danger."[25] It was essential for both personal and group safety that "a properly qualified individual or agency, such as a psychiatrist, psychologist, hospital, or clinic," be part of the movement, not just for emergencies but for longer-term care.[26]

Trying to find local mental health care for civil rights workers, however, immediately revealed the abject state of affairs in existing psychiatric facilities and raised broader concerns for the mental health of local Black communities in Mississippi. Two examples demonstrate this struggle and the intersection between psychiatry and civil rights activism. MCHR nurse Josephine Disparti encountered these issues firsthand while dealing with the behavior and problems caused by a Council of Federated Organizations (COFO) volunteer. Mr. S. had been behaving erratically, talking incessantly during planning meetings, and had been arrested for disorderly conduct. Disparti met with him and found him "very depressed and unable to respond coherently to my questions. He made inappropriate references to various happenings in Columbus and the general ill state of the world."[27] She was able to get him to see Dr. Bob Smith, who felt he was definitely in a deep depression and had possibly suffered a psychotic break. Dr. Smith prescribed and supplied some Thorazine and then persuaded Mr. S.'s parents not to have him committed to the Mississippi state institution, arguing that he would be better served at home.

After some to and fro, the parents agreed to pay for Mr. S.'s flight home as well as a return flight for a companion. Disparti herself accompanied Mr. S. on a tumultuous and long journey from Jackson to Atlanta to New York that required Student Nonviolent Coordinating Committee (SNCC) volunteers to meet them at the Atlanta airport to keep Mr. S. out of trouble. Once in New York, Mr. S. was seen by Dr. Israel Zwerling at Yeshiva University, who uncovered a long history of drug use and mental health hospitalizations.[28] Dr. Zwerling wrote back to Bob Smith, who forwarded the report to Bob Moses, program director of COFO. Both Dr. Zwerling and Dr. Smith strongly argued that while they could not keep Mr. S. out of Mississippi, it would be necessary for COFO to refuse to acknowledge or countenance Mr. S. as a volunteer again.[29] Their feeling was that he not only was unsuited to the work for his own psychological and emotional reasons but also posed a danger to the movement itself with his conspiracy theorizing and inability to maintain confidentiality. For this reason, at the end of her report, Disparti wrote, "Perhaps COFO can be made now to realize the importance of screening (and relying on the interview info)."[30] All of this correspondence, and the incident surrounding Mr. S., spoke to the difficulty of making sure that volunteers were ready for civil rights work and for the provision of mental health care once they were in the field.

The strain of life in Mississippi, especially for Black volunteers, was also made evident in the evaluation of a SNCC worker, Mr. B. In August 1964, Mr. B. was seen by Dr. Greenwood.[31] In his notes, the doctor wrote that he had seen the twenty-five-year-old Black man because he had

> complained his "nerves are shot." . . . He related how he had been "thrown out" and rejected by his family when he began to devote himself full time to [the] Student Nonviolent Coordinating Committee (SNCC) three years ago. He has been, along with Bob Moses, a pioneer in SNCC in the state and has a distinguished record of service. During this period he has had many harrowing experiences, has been beaten by police and local whites many times and has lost the sight of one eye . . . as a result of these beatings. He has been arrested and imprisoned about 25 times including a six month stretch at the State Penitentiary.[32]

All of these imprisonments, including six months at the notorious Parchman, were for Mr. B.'s "crimes" related to civil rights work and resisting white authority—breaches of the Jim Crow routine.

Mr. B. went on to explain to the doctor his deep sense of responsibility to the cause and to his partner and newborn child but also struggled with "anorexia, insomnia, anxiety, sense of loneliness, bouts of depression." Mr. B. spoke about wanting to get married, to leave Mississippi and pursue his education elsewhere, and to provide a stable life for his partner and child, and his realization that he would continue to return to SNCC as long as he lived in Mississippi. The guilt he felt at potentially leaving the cause was almost crippling.

Dr. Greenwood expressed deep sympathy for Mr. B. and recommended "immediate withdrawal from the battlefield and start of [a] small b.i.d. Stelazine dose," as well as a plan for ongoing therapy. Dr. Greenwood noted that he had made a follow-up appointment with Mr. B., but he did not return. There is, however, a handwritten note from a Dr. Redler dated August 8 stating that "plans are being made for follow up (withdrawal from Miss., help in planning schooling, rest and psychiatric treatment)." This concern for Mr. B. and the actions taken demonstrated the importance of psychiatric work in the civil rights movement and the ability of the MCHR to mobilize its national networks. At the same time, Mr. B.'s experience spoke not just to the mental health toll of civil rights work but to the very real trauma of being Black in Mississippi when a person chose to defy the usual protocols of the Jim Crow performance.

Although the MCHR volunteers were under strict orders not to offer clinical services to local patients, it was impossible to draw a hard line between civil rights work and clinical practice, not least because it was actually local people who were the civil rights volunteers.[33] For most people that the MCHR encountered, there was no separate space between everyday life and civil rights work—civil rights work *was* everyday life in the Jim Crow South. Therefore, concern for the mental health of civil rights volunteers was also concern for the mental health of people living under the regime of white supremacy, and so psychiatry intersected with civil rights work both at this level of the self and at the level of legislative enforcement. This meant that sometimes clinicians or volunteers involved with MCHR were also directly involved in providing psychiatric care or advice to patients, and those encounters also helped volunteers gather a broader picture of the state of services and the difficulties being encountered by local families trying to get help.

For example, in July 1966, MCHR volunteer Charles Meyer, working in Greene County, Alabama, submitted a report about his encounter with a fifteen-year-old child, who was the nephew of a local Southern Christian Leadership Conference (SCLC) member.[34] The boy's aunt asked for help from Meyer, who managed to examine the boy and talk to his mother. The boy had a history of mental illness and had been experimenting with concoctions of local "dope." When Meyer saw him, he was thin, lethargic, and slightly feverish, and had not eaten or drunk anything for about sixteen hours. His mother and Meyer managed to get him dressed so he could visit a doctor, but he disappeared. Meyer noted that "it had been suggested that I should not take him to see Dr. Smith since he is hostile to CR workers," which demonstrated the double bind that volunteers and local families were under when it came to seeking help in the context of the backlash to civil rights and the hostility of white doctors.[35] Meyer wrote, "[I intend] to look into psychiatric treatment for the boy through the county health department. This will serve both the purpose of introducing me to Health Department officials and the primary goal of helping the boy. The mother was quite willing even when I mentioned the possibility of hospitalization. She feels that something has to be done."[36] In this sentiment, the boy's mother was much like Mrs. Hurston, desperate for help but abandoned by a segregated and racist system and its practitioners, to the point that even a visit to the local doctor was dangerous.

Meyer may have mentioned hospitalization without full knowledge of what that may have entailed in Alabama, but the MCHR administration was certainly aware of conditions for Black patients in Alabama and Mississippi. Sometimes that information came directly from patients themselves, who were cognizant of the many ways in which their civil rights were being breached through the mechanisms of psychiatry.

In February 1965, the MCHR office in Montgomery, Alabama, received a typed letter from a Mr. Edward Jones, who had in his possession an original handwritten letter from Dr. H., who was being held against his will in Searcy Hospital in Mobile.[37] Dr. H. had a PhD from Howard, a master's degree from Atlanta University, and a bachelor of science from Tuskegee. Despite his qualifications and stellar academic record, Dr. H. had been intermittently confined, in one form or another, since 1945, when he applied to the University of Alabama Law School. The letter does not state how or why Dr. H. came to be at Searcy, but it speaks to the way that psychiatry was used to patrol the boundaries of the Jim Crow routine.

For Dr. H., his commitment was clearly part of a white supremacist conspiracy in which he had been persecuted, run out of his hometown (Tuskegee), and "been subjected to extreme economic pressure for nineteen years." Dr. H. saw his confinement as a civil rights issue stemming from white supremacy and listed the full history of the laws that were being broken by his involuntary commitment. As he argued, "All of my constitutional rights have been violated. . . . I am held in a hospital while in excellent mental health." Mr. Jones, who had received Dr. H.'s "smuggled" letter from Searcy, added that there was a list of names included, consisting of superintendents and other Alabama officials that the MCHR might be interested in investigating. There is no mention of any follow-up to Dr. H.'s letter directly, but it was certainly the case that volunteers were using their contacts and access to services in order to document the nature of mental health services as well as the many ways they were in breach of the Civil Rights Act.

There are few reports in the MCHR files about actual psychiatric hospitals, but the ones that do exist are telling. In a report titled *Psychiatric Facilities in and around Clarksdale and Mound Bayou*, dated August 29, 1964, Dr. William Sykes documented the lack of community-based services and the intersection between the carceral and mental health systems.[38] For example, "When a person becomes mentally ill here," he wrote, "they must be treated by the local MDs if they are to be treated on an outpatient basis. All others eventuate to the State Mental Hospital." There were implications in this system for both local people and civil rights volunteers. Dr. Sykes wrote, "The usual route to the State Mental Hospital is as follows: the patients are taken to the police station and then to jail. Sometimes they are examined in jail by the county doctor. If he concurs in the diagnosis, the patient is then taken to the State Hospital by a relative or the Sheriff. (N.B. Implication of this procedure for possible COFO workers who have acute mental illness.)" Dr. Sykes spoke to various local physicians, who detailed the ways that the state hospital acted as a catchall for people who suffered largely from the psychological burden of social problems—"the poverty, over-crowding, poor and unregarding working conditions which I am sure must have repercussions psychologically—nevertheless, there are meagre facilities for people with mental illness."[39]

Interestingly, Dr. Sykes also documented two important work-arounds to the jail-to-state-hospital system. One involved sending patients to Vicksburg, where a Jewish doctor by the name of Dr. Fuerst "had a large psychiatric practice (mostly shock-treatment, who usually charged a $20.00 fee but would scale his fee down and who did accept Negro patients)."[40] Dr. Fuerst was also considered the first port of call for children, whose other option was a referral to New Orleans to "the University affiliated out-patient clinics." Dr. Sykes does not specify which university or whether Black children were accepted, but out-of-state care for working-class Black families like Mrs. Hurston's, for example, would surely have been prohibitive.

The other work-around to the jail-to-state-hospital system was a different form of community-based care, which involved avoiding the medical system entirely. This was especially the case for cognitively impaired people, who, it seemed to Dr. Sykes, "do not usually require treatment in a community such as this, since the community tolerates them and does not make demands which they cannot meet."[41] This observation gives some weight to my earlier analysis of the different rates of service utilization in Georgia, which were not simply about differences in diagnostic rates but also about an active refusal to engage with the state system and a different way of caring for and about community members that did not rely on their categorization as dangerous, criminal, or unproductive.

Another report submitted to the office in Jackson was written by Mildred Beldoch, PhD, and Clarice Whelan, RN, who visited the East Mississippi State Hospital in Meridian.[42] They quickly learned what everyone else knew about the Meridian facility—that even though it had initially accepted both Black and white patients, it had been firmly closed to Black patients and staff since 1905. They noted that they were directed to the facility by a local "Negro boy . . . who knows the local situation well [and] said that he could not even accompany us on the grounds, so evidently there are no Black personnel on the grounds."[43]

The boy's fears were well grounded. Meridian was a hotbed of Klan violence, and it was no coincidence that the state hospital there maintained heavily policed racial lines.[44] East Mississippi State Hospital was therefore dedicated primarily to the care of older white people with senile dementia, and even then there were not enough spots for the demand. The two women were able to spend half an hour with Dr. White, "the director" (he was simply the head physician), who told them that he had a long waiting list and cared for 900 patients on $2.51per patient, per diem. No children under sixteen were admitted "unless placing them in a ward with adult psychotic[s] would be [a] clear improvement over any other choice." The nature of the patients meant that active treatments like electroconvulsive therapy (ECT) or insulin shock were rare, but "Thorazine, Mellaril and the like are in heavy use," which reflected the chronic understaffing and lack of psychodynamic or therapeutic programs. Dr. White told the women he had plans to apply for $100,000 from the NIMH to improve staffing and equipment, but they wondered, rightly, "Can they do this in a non-integrated facility?"

The answer would prove to be no, but this thought barely seemed to occur to Dr. White, who had his hands full dealing with the white people he already had. As the women writing the report noted, in a situation "where the white community is getting little in the way of adequate mental health coverage, it is no wonder that there seems to be a complete lack of interest in the mental health of the Negro community."[45] This comment reinforces the idea that exposés, investigations, and even new federal legislation like the Community Mental Health Act deliberately focused on concerns for white patients, rendering the situation for the Black patient and family largely invisible. Grassroots activists used two particular tactics to increase that visibility: lodging complaints with HEW and reporting conditions in civil rights newspapers.

Lodging Complaints with HEW

Activists widely believed that the best way of improving conditions for Black patients was integration (which was also the law), and this belief sustained the campaign to enforce the nondiscrimination requirements of the Civil Rights Act. After Freedom Summer, the MCHR hired Black psychiatrist Dr. Alvin Poussaint as its director of Southern projects. Under Poussaint's leadership, the MCHR used its network of volunteers and visitors to monitor civil rights breaches in hospitals across the South and report those conditions back to the Department of Health, Education, and Welfare. This was not simply a by-product of their clinical support work but became an overt mission of the MCHR and its volunteers.

In August 1965, the MCHR offices in Selma and Jackson circulated a memo to "all interested parties or groups," along with a three-page guide on how to collect information and compile a report documenting the existence of segregation in facilities, wards, clinics, and staffing. Sample reports were included, which demonstrated the multitude of ways in which hospitals across the South continued to defy the federal order to integrate: segregated lunchrooms for staff; specialist training programs for white employees only; Black physicians not allowed to use the same parking lot as white physicians; Black patients seen only after white patients or on alternate days; free clinics for white children and not for Black children; Black patients addressed by first name, and white patients addressed as Mr. and Mrs.; and so on. The continued belligerence of white staff was also actively documented, such as the nurse at one clinic who told a civil rights worker she "would not give him any information about welfare regulations or clinic hours because she considered him a 'bad influence in the community.'"[46] This kind of hostility was a perfect example of the attitude of many white clinicians, who continued to defy the law and use their moral authority and positions of power to provide medical help unequally.

At the end of the memo was a note clearly stating that HEW would not "investigate any facility unless they get complaints" and that complaints were kept anonymous to protect those gathering information. Complaints were filed from the MCHR office in Jackson along with a cover letter. The memo also pointed out that the volunteers compiling the complaints did not need to know the funding status of the segregated institution, making the astute observation that even if the facility was not receiving federal funds at the moment, "they may ask for them in the future."[47] At this point, the MCHR volunteers and HEW itself were relying on the nondiscrimination clause in Title VI of the Civil Rights Act as the basis for complaints against hospitals receiving Hill-Burton funding, but MCHR was unhappy with the progress of integration.[48]

By May 1966, Dr. Alvin Poussaint had had enough. In a terse letter addressed "Dear Congressman," Poussaint pointed out that only 5 out of 140 hospitals in Mississippi had voluntarily complied with Title VI of the Civil Rights Act.[49] He noted that Southern governors were being particularly active in trying to find ways to disburse incoming Medicare funds to blatantly noncompliant hospitals and argued, "Our Negro citizens are again being threatened with being short-changed on equal access to health facilities by the federal government."[50]

Poussaint made a direct reference to the potential power of Medicare funding to bring about the required change, stating, "Our patience is indeed wearing thin, and we urge you to do all in your power to see that Medicare funds are withheld from hospitals which are still in violation of Title VI. If Medicare money is dispersed to non-compliant hospitals, we have no other choice than to go on a direct action campaign of demonstrations etc. against these facilities."[51] Poussaint's position was reinforced and supported by local student activists who were on the ground as part of Freedom Summer and were determined to use the press to highlight conditions for Black folks across the South in the face of an apathetic Northern and mainstream press and the continued lack of government action.

The Southern Courier and Psychiatric Civil Rights

The link between civil rights and mental health was a prime target for the short-lived but important civil rights newspaper the *Southern Courier*. Established in 1965 by journalism students from Harvard who were keen to circulate pro–civil rights information out of the South after Freedom Summer, the *Courier* had strong connections to the Medical Committee for Human Rights, not least because one of its journalists, Gail Falk, was the daughter of Dr. Leslie Falk. During its four-year run, the *Courier* published several stories about issues related to the psychiatric hospitals in Alabama and relied on local civil rights networks for information.[52]

In its organization files, which are housed at the Tuskegee University Archives, there is specific reference to Dr. Al Payman at Bryce Hospital, who was sympathetic to the *Courier*'s cause and was "willing to talk," and this undated file also includes the note "Desegregation of mental hospitals in state with Bryce as target," listed as a possible story.[53] The paper ran the first part of the story on January 23, 1966, with the headline "Alabama Mental Hospitals Say They Will End Segregation."[54] The article contains information from LeFlore and the Atlanta office of the Public Health Service about a preliminary agreement that had been reached with Alabama to desegregate the hospitals. According to the article, the PHS was working with the state representatives who administered the hospitals and would rather move slowly to reach compliance rather than withdraw funding if it could be avoided. The article set out how much money the hospitals received from the federal government—"huge amounts of government surplus food . . . sizeable grants from HEW for new buildings and various projects. . . . Bryce alone has in operation a $300,000 project to study a certain mental illness and a $25,000 in-service training program."[55]

But the article noted the vast discrepancies in conditions and treatment for Black versus white patients and staff, including the disparity in pay between Black and white attendants, where the most a Black attendant could earn would be $236 a month, which was the starting salary of a white male attendant. And Black attendants were treated worse than white ones. As one Black hospital worker reported, "It seems like they pick out the worst food to give us. We get left-over salads and desserts, and the food is almost always cold. And if there is a dirty job to be done and a white and [a] Negro attendant are nearby, the Negro will get the job."[56]

For patients, the spending was significantly lower, and the differences particularly showed up "in the 'extras' Bryce has—better materials for occupational therapy classes, more elaborately kept grounds, more variety in facilities." These discrepancies could be eliminated with desegregation, the *Courier* argued, not least because it would raise salaries for Black employees and attract more people. "If attendant jobs in all the hospital wards were open to Negroes as well as whites," the article suggested, "part of Bryce's staffing problems might be solved."[57]

The cautious optimism of this article soon gave way to frustration with the state's delaying tactics and the ever-worsening conditions for patients. Throughout 1967, the *Courier* ran a series of articles detailing the abject treatment and conditions of Black patients at Searcy in particular. In June 1967, the newspaper picked up the story of Miss Inez Pruitt, who was committed to Searcy against her will.[58] Miss Pruitt had made inquiries at the Mobile County welfare office about what she believed was a welfare check owed to her. Miss Pruitt had recently been hospitalized with pneumonia and also lived with a disability in her left leg but had been working as a housekeeper for a local white family. When the welfare officer denied that she was owed any money and accused her of "faking," Miss Pruitt reported, "She made fun of my condition. . . . She raised a leg to kick me, I lost my temper and hit her with my umbrella. I apologized later."[59]

Even though the welfare officer said she was not hurt by the umbrella (she also denied the abuse allegation), four days later Miss Pruitt was picked up by the police and taken to Mobile General Hospital, where she was examined by Dr. Thomas. He "looked her over and classified her a paranoid schizophrenic" and in the same breath said, "But of course I'm no psychiatrist."[60] From there, Miss Pruitt should have been seen by a psychiatrist at Mobile General but instead she was transported to Searcy. When questioned about this process, the Mobile County welfare office said that it was doing her a favor. Under Alabama law, people were not entitled to welfare unless they were considered permanently disabled, and in pursuing committal to and a diagnosis from Searcy, the welfare office argued that they were trying to get "medical evidence that can get her on welfare for the rest of her life." Yet, the reporter noted, patients who had been committed to a mental hospital were not in fact entitled to welfare assistance at all.[61] In one move, the local medical profession had rid themselves of a troublesome Black woman seeking assistance and put that assistance itself out of her reach. More than that, they had condemned her to trauma, violence, and abuse.

In Searcy, Miss Pruitt was denied medication for her blood pressure and was not able to control her diet.[62] In a follow-up article three weeks later, the *Courier* reported that Miss Pruitt had been released from Searcy but not before she was strapped down and subjected to three rounds of electroshock treatment "against her will."[63] This article detailed the way that Miss Pruitt's sister and a white friend, Mrs. DaPonte, had been to visit her multiple times and also conducted "a stormy interview with Dr. Harry Rowe, assistant superintendent at Searcy."[64] Echoing his earlier comments to Ms. O. about her "troublesome" daughter, Rowe was unwilling to release Miss Pruitt without signed letters to the effect that her sister would be accountable for her and that no one at Searcy would be held responsible for her future behavior. Rowe claimed that she had been violent against staff and "did cause quite a bit of disturbance. . . . But she was improving."[65]

Her defendants claimed that her acts of violence against staff were actually her fighting the forced electroshocks, which they claimed were illegal, but Rowe's counterargument demonstrated the circular logic of carceral psychiatry when he claimed that "after a patient is legally committed, we give them the treatment we think they need."[66] The fact that Miss Pruitt's commitment, and that of so many others like her, was subject to the whim of local white practitioners, with no legal due process or recourse, appeared to escape Rowe's mind. As the assistant superintendent, his word was the only one that mattered.

Miss Pruitt was released in June 1967, and in August of that year, she received a letter from the welfare department stating that she would receive sixty dollars a month "for being 83% disabled," a decision facilitated by Robert Feinstein, a law student from New York. Miss Pruitt's case demonstrated the active relationships between families and communities and Searcy Hospital, and the importance of the agitation of her sister and her white friend. It also demonstrated the broad reach and concerns of *The Southern Courier*, as well as its connections to law students active in the South as a result of Freedom Summer and other civil rights internships and programs. But for every Miss Pruitt, there were hundreds if not thousands more patients held without recourse to appeal, and the *Courier* continued to document their situation and argue that integration was the only solution.

In a long article in August 1967 (see figure 7.3), the *Courier* reported in minute detail the everyday conditions of life at Searcy, which reinforced what LeFlore and his team had long been documenting.[67] The main point in this article was the lack of Black professional staff, like social workers and nurses, and the abusive behavior that came as a result. The most egregious example of this was the reliance on electroshock as a form of

Former Patient Tells What Life Is Like Inside Searcy State Mental Hospital

'If You Have Your Sanity, You Will Lose It'

(The author of this article was formerly a patient at Searcy State Mental Hospital in Mt. Vernon. This is her story of what life was like inside the hospital—and her ideas on how it could be improved.)

MT. VERNON, Ala.—When you enter the door, it looks very pleasant. But the worse will come. Although all of the patients are Negroes, most of the attendants are white. There are only a very few Negro attendants. All of the social workers are white.

After arrival at the hospital, all persons are carried to the receiving section. For women it is Ward 4N and for men it is Ward 3S. When received, you are met by an attendant and another patient who has been there a long time.

Sometimes the patient who has been there a long time is a criminal who can't be released unless the court tells the hospital to set him free.

All of your clothes are removed to be marked. Sometimes they are given back to you a few days later. Sometimes when you ask about your clothes, you are told they were misplaced.

Next you are sent into the shower. If you don't go in, you are pushed or sometimes slapped and cursed and given a bath by some of the patients. If you are in a rage after the bath, you are locked up.

You are given just two items of clothing to put on. Sometimes they are good, sometimes raggy—but always un-ironed. A lot of the women are not given panties, and the men wear no undernants.

If you ask too many questions you are locked up for worrying them. Some patients are locked up because they go to patient canteen or other wards without asking. If there are court charges against you, you may be locked up.

When you are locked up, you are let out at certain times to get water. There are no toilet facilities in the room where you are locked up, so you must eat and use the bathroom there.

At Searcy, all the food is served in eight hours, early in the day. Breakfast is between 6:30 and 7:30 a.m., dinner between 10:30 and 11:30 a.m., and supper between 3 and 4 p.m.

Breakfast is always grits or something resembling oatmeal, with gravy. There is watery coffee, sometimes sweet and sometimes not. Bread can be day-old rolls, if not, sometimes there is sliced bread or cornbread.

You get no meat at breakfast—unless you find it in the gravy. No butter either, However, the employees have butter for their breakfast.

Dinner is varied. The vegetables are whatever is raised on the farm. Sometimes we have beans and peas mixed, or squash with cucumbers and hot peppers mixed. Greens are cooked sometimes in plain water, sometimes with meat. Sometimes they are not even washed clean.

At dinner, we have powdered buttermilk to drink. Most days we have salt meat sliced. Some days it is chicken, sometimes pork chops. Very rarely, it is weiners and bologna. On Friday we have some fish that is never cooked done.

Our supper is always boiled potatoes in the skin (not even washed clean), some cereal, and sausage boiled in water. There is never enough for all to get some. Dessert is dried fruit, such as prunes or peaches, with never enough sugar on it. The powdered sweet milk is sometimes sour.

In the summertime, fresh fruits like peaches, plums, pears, watermelon, and cantaloupes are given as long as the garden supply from the field lasts.

You can buy food at the patient canteen. The canteen is run by white people. The food you get there is thrown—not handed—to you, like you were a dog. Some patients volunteer to work, but others are forced. They carry clothes on their backs to the laundry, rain or shine. If they are not there, they are looked for as if they were paid to work.

Men and some women go to the field to work the garden. About two of the patients work for Dr. Harry S. Rowe, the assistant superintendent. He gives them a very, very small salary.

There is recreation daily, and it is the only thing at Searcy that is supervised by Negroes. It is helpful to many. But usually, some patients are being punished, and can't go.

Some patients come to recreation dirty. The women are kept much cleaner than the men. Some of the wards are cleaner than the others.

If you talk back to an attendant or sass them (as they call it), you are given an electric shock treatment. All the attendant has to say is, "I want this patient shocked," and the patient is taken in for a treatment. The usual treatment is ten shocks, but sometimes it is more.

If patients refuse to eat the half-cooked or dirty food, they are sometimes given shock treatments. A lot of patients have been shocked and never awakened again.

When patients walk to the attendants and tell them they are sick, the attendants most times say, "You off and crazy." Patients have been kicked, slapped, and even stomped by some of the attendants. But other attendants are kind and understanding.

There are no psychiatrists, psychiatric nurses, or clinical psychologists at Searcy Hospital. Many doctors are Cubans studying to pass the Alabama medical examination.

The kitchen has no dietitian or dietitian's aide to prepare the food. The head man over the kitchen received his experience in the army. All the help besides a few white bosses and a white truck driver are Negroes. They put the food together as ordered by the headman over the kitchen. Just a few of the Negro help stay long.

Searcy is a place that, if you are sent with your sanity, you will lose it. Some patients die of starvation or for lack of medicine.

To improve Searcy, it must be integrated. It should have trained nurses, attendants, and dietitians. It should employ more people trained for treatment of the mentally ill. The hospital should hire Negroes as social workers and secretaries, and for other responsible positions.

SEARCY HOSPITAL

punishment and behavior control, which belied its use as a therapeutic technique.

In the article, which was written entirely from the perspective and experience of a former patient, the author noted, "If you talk back to an attendant or sass them (as they call it), you are given an electric shock treatment. All the attendant has to say is, 'I want this patient shocked,' and the patient is taken in for a treatment. The usual treatment is ten shocks, but sometimes it is more. If patients refuse to eat the half-cooked or dirty food, they are sometimes given shock treatments. A lot of patients have been shocked and never awakened again."[68] This comment goes some way to explaining my interpretation of the ECT statistics I outlined in chapter 3, where the technique was disproportionally used on the Black patients at Searcy compared to the white patients at Bryce.

But it is just one marker of the awful reality of life for Black patients at Searcy, where they were forced to work in the fields, laundry, and coal pile; where the food was watered down, half rotten, dropped on the floor, bland, and devoid of nutrition, "thrown—not handed—to you, like you were a dog"; where people were forced into showers and personal items and clothes removed, as if they were prisoners; where any form of resistance resulted in being shocked, locked up, "kicked, slapped, and even stomped." If people were dying from ECT, they were also dying of "starvation or for lack of medication," criminal behavior for a facility that was called a hospital yet employed "no psychiatrists, psychiatric nurses, or clinical psychologists" and where "many doctors are Cubans studying to pass the Alabama medical examination."[69]

The article finished with a clear call for desegregation. "To improve Searcy, it must be integrated," the author argued. "It should have trained nurses, attendants, and dietitians. It should employ more people trained for treatment of the mentally ill. The hospital should hire Negroes as social workers and secretaries, and for other responsible positions."[70] But student newspapers could only do so much in the face of federal inaction and populist politics, which characterized the massive resistance to the civil rights movement organized by white supremacist groups. These groups had very specific (and odd) things to say about the threat of integration in psychiatric hospitals.

(*opposite*) FIGURE 7.3 "If You Have Your Sanity, You Will Lose It: Former Patient Tells What Life Is Like Inside Searcy State Mental Hospital," *Southern Courier*, August 5–6, 1967.

Mental Health and Massive Resistance

The situation in psychiatric hospitals cannot be understood separately from the prevailing environment of massive resistance to civil rights. Much has been written about the activities of white supremacists in relation to educational integration and voting rights, as well as the work of formal organizations dedicated to segregation, like the Citizens' Councils and the Mississippi State Sovereignty Commission (SovComm).[71] But little has been written about their attitudes toward mental health or integration of hospitals. But given the fascination of white supremacists with the allegedly primitive and criminal nature of the Black personality, it should not be surprising to find that the commission was watching the situation at Whitfield closely.

Established in 1956 in direct opposition to federal laws aimed at racial integration, SovComm was posed as an agency authorized "to do and perform any and all acts and things deemed necessary and proper to protect the sovereignty of the State of Mississippi, and her sister states, from encroachment thereon by the Federal government."[72] As Yashuhiro Katagiri has argued, the phrasing of the legislation that established the commission never used the words "race" or "integration," but it was well understood that what the commission sought to protect was not simply the Jim Crow routine and the Mississippi "way of life" but "the purity of the bloodline of our Anglo-Saxon race."[73] It was this eugenic concern with bloodlines that provided the justification for arguments against integration of patients in hospital and other medical settings. In employment relations, it was an issue of power and authority, in which the white boot needed to be kept firmly on the Black neck.

SovComm was particularly interested in employment relations and the potential threat posed by Black workers with any kind of authority over white workers. There are two reports in the commission's papers specifically about Dr. William Jaquith and his workforce at Whitfield.[74] The first report, submitted on January 10, 1961, was written by Tom Scarbrough and Virgil Downing and concerned a new Presbyterian chaplain hired at Whitfield, the Reverend Wallace Carr. SovComm had received a complaint about Carr from the secretary of the Citizens' Council in Monroe County, who alleged that Carr had been a proponent of integration in his previous parish in Pulaski, Tennessee. SovComm made inquiries with the chief of police in Pulaski about Carr's history and were assured that he was "alright."[75] The investigators also received a letter from Robert Story, from the board of deacons in Pulaski, who stated that the reverend was "a Christian, a fine citizen," and that the allegation that he had integrated a church camp was false.[76] They also spoke to John Rayburn, representing the Presbyterian Church, who "gave testimony refuting charges that Reverend Carr ever preached or advocated the mixing of the races."[77]

Scarbrough and Downing then requested a meeting with Dr. Jaquith, who assured the investigators that he had performed a thorough background check on the reverend, which had revealed no red flags, and that he was of exemplary qualifications and character. Jaquith's approach to SovComm was one of quiet collaboration if not outright endorsement—in this instance, he went so far as to thank the investigators for their information and concern, and assured them that "he would watch him [the Reverend] more closely." While Jaquith reminded the investigators that it was his job and responsibility to ensure the good conduct of his employees, he did tell them that "if Reverend Carr ever preached or advocated integration in any shape, fashion or form, he would dispose of his services immediately."[78]

The investigators finished their report with the observations that "Dr. Jaquith was very cooperative, and expressed his appreciation for our visit," and that they felt that "Dr. Jaquith will take care of any integrationist preacher out at Whitfield."[79] This investigation is particularly interesting in light of the fact that Dr. Jaquith did operate a fully segregated service for Black patients, which had at times included Black doctors and a Black chaplain.[80] SovComm was not concerned with a segregated service existing at the same location, however. Its concern was ensuring that the segregation held firm and that no Black employees had any contact with white staff or patients unless it was a contact of subservience.

This position was reinforced a year later when the director of the Sovereignty Commission, Albert Jones, ordered an investigation of Whitfield's employment of Black people, especially "regarding two Negro employees of the hospitals as having positions of employment in the general hospital that places those two Negroes in a position that they are over some of the white employees of the hospital."[81] The investigator was again Virgil Downing, who met again with Dr. Jaquith to discuss the circumstances of the two employees, Rubye Smith and Robert Crosby. Both of these employees worked in the general hospital on-site at Whitfield, where patients with diseases or illnesses other than their psychiatric ones were treated.

The complaint about Ms. Smith and Mr. Crosby was not that they were in contact with patients or even other employees but that they might be in positions where they earned more than or had supervision duties *over* white employees. Dr. Jaquith explained that Ms. Smith, who had been a maid at the hospital for eleven years, now earned $100 per month, which had increased in the same way as it had for all employees over that length of time. As a maid, Ms. Smith was working in the supply room, where at times she might be required to hand items out to white nurses when other white nurses were not present.

As an orderly in the operating room, Mr. Crosby had only been employed less than a year, and his salary had risen from $75 a month to $80 per month after his first three months, which was hospital policy for all employees. It was not clear to Dr. Jaquith what kind of complaint could be made about Mr. Crosby. Jaquith reported "that it was hard to keep a white man doing orderly work at the hospital," that Mr. Crosby was dependable and hardworking, and that he had no knowledge of "this Negro man being over white employees of the hospital."[82]

To put Mr. Downing's mind at ease and to get the commission out of his hospital, Jaquith made it clear that integration was not on his mind for Whitfield, and that if federal money was used to force integration, it would make no difference because Whitfield did not receive any federal money "with the exception of a small grant . . . for a sewage line."[83] But Jaquith also supported this link between no federal funding and continued segregation—it was a line he would maintain for the next five years, even under threat of suspension of Medicare funding. Director Jones seemed satisfied with Mr. Downing's report on Whitfield, and there are no more reports about Jaquith or Whitfield in the available files.

Not to be left out, the Ku Klux Klan also made their opinions known about integration at Whitfield. The KKK in Mississippi was not necessarily as well organized or as unified as its counterparts in other states, with the White Knights of the Ku Klux Klan not formed locally until 1964. However, the United Klans of America (UKA, founded in Alabama in 1961) had a strong presence in the state. David Cunningham has documented in minute detail the known locations and density of the UKA and the White Knights of the Ku Klux Klan (klaverns across Mississippi).[84] Cunningham's maps demonstrate that in key counties and regions where community-based services were being planned, such as Pike County on the southern border with Louisiana, and Washington County in the Delta, Klan presence was extremely high. This was also the case in Hinds and Rankin Counties, home to Jackson, the capital, and to Whitfield Hospital, respectively. There is no coincidence here, of course: Pike, Washington, and Hinds Counties were also home to major elements of the civil rights movement, and so the Klan was active in response to anything that challenged white supremacy.

Various klaverns undertook violent activities that ran alongside, and sometimes at a tangent to, more formal bodies, like the Citizens' Councils or the Sovereignty Commission, taking actions that "respectable" state bodies could not be seen to endorse.[85] In an undated document contained in Governor Johnson's files, the UKA took aim at Rankin County as a cesspit of moral degeneracy, alcoholism, and corruption, and then focused specifically on Mississippi State Hospital.[86] In a long detailed paragraph, they accused Dr. Jaquith, a known Catholic, of not only submitting to the federal government for the "small sum of two hundred and fifty thousand dollars in commodities" but practically rolling out the red carpet for Black control at the hospital.

According to O. O. Buckshot, the author of the four-page diatribe *Your Children's Future Is Being Made Today: What Are YOU Doing?*, not only had Dr. Jaquith capitulated to the federal government, but "his assistant, Dr. Head, escorted a group of Negroes into the White cafeteria and ate at the same table with them." Soon, he claimed, "the attendants on all wards would be mixed, including in the living quarters, as would the patients. Worse still, the Negro doctors are to practice on white patients, including white women." Meanwhile, white female attendants and nurses would be caring for Black male patients, "starting with combing their wool and bathing their privates properly." For Buckshot, the future at an integrated Whitfield was nothing short of apocalyptic. "Can you think what it will be like with white insane patients, a large portion white women, and all Negro employees? Christians, does God mean for you to do nothing?"[87] Rankin County was home to three klaverns of the UKA and at least one of the White Knights, but I have no evidence of any direct action taken against Whitfield. It did, however, create an environment of fear when it came to planning for either community mental health or integration and also shaped the responses of policymakers and administrators.

The concerns voiced by groups like Americans for the Preservation of the White Race and the Klan are easy to dismiss as kooky or extreme, but in a way they reflected the legacy of the internal racism of psychiatry itself. For white supremacist groups like those in Mississippi, the integration of psychiatric facilities was framed as a social threat of the greatest order, based on fears of miscegenation that spoke to the basic eugenic rationale behind both white supremacy and psychiatric confinement. The idea that "Blackness" and "madness" were already synonymous was made even worse when that madness was posed as a threat of violence. These fears then informed populist governors, who used them to continue to avoid the mandate to integrate, arguing that psychiatric patients were especially vulnerable and that integration would cause violence between them.

These arguments found little purchase with legal activists both within and outside the federal government as they sought to enforce compliance either voluntarily or through the court. Throughout 1965 and 1966, John LeFlore continued to pester anyone who would listen, writing repeatedly to James Quigley at HEW, reminding him about the petition and reiterating that the Civil Rights Act gave HEW the capacity to withhold federal assistance for noncompliance.[88] LeFlore rebuked Quigley for the lack of action and demanded that HEW move toward withdrawing federal funds "for the operation of all Alabama mental hospitals."[89]

The Medical Committee for Human Rights took the same line. Representatives from the MCHR and the NAACP Legal Defense Fund corresponded and met with representatives of HEW, but made little real progress. On June 10, 1965, David French, chair of the Washington metropolitan chapter of the MCHR, sent a telegram to Assistant Secretary Quigley stating, "It is our understanding that Federal funds are still granted to the Alabama welfare department although they have not filed a statement of compliance with the Civil Rights law. Will HEW now withdraw the funds?"[90]

If voluntary compliance was the preferred tactic from HEW, for activist groups like the MCHR and the NAACP LDF, a broad threat of funding withdrawal was considered more powerful. They had argued and agitated, written letters, organized petitions, published newspaper stories, and still segregation remained. This segregation was clearly understood as not simply a form of oppression but also a threat to Black life itself. Even though the legal precedents for medical integration now existed, it was the threat of withdrawal of Medicare funding (and other construction and grant money) that was seen by both the government and legal activists as the best tactic for securing an end to segregation. The ways in which various state governments responded to this threat is the subject of chapter 8.

8   Enforcing Civil Rights

April 22, 1966

Dear Sir
I was born in Alabama in 1888 have never lived anywhere else. Have and have had Negro friends all my life but have not known any of them who felt equal to white people, so I don't feel they are equal to white people. I want to commend you for speaking out for segregation and for practicing what you preach, I'm referring to ordering the mental patients that had been moved, moved back to the hospitals provided for them by ala officers and taxes. . . . I feel negroes are not citizens. They didn't help write our laws, are they or their present promoters Americans?
—Mr. G. V. McCarn to Governor George Wallace

I almost missed Mr. McCarn's letter in the Alabama Department of Archives and History because it was in the last file in the last box I looked at after a long, frustrating day in December 2017, and that file was named "Partlow State School," which was not an institution I was specifically concerned with at the time.[1] But written in pencil on the tab of the file was the word "Integration," so I pulled it out and there they were, fourteen letters in total like this one, expressing varying levels of support for Governor Wallace's refusal to integrate the psychiatric hospitals in Alabama. McCarn's letter is written in long sloping text, pencil on thin notepaper, and someone in Wallace's office had taken the time to decipher his text and address and find out his full name before sending a "thank you for your support" response.

Mr. McCarn's letter is symbolic of the type of popular resistance to integration that governors like Wallace manipulated for political gain and, in the process, wasted taxpayer money on legal battles and failed to develop adequate mental health services. All the work in the Alabama Comprehensive Community Mental Health plan came to nothing in the face of this "crippling preoccupation with race," as Mr. McCarn and so many others like him would rather have had no money than admit that their Black friends and neighbors were even American.

I am not sure why these letters were in a file marked "Partlow"—the hospital and school for disabled children—given that the letters had nothing to do with that institution. This was my first visit to the ADAH and my first attempt to try to understand the history of underfunding in Alabama's mental health system, and so my whole story began with this file. That story, and this chapter, became the first piece I wrote about the attempt to desegregate the psychiatric hospitals in Alabama, which I published as a stand-alone article.[2] Since then, I have worked my way backward to try to understand the broader and comparative approach to the implementation of the Civil Rights Act at the intersection with psychiatry. That work led to the other chapters in this book.

This chapter expands on the published article to take a deeper look at each state's official responses to the mandates of Title VI and its implementation in their psychiatric facilities, beginning with Georgia's voluntary if reluctant compliance and Mississippi's passive-aggressive resistance. It focuses on the work of the lawyers in the Office of Equal Health Opportunity (OEHO) and travels with special counsel Marilyn Rose on her visits to Dr. Jaquith at Whitfield and Dr. Rowe at Searcy. And finally, it follows Alabama to court. Alabama's belligerent resistance to integration and the subsequent court action exposed the lie at the heart of medical justifications for segregation and demonstrated the importance of federal judges like Frank M. Johnson in the fight for medical civil rights.

This legal battle in Alabama was not fully settled until the 1970s and demonstrates the long reach of racism in mental health, which worked to limit both integration and community-based mental health. In this long-range analysis, I argue that there are direct links between the resistance to psychiatric integration and the mass incarceration that plagues Southern states today.

Securing Voluntary Compliance in Georgia

Given that Georgia had been actively working with the National Institute of Mental Health (NIMH) on improving conditions prior to the Community Mental Health Act (see chapter 6) and given the political context of not wanting to be seen as too extreme in opposition to what was now federal law, state officials were well primed to move on voluntary compliance.

In early January 1965, there was a flurry of correspondence between the office of Addison Duval, director of the Division of Mental Health, and John Venable, director of the Department of Public Health. In a memo dated January 4, 1965, Dianne Stephenson listed all the behavioral and mental health services that were in active receipt of federal funding, had grants pending, or were planning to apply. The Georgia Mental Health Institute was requesting the greatest sum, $750,000 in "research construction," with Milledgeville State Hospital requesting more than $350,000 in training, residency, and improvement projects. Gracewood, the state school for disabled children, was requesting over $217,000, and the Alcohol Rehabilitation Service had more than $280,000 in grants pending. Each of these institutions was also requesting $100,000 specific to "hospital improvement," which would have drawn on Hill-Burton funding and was therefore immediately subject to civil rights compliance.[3] This total of more than $1.5 million in federal funding was a significant amount of money that the state could not afford to play around with.

The planning for voluntary compliance began immediately. Not two days later, on January 6, 1965, Dr. Venable received a memo from Dr. Charles Bush, assistant to Dr. Duval in the Division of Mental Health. This memo set out detailed considerations of the ways the state might respond to the December 23, 1964, memo from the Office of the Surgeon General regarding implementation of Title VI. Despite the work associated with planning for community mental health, Dr. Bush noted that "services to patients at the Milledgeville State Hospital and the Gracewood State School and Hospital in general are completely segregated at this time."[4] Dr. Bush noted that if the state was going to comply with both the spirit and the word of the surgeon general's memo (rather than looking for loopholes, like Mississippi and Alabama were), then it would need to bring about a complete integration of staff and patient services throughout the mental health program, not just in single facilities.

In an institution the size of Central State Hospital (Milledgeville), this would not be an easy task. Dr. Bush was concerned that "this cannot be done quickly without getting patients upset and thus adding to their emotional problems. If the transferring of patients can be done in connection with other changes, methodically and giving people, both patients and employees[,] time for adjustment, integration can be accomplished in a wholesome manner."[5] Dr. Bush suggested that this might take as long as twelve months at Milledgeville, given that there were more than 12,000 patients to consider.

Bush's memo mentioned some potential issues in regard to ending discrimination among the staff and personnel as well, most notably the huge cost of bringing about salary parity between white and Black staff, noting that "to upgrade all nonwhite employees at Milledgeville to the same step in grade would cost an additional $16,000 a month and no additional funds have been provided." This is a telling admission about the economic consequences of segregation for Black workers. The hospital had only been able to bring pay parity to the employees at the very lowest grade by not filling vacancies in the same period, meaning that the hospital continued to be chronically understaffed. Pay was not the only problem for staffing integration, however. Dr. Bush's memo noted that even though the dining rooms at Milledgeville were already informally integrated, "few of the nonwhite have taken advantage of this situation, preferring to eat on a segregated basis."[6] This spoke to a culture at Milledgeville where it seemed likely that de facto segregation would continue regardless of the law.

To overcome any potential difficulties in managing both patients and staff at Milledgeville, Dr. Bush recommended taking advantage of the changes that were already underway as a result of the community mental health planning process, as well as pursuing a very strategic communication plan. He suggested that small groups be arranged, beginning with the highest "echelons" of staff, to communicate the required changes and give people a chance to discuss and ask questions. He cautioned that "until the lower echelons have been fully appraised of the situation, no movement of patients should be attempted." Once all staff were on the same page, the move toward "units" based on type of illness or disability would facilitate integration among those groups, "then the balance of patients would be divided into geographical units. Integration of these groups could be accomplished as they are separated from the main groups of patients. At the same time, newly admitted patients would be assigned to receiving wards without regard to race, color or national origin, and the medical-surgical service would assign patients to rooms according to diagnosis."[7] In this suggestion, Dr. Bush was speaking directly to the advice already given to Central State administrators by the NIMH inspectors, specifically their suggestion to eradicate a dual service. For both community mental health planners and hospital administrators, the organization of the population along a mix of diagnostic and geographic grounds was considered enough to force integration of the entire population, at least in writing.

Dr. Bush's memo was followed by a series of fourteen meetings with various facility and department managers in February 1965, who all agreed to forward assurances of compliance to the Public Health Department by March 1. This process was set out in a public statement issued by Governor Sanders, who stated that "in commenting on the quick approval of Georgia's statement of compliance, Dr. Venable noted 'we felt that we understood what Health, Education and Welfare wanted, and we did what we thought was required.'"[8] The statement of compliance makes for interesting reading; it sets out clearly which services in the state were not integrated and gives a timeline by which they would be.[9] The section related to Milledgeville clearly states that the hospital was not currently in compliance and would need to adopt a staged approach to integrate all aspects of the facility. The statement was cautiously optimistic that the changes could be effected quickly, although concern was again expressed for the well-being of patients: "The major consideration which must be given in the integration of so large an institution is the best interest of the mentally ill patients and an effort to program changes in such a way as to minimize the disturbance of patients."[10]

The plan was to integrate shared therapeutic and entertainment programs by April 22, 1965; classrooms by June 15, 1965; children and adolescent units by August 15, 1965; and the remaining population by November 15, 1965.[11] Specific references were made to the fact that integration was being linked to the reorganization of units along geographic lines: "The hospital is presently in the process of reassigning patients between units so that a particular unit will house patients from a designated geographical area of the state. Integration has begun with the transfer of patients and employees from the wards of two units at a time." It was noted that this integration applied to staff as well as to patients, and as the units were reorganized, so were the staff, some of whom stayed with their existing unit and some of whom were transferred to other units to ensure racial parity. Once this reorganization was complete, "employees will be assigned in such a manner as to prevent distinction on the grounds of race, color, or national origin."[12] This particular assurance was significant, as it signaled a commitment to meaningful and affirmative action and not a fallback to de facto segregation through regionalization.

The original statement of compliance was submitted to HEW on March 12, 1965, and the statement from the governor reported that it had been accepted without prejudice, making Georgia's health department "one of the first three states in the nation to have their compliance schedules approved." Dr. Venable was quoted in this statement as saying, "We are pleased to know that there will be no lapse or delay in the receipt of some 15 million dollars in federal funds used by the Department and its affiliated agencies."[13]

But it seems as if both Dr. Venable and the governor spoke too soon. The date on the statement of compliance I have been quoting from lists March 12, 1965, as the original submission date, and then immediately underneath that is typed "4/22/65 (Revised Statement Date)." Without the very first submission, which I have not found in the archives, it is impossible to say what was changed, but it is telling that also in this file is a copy of a telex transmission from Dr. Harald Graning, head of medical facilities in the Public Health Service (PHS), to the regional office of the PHS in Atlanta. In the telex, Graning wrote, "In implementing decision by department that signature on 441 means statement of fact rather than intent . . . this confirms that effective immediately approval of a part 1, 2, 3 or 4 of a Hill-Burton application involving additions to or modernization of an existing facility should not be made unless you or a member of your staff has either personally visited hospital or feel certain beyond reasonable doubt that there is in fact neither discrimination nor segregation because of race, color, or national origin. This should be applicable to patients, professional staff, interns, residents and all students in training."[14]

This note would potentially have direct implications for the $100,000 pending requests for "hospital improvement" at Central State (and other facilities). In other words, HEW would not be satisfied with empty promises about what a state or hospital might intend to do in the future. It expected that hospitals would be fully integrated *before* any more funds were dispersed, which likely hastened things along in Georgia's case, given the desperate need for construction funds, let alone research and training grants, as well as public pressure to improve mental health services.

At any rate, there is no more correspondence related to delays concerning Central State Hospital, but in May 1965, Dr. Venable received a memo from Richard Lyle, Regional director of the Public Health Service, warning him that complaints had been filed about a number of hospitals and clinics across Georgia that were still not in compliance with Title VI of the Civil Rights Act. This included major institutions like Macon City Hospital, University Hospital in Augusta, Grady Hospital in Atlanta, and a number of county and regional hospitals that were important providers in their region, such as Phoebe Putney in Albany and Memorial Hospital in Savannah.[15] Documenting their progress toward integration is beyond the scope of this book, but the fact that eleven major providers in Georgia continued to discriminate indicates the difficulty of securing voluntary compliance and the importance of the follow-up complaint process. This was particularly true in the cases of Mississippi and Alabama.

Passive-Aggressive Resistance in Mississippi

It would be hardly surprising to learn that Mississippi adopted a strategy of initially passive resistance to the mandate to integrate its hospitals in that it simply largely ignored the nondiscrimination requirements of Title VI. That resistance became more aggressive and active as HEW tightened the screws and hospital administrators, aided by segregationist Senator John Stennis, looked for loopholes in the legislation. Stennis's archives are full of letters and memos from local constituents and service directors complaining about federal overreach and the impact of the Civil Rights Act on their funding.[16] The content of this correspondence is a classic example of the way the Jim Crow routine was performed in the context of hospital segregation.

For example, in a letter to Stennis dated April 26, 1965, Foster Fowler, the executive director of the Mississippi Commission on Hospital Care, complained about the multiple ways that the Public Health Service was to blame for the delay in Hill-Burton funding approvals.[17] Rather than accept responsibility for their own refusal to follow what was now federal law, Fowler argued that the Public Health Service was determined to assume that all hospitals in the South were "guilty of discrimination until proven innocent," which he found particularly offensive because Mississippi had a wonderful record of providing nondiscriminatory health care for Black patients, predating the Hill-Burton Act.

The appeal to Hill-Burton was disingenuous, as it actually and actively allowed for segregated facilities so long as "equal" services were available to Black patients. Under this interpretation, Fowler could claim that only 3 of Mississippi's 118 short-term acute-care hospitals were for white people only. "This is not surprising to people who know Mississippi," he stated, "since the custom of caring for negro patients in Mississippi hospitals antedates the Hill Burton Act itself. This custom is some 30 to 40 years older than the Civil Rights Act itself which is being used to make us a whipping boy."[18]

In this line of argument, Fowler is relying on the rhetoric of paternalistic benevolence so central to the Jim Crow routine, and he goes on to explain that the state should be held up as a beacon of progress for how many Black physicians they "allowed" to practice, with the caveat, "where they were suitably qualified." The issue, for Fowler and the Mississippi Commission on Hospital Care, was one of politics, where "the Public Health Service has been led so far afield from the primary purpose of the Hill-Burton Act, which is providing needed health facilities, in an effort to win glory for themselves in the field of race relations."[19] Of course, the primary purpose of the Hill-Burton Act had deliberately been to provide *segregated* healthcare facilities, which notoriously did *not* equate to equal services for Black patients, so in this sense Fowler was correct in his assessment of the PHS's stance. Integration was now the goal and the law, and the PHS intended to pursue it.

The complaints about delays in funding, and the link between federal funding and integration, was a subject of frequent complaint, especially regarding the introduction of Medicare in Mississippi. Stennis received a plethora of correspondence objecting to the need for white patients to be placed with Black patients in order to qualify for Medicare or Medicaid, even when that funding was desperately needed. Here, the rhetoric became one of freedom of choice, equality based on ability to pay, and the potentially disturbing effects of integration on the health and well-being of white patients.[20]

For example, Dr. W. K. Purks, chief of staff at Vicksburg Hospital, argued that the hospital considered itself completely desegregated but was having funding threatened because of a refusal to place Black and white patients in the same room. "We are now informed," he complained, "that we fail to comply because . . . we have not as yet forced white patients and colored patients to be housed in the same two-bed room. Forced compliance with this apparent 'guideline' is medically unsound in every respect and not in the best interest of the patient, either white or colored."[21]

This idea that integration was medically problematic appeared as frequent justification, with no scientific rationale or any evidence that the patients themselves saw it that way. At the same time, many of these hospitals charged a fee for service, which they stated was their only criteria for admission, arguing that this was "freedom of choice" and not discriminatory. Of course it was, and they knew it. Writing about Mercy Hospital in Vicksburg, Dr. Augustus Street noted that if they were forced to integrate Black and white patients in the same room, the white patients would exercise their freedom of choice to go elsewhere, while the Black patients would have no choice but to stay. "If we try to put white and colored patients in the same room, we would automatically convert the hospital into one for colored only," he argued.[22]

Dr. Street's comment demonstrated that the real nature of the problem was not medical vulnerability but white racism. Integration was a problem because it brought with it the threat of white flight and the loss of white dollars, a problem for which Black patients and their advocates would be blamed.

The ability of white supremacist groups to blame poor services or underfunding on integration rather than on their own resistance to federal funding was a particular quirk of the medical Jim Crow routine. In June 1966, Stennis received a copy of a statement from the Executive Committee of the Association of Citizens' Councils of Mississippi, who bundled civil rights with communism. The statement urged hospital administrators to "join in a united effort to deliver our citizens from the blight of socialized medicine by refusing to comply with the unreasonable, unworkable, and inhumane guidelines" that were being imposed by HEW.[23]

The Citizens' Councils would rather have no federal funding than be forced to lose the perceived "freedom of choice." Its members were in fact not interested in Medicare, arguing that the "rights of our citizens should not be bartered for a few federal dollars" and that the burden of Medicare would fall on taxpayers who would then be underwriting a "flood of patients not really needing medical attention, but insisting on their rights to 'free' services."[24] This argument of course neglected the fact that all Mississippians stood to benefit from Medicare, but this antipathy to the poor can also be read as antipathy to providing subsidized services for the Black community.

The Citizens' Councils also argued that white fragility posed as medical vulnerability was a reason to resist integration in the state psychiatric hospitals. In their statement, they wrote, "Forced integration in our mental institutions can have only an adverse effect on the mentally disturbed patients and obstruct their early return to society."[25] While Stennis did not reply to this statement, he did use medical justifications for segregation explicitly in his active campaign to find loopholes in the Civil Rights Act. On this front, he worked with fellow senators Richard Russell in Georgia and Lister Hill in Alabama to badger HEW officials about the terminology and wording of compliance guidelines in relation to hospitals.

Through the auspices of a Committee on Appropriations (Lister Hill was chair of the Subcommittee on Labor and Health, Education and Welfare and Related Agencies), the three conservative senators made an amendment to Section 206 of the HEW Appropriation Bill (H.R. 14745). That amendment, passed by the Senate on September 27, 1966, stated, "No funds appropriated by this Act shall be used to impose or enforce any requirement and responsibility so far as certified patients are concerned on any hospital or other medical facility as to an individual beneficiary or other medical facility which is contrary to the beneficiary's physical or mental well-being."[26] The senators met with secretary of HEW John Gardner in October 1966 to clarify the particularities of ward assignments for patients, specifics about timelines for compliance, and procedures for hearings regarding noncompliance.

There is a lot of intricate detail that is not necessary to repeat here, but the meeting resulted in a series of memos from John Gardner and Wilbur Cohen, the undersecretary, in which the federal administrators sought to placate the Southern segregationists. They assured the trio that administrators of the Civil Rights Act "will honor determinations made by physicians that are based on a valid medical reason for making room assignments in a hospital on a segregated basis. We will consider this determination to be conclusive as it applies to a specific patient. We will disregard patients assigned on a segregated basis as a result of a medical determination in evaluating the hospital's compliance with the provisions of Title VI of the Civil Rights Act unless it appears that over a period of time segregation is being practiced as a matter of policy under the guise of a medical determination."[27] This last sentence was the catch—how would the department decide if segregation was medically justified or being used as an excuse? This whole scenario reads like a disappointing capitulation from HEW and signals their own lack of fortitude when it came to enforcing the nondiscrimination requirements of the Civil Rights Act in medical settings.

This was, to some extent, a frustration also felt within the department itself. As a response to repeated complaints about lack of compliance, the Civil Rights Unit in HEW formed the Office of Equal Health Opportunity (OEHO), which reported to the Office of the Surgeon General. David Barton Smith has written extensively about the work of the OEHO and its leader, Robert Nash, who was a dedicated civil rights advocate who was frustrated by the lack of progress in medical settings. In his book *Health Care Divided*, Smith has argued that the state psychiatric hospitals that remained segregated in the South constituted fairly "easy targets" for OEHO except for those in Virginia, Alabama, and Mississippi.[28]

For example, Virginia tried to pursue a ridiculous "freedom of choice" line (ridiculous given the reality of involuntary commitment, which by definition ruled out the possibility of free choice about anything), which was relatively easily to overturn when the University of Virginia School of Medicine also had its funding threatened.[29] While "reason" may have eventually prevailed in that state, "the governors of Alabama and Mississippi saw them [the state hospitals] as emotional symbols that could be manipulated for political gain."[30]

In Smith's assessment, "Mississippi . . . represented the most difficult test for OEHO," but my own research suggests that in fact Alabama was the hardest nut to crack. Smith largely uses the memories and testimony of ex-OEHO worker and special counsel Marilyn Rose to make his argument and ends his short section on integration of state hospitals with her experience in Mississippi. In the section that follows here, I want to flip the timeline a little by starting with Mississippi and ending in Alabama, and I will add to the case Smith makes by supplementing Rose's memories with material from the archives in Mississippi and, significantly, from records associated with two combined court cases in Alabama.[31]

Rose visited Mississippi in May 1967, taking with her three OEHO staff members and a consultant psychiatrist.[32] The group visited Whitfield near Jackson, East Mississippi State Hospital in Meridian, and Ellisville, the state school for children. All three hospitals were (and still are) in the southern or eastern part of the state—Meridian literally on the border with Alabama on Highway 20; Ellisville about sixty miles southwest of Meridian on Highway 59, forming the bottom point of an inverted triangle; and Whitfield eighty miles to the northwest. At the time of the investigation, Eastern State Hospital in Meridian (completely white-only until October 1965) had admitted thirty-five mentally ill Black people (but twenty-eight of them were out on leave) and four Black "mentally retarded" people, while Ellisville had admitted thirteen Black children into its vocational rehabilitation program.[33] These small numbers of Black patients were one way that hospitals claimed integration on paper while maintaining beds for mostly white patients. Case in point: There were also 1,124 white children at Ellisville.

The team documented that "Whitfield is a strictly segregated institution, in which the Negro patients have separate and unequal facilities and services. . . . Negro mentally retarded persons are admitted to the Annex at Whitfield where there is no education or vocational rehabilitation program and they are kept in custodial care."[34] These notes about the differences in treatment and activity programs were important evidence against the state's stance that they were providing separate but equal facilities as required under Hill-Burton funding. That is, the fact of segregation was not the only problem; it was the lack of treatment and care that occurred under segregation that was also the issue.

This report also documented the amount of federal assistance each of these institutions stood to lose: $25,000 each for Whitfield and Ellisville for training programs, $100,000 for Ellisville for a hospital improvement grant, about $120,000 worth of surplus food commodities, and 75 percent of $146,000 for the vocational rehabilitation training program at Ellisville.[35] This was above any pending Medicare support or community mental health construction money—not a lot (about $400,000 in total), but enough to make a difference in a state with so little mental health funding.

Rose also met with Seth Hudspeth, the commissioner of mental health, and Dr. Jaquith, the director of Whitfield. The OEHO team initially proposed a plan for implementing desegregation, but Dr. Jaquith was not happy and "indicated at the negotiation meeting that he feared desegregation would lead to riots. He made some mention of broken coke bottles being a possible weapon."[36] This threat of violence went beyond the state line of concern for patient well-being and placed that concern fully in the context of the racial violence occurring in Mississippi at the time. The real danger that Jaquith was hinting at was more likely to be Black patients facing potential white violence. Of course, the OEHO inspectors, one of whom was a Southerner, reminded Jaquith that if "broken coke bottles would be the weapons, they would have to have been supplied from within and that the Director had the responsibility to see that did not happen. The director backed off."[37]

Jaquith's attitude was all bluster; he had been repeatedly requesting more money from the state to improve facilities and programs at Whitfield, and he knew how important this federal money would be. This political posturing was endemic to all the negotiations OEHO attempted in the South. For example, Rose documented that even if the OEHO plan was designed to give the state reasonable time in which to make the requisite changes, "Hudspeth actually advised us that he could not go forward to adopt the plan unless he was served with a Notice of Hearing, and that was made known to higher officials in HEW."[38] This tactic was purely political gamesmanship—Stennis, Governor Johnson, Hudspeth, and Jaquith alike all knew that integration was likely, that they needed Medicare funding, and that they needed the pending grants for improvements and training, but they could not be seen to give in to the federal government too easily.

Hudspeth got his notice of hearing, but not until December 1967. This delay was through no fault of Rose's. In the report attached to the letter from Peter Libassi, general counsel at HEW, a paragraph at the end documented "attempts to secure compliance by voluntary means," which set out the many steps the federal government had taken to inform and support administrators in Mississippi to integrate their mental health facilities. It was noted that as early as the fall of 1965, representatives of the regional NIMH office in Atlanta had visited and worked with the Board of Trustees of Mental Institutions in Mississippi to develop a plan that had been scheduled to be put in place in June 1966 but was not. Libassi's report documented the OEHO team visit in May 1967, which had led to a new plan for compliance dated June 2, 1967, which received no response. Neither did a follow-up letter sent in September 1967. "By telephone HEW was informed that the plan could not be instituted," the report stated.[39]

But this is not quite how Marilyn Rose remembered things. In her interview, she recounted how she had returned to Washington, DC, and immediately prepared a notice of hearing and had been cleared to send it, but she needed a signature from Robert Nash, who was out of town. His deputy had taken the papers back to his office, where he stated he needed to review them. When Rose asked him for the papers, he refused, and then Wilbur Cohen, the undersecretary of HEW, agreed to stop the notice from going forward "in response to some promise (or threat) to the welfare appropriation."[40] It is possible that Cohen was referring here to the loopholes about medical justifications for segregation that Stennis, Russell, and Hill were working on.

Rose and Nash were angry and frustrated by the delay—"angry that the civil rights considerations would take a back seat" and frustrated by the way that the department continued to negotiate with the Southern senators, who themselves used the position of resistance as political ammunition. Rose's final recollection of the situation in Mississippi is particularly telling: "When I finally sent the notice out, Hudspeth called me, and asked, 'What took you so long?' I responded, 'You know, and I know, and Senator Stennis knows, what took us so long.' He laughed and said, 'Well I couldn't do anything until I got it, you knew that.'" After that incident, Rose recalled, "Once I was given the go-ahead to send out notices of hearing, I made sure they were sent out as quickly as possible and would not even use the mail room, but had my secretary mail the notices in U.S. mail boxes outside the building."[41]

There is no evidence beyond this point that Mississippi continued to drag the proverbial chain—Whitfield and Meridian and Ellisville were all slowly integrated from that point on—but there is certainly plenty of evidence to indicate that integration itself did not solve the broader problems of lack of funding for public mental health services in the state, which remained the subject of public scrutiny for some time.[42]

Running a Southern Plantation: The OEHO in Alabama

While the notice to Mississippi might have been the last notice of hearing for a psychiatric hospital Rose needed to send out, it was still the case that integration was far from achieved in Alabama. Rose and her team from OEHO had visited Bryce and Searcy Hospitals in the summer of 1966 and had been horrified by what they found. In an interview some thirty years later, Rose remembered the visits in detail. Her impressions are worth repeating in full, not least because they support and replicate the conditions that LeFlore and the reporters from *The Southern Courier* had already documented:

> While the staffing and services at Bryce as a whole were a mixed bag, services for patients at Searcy were custodial, and the general wards were horrid. There were only 5 doctors, 4 of whom were foreign (whose primary language was not English); they were not licensed in the United States and did not have credentials as psychiatrists in their native country. The fifth psychiatrist was the Administrator, obviously not conversant with modern psychiatry, and seemed to be running a southern plantation. A visit to the wards suggested to me what one might have found in the nineteenth century, at a time when mental patients were warehoused. The wards looked like prison cells. It was a scene out of a Kafka play.[43]

These horrors were not confined to the adult hospitals. Rose also visited the Partlow State School and Hospital in Tuscaloosa, which took both Black and white children but segregated them from each other in the same building. She recalled, "We went into the day room of one ward of black patients who were profoundly mentally retarded, with physical handicaps as well; many of them were sitting and/or lying on the floor in their own excrement. . . . There was no ward for white profoundly retarded to match the depth of despair and mistreatment as this one for blacks."[44] Rose's observations demonstrate that "separate but equal" was never a reality in medical or psychiatric facilities. Instead, the practice had created a space where people could be removed from visibility entirely, and where Black patients existed in a complete vacuum of approaches to treatment or care.

Exposing these conditions was not without risks. Like many civil rights activists working in Alabama at the time, Rose and her colleagues found themselves the subject of intimidation, harassment, and violence. Their visits attracted significant media attention, and they were frequently followed by Federal Bureau of Investigation agents. Witnesses in the cases were given the lawyers' home phone numbers after someone fired a shot into a witness's home. Two of Rose's fellow investigators in Demopolis, Alabama, were arrested on a bogus stolen vehicle charge. Rose herself was lucky to emerge unharmed from an incident in Tuscaloosa in which the lugs of the front wheel of her rental car were removed while it was parked outside Bryce Hospital.[45] She remained undeterred, however, and prepared a brief for the surgeon general and HEW, articulating the many ways in which the state of Alabama's provision of mental health services breached the Civil Rights Act.

The evidence Rose presented was a litany of horrors. At Bryce Hospital, 400 Black patients were housed in either Treatment Center Number 2 (the Jemison Center), located eight miles from the main complex, or Ward X and the Lodge "for the purposes of performing work at or around these facilities."[46] Rose noted that "Ward X is particularly unsatisfactory. Negroes are housed in the old, dimly lighted building solely to work in the laundry and certain kitchen areas at Bryce. The building is adjacent to the laundry, is set off from the rest of the complex, and has a living space comprised of one large room with approximately 87 beds in close quarters. The Lodge apparently is a converted stable and is located at the rear of the main complex."[47] At Searcy, the 2,500 Black patients were subjected to facilities that were "very old and crowded, have no day rooms, and have bare cement floors and seating consisting of backless wooden benches. Bryce has many recreational and occupational programs and craft shops, Searcy has a television set, dominos and cards if requested, and a weekly visit from the recreation department."[48]

While the documents do not detail the specifics of treatment, they do note that no Black patients were part of the large PHS grant for young men with schizophrenia, and that inferiority in treatment and care was compounded by discrimination and lack of spending in staffing. They also noted that there were no Black professional staff members, such as physicians, psychologists, and nurses, at the three institutions. While Bryce Hospital offered extensive nurse training for schools throughout the state, which supplied ready labor, no nurses' training program had ever existed or been sought at Searcy. Similarly, expenditures at Searcy were proportionately lower per patient than at Bryce, and Searcy had never applied for any PHS grants. Rose also noted that "the Negro employees of the state institutions execute their functions under segregated, unequal, and inferior working conditions."[49] This included separate dining areas and a pay system that had previously discriminated based on race but was now focused on the dubious idea of "merit," which would not see pay parity achieved until 1973.[50] Based on these findings, Rose was given permission to issue a notice of administrative hearing.

The hearing itself took place in Washington, DC, in the spring of 1967. Rose organized HEW's case and called on expert testimony from psychiatrists from New York and Baltimore, as well as local psychiatrists from the University of Alabama. She was deliberate with her witnesses, choosing people from both the North and the South who could argue against Alabama's position that "it would be medically detrimental to integrate white and black patients and could cause riots."[51]

Dr. Robert Hunt from New York State Hospitals department argued that even though he had no personal experience of working in a segregated system, he knew many "deep south psychiatrists" who had told him that they see "no clinical grounds for separating treatment of patients on racial grounds."[52] Dr. James E. Carson from the Department of Mental Hygiene in Baltimore, a native of South Carolina, argued that he thought he "knew what a Southerner was" and saw no reason why the South should continue its segregated practices. He related the experience of a state hospital on Maryland's Eastern Shore that had been segregated until 1963 but now had an integrated staff and treated all patients, regardless of race.

Despite the institution's location in a region of Maryland that was historically "similar to the South in cultural attitudes" and had experienced widespread civil rights–era strife, there were no problems within the hospital itself. He also pointed out that there were no contraindications from integrating patients, including among the "white patients placed in the hospital which formerly had been all Negro."[53] That is, the argument that white patients would be harmed in some way was groundless. Importantly, Dr. Carson, under cross-examination, pointed out that integration had not proven a barrier to recruiting staff.[54] This testimony actively rebutted the state of Alabama's arguments that cultural norms should be maintained for safety and that broader civil rights unrest would prove dangerous to the patients themselves.

These pro-integration arguments were reinforced by three influential psychiatrists from within Alabama: Dr. Patrick Linton, Dr. James Folsom, and Dr. John Carter. Linton was associate professor of psychiatry at the University of Alabama at Birmingham and a consultant to the Birmingham VA Hospital. He was a progressive psychiatrist, at the vanguard of new treatments that departed from older ideas about racial difference, and testified that there was "no therapeutic counter-indication from treating psychiatric patients in an integrated hospital."[55]

Similarly, Dr. James Folsom saw "no therapeutic disadvantage of integrating white and Negro patients."[56] Significantly, Folsom pointed out that the belief in the inferiority of black mentality had no scientific justification. Rather, he argued, any difference in IQ between Black and white patients was "due to social-economic factors, not to race."[57] These ideas were reinforced from the African American perspective by the testimony of Dr. John Carter.

Carter had been a psychiatrist with the Tuskegee Institute and the Tuskegee VA Hospital since the 1950s and was now working at the Salisbury VA Hospital in North Carolina. As he pointed out, the VA Hospital at Tuskegee had always taken white patients and had never experienced any problems, and neither were there any at his current hospital. He stated that Tuskegee employed Black staff to care for white patients "from deep south" areas, and this too had caused no problems.[58]

The testimony of the psychiatrists at the hearing is interesting because it runs counter to the long narrative of racial difference that had underpinned American medicine and reveals the shifts in psychiatric thinking that had begun to take place outside the South.[59] At the same time, white psychiatrists from Alabama had also been part of the segregated system they now sought to critique. Their willingness to testify and the strength of their evidence indicated a shift in psychiatric thinking that put the state's continual reference to "medical justification" on unstable ground.

The hearing also revealed the way that debates about justifications for segregation were largely knowingly disingenuous and part of the usual performance of Jim Crow politics for segregationist governors. The rights of patients to more and better services came very low in the list of gubernatorial priorities and were easily sacrificed on the altar of states' rights rhetoric, which Alabama used to justify its continued resistance to the legal mandate to integrate.

"Alabama Dares Defend Its Rights"

When you drive along I-85 from Atlanta, Georgia, to Montgomery, Alabama, there is a rest stop just across the border. I stopped at it many times during my research trips to the Alabama Department of Archives and History or to the Tuskegee University Archives. The semi-confederate state flag flies above the blond concrete building, and there is a little stone marker with the phrase "Alabama Dares Defend Its Rights" etched into it. This statement seemed a direct reference to the recalcitrance and defiance I would always find in the archives but at the same time a sad reference to the cost of that defiance. Nowhere is that cost more clearly demonstrated than in the state's stance against integration of its psychiatric hospitals, which continues to cause major problems for the provision of mental health care in Alabama today. In this section, I look at the way this belligerence against federal interference manifested in the state's initial approach to operationalizing integration in its psychiatric facilities, and how this performance led to a long and expensive court case.

The campaign for medical integration largely paralleled the governorship of George Wallace, who was no stranger to the fight against civil rights and a master at manipulating public perception for political expediency.[60] His approach to desegregating psychiatric hospitals was no different from the way he had approached educational integration or any other matter related to racial equality. As per usual, he relied on denial, obfuscation, and public blustering to resist integration.[61]

As had been the case in Mississippi before HEW had begun its investigation, Wallace's strategy with psychiatric hospitals was to wait and see; on June 4, 1965, Wallace sent the superintendent of Alabama State Hospitals, James Tarwater, a memo thanking him for their fruitful meeting "the other day" (see figure 8.1). In reference to "the matter we discussed," Wallace made vague suggestions about "the movement" and "let's see what will happen."[62]

As far as I can tell this is one of the very few times that Tarwater ever met with the governor, and he would not have done so over a trifle. It seems safe to assume that they discussed integration and had agreed to a transfer of patients, and that Wallace decided to say nothing public about it. Both Wallace and Tarwater knew something had to give—Tarwater had been under constant siege from HEW and the Public Health Service regional office in Atlanta for months.

As the director of the Alabama Mental Health Board, which oversaw all mental health and psychiatric facilities in the state, Tarwater was asked to prove these services' compliance with the Civil Rights Act. In July 1965, he sent a series of memos to various facility and clinic directors asking them to verify their compliance in writing.[63] The process of establishing written compliance revealed that the state hospitals were clearly not compliant. The PHS constantly reminded Tarwater that he needed to do more than simply submit a form.[64] William Page, the director of the PHS in Atlanta, stated that the department would not hesitate to take legal action if desegregation

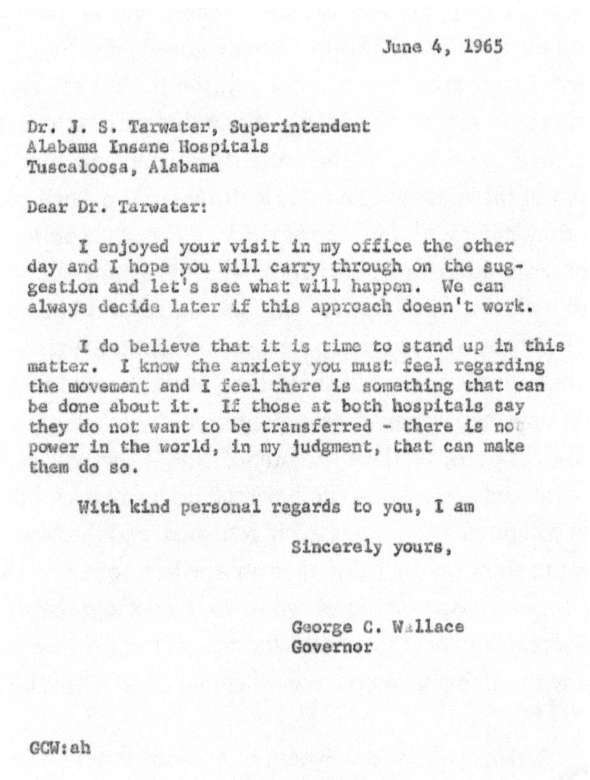

FIGURE 8.1 George Wallace to James Tarwater, June 4, 1965, box SG021951, folder 18, Alabama Governor State Institutions Files, 1963–1979, ADAH.

> June 4, 1965
>
> Dr. J. S. Tarwater, Superintendent
> Alabama Insane Hospitals
> Tuscaloosa, Alabama
>
> Dear Dr. Tarwater:
>
> I enjoyed your visit in my office the other day and I hope you will carry through on the suggestion and let's see what will happen. We can always decide later if this approach doesn't work.
>
> I do believe that it is time to stand up in this matter. I know the anxiety you must feel regarding the movement and I feel there is something that can be done about it. If those at both hospitals say they do not want to be transferred - there is no power in the world, in my judgment, that can make them do so.
>
> With kind personal regards to you, I am
>
> Sincerely yours,
>
> George C. Wallace
> Governor
>
> GCW:ah

was not actively pursued.⁶⁵ The Alabama Mental Health Board was not in a hurry to comply, and it was not until December 1965 that it finally resolved to take action, which still took months to enact.

Eventually, on March 14, 1966, Tarwater ordered that thirty Black women from Searcy Hospital be transferred to Bryce and, in exchange, thirty white women be moved to Searcy. It seems likely that the patients being "transferred" were the ones referred to in Wallace's memo from some ten months earlier, although this is never explicitly acknowledged. The *Montgomery Advertiser* ran a story the next day titled "Mental Facilities Desegregated," in which it reported, "One of the few remaining areas of racial discrimination in Alabama tumbled Monday with the announcement that the state mental facilities are being desegregated July 1."⁶⁶ While Mental Health Board member Dr. Robert Parker admitted that the move "was a bitter pill to take," he also made clear that the threatened withdrawal of federal funds had compelled him and his colleagues to "vote unanimously for compliance with the Civil Rights Act of 1964."⁶⁷

Governor Wallace was notably quiet on the issue. There was no public comment from him until the relatives of a white woman named Pearl Stokes, who had been transferred to Searcy, organized a petition for her release, which they sent directly to US senator Lister Hill. When this petition made the news, Wallace claimed ignorance of the patient transfer and sent a telegram to all members of the Alabama Mental Health Board on April 26, 1966, demanding that they meet with him the next day. Given the communication with Tarwater from almost a year before, we can assume that in fact Wallace knew full well that the transfer was scheduled and had remained silent about it until the Stokes family went to the senator registering their dissatisfaction with the move. At that point, Wallace used false outrage to capitalize on popular support for resegregation.

At the meeting with the board, Wallace threatened that if they did not move the patients back immediately, he would have the highway patrol do it for them.[68] The board complied, the patients were returned, and the *Montgomery Advertiser* ran that story on the front page on April 27, 1966.[69] As a result of the reversal, Tarwater was forced to report to the regional office of the Public Health Service on June 20, 1966, that the state of Alabama would not be taking any more formal steps toward compliance with Title VI of the Civil Rights Act.[70]

During this back and forth, Wallace received a number of letters from his constituents demonstrating the type of support that existed for segregation. On April 4, 1966, Wallace received a copy of a letter that Mr. J. S. Haddock had written to Tarwater to which he added a note for the governor.[71] Haddock complained that the patient transfer was "the most damnable thing possible for poor, innocent, helpless people, especially a Southern Educated Woman who has suffered the misfortune of a sick mind . . . AND NOW SHE IS TO BE PLACED WITH NEGROES. You are sentencing her to death" (emphasis in the original). Here, Haddock was drawing on well understood ideas about the danger that the "Angry Black Man" posed to the "innocent white woman," the fear of bodily contact, miscegenation, and the invasion of intimate (white) spaces by the Black body.

Haddock also placed his concerns in the context of anti-federalism when he argued, "And now, we are to be taken over by and ruled by JOHNSON, Negroes and Communists." The rhetorical linking of progressive President Johnson and civil rights with communism was a familiar trope in the rhetoric of anti-integration groups and would have made perfect sense to Wallace.[72] Equally powerful was Haddock's reminder to Wallace of his vote, which he expected to be in service of "states' rights": "It appears to me, we are being force [sic] to surrender, or sell our birth rights, for Federal Aid Money? We may suffer for a while, but any and every sacrifice, will prove beneficial."[73] This is the same attitude that public health officer Dr. Ira Myers had lamented in his community mental health plan and represented the anti-federalism that undercut Alabama's willingness to subscribe to any federal grant scheme that would in fact have benefited all Alabamians.

Wallace replied to letters like the one from Mr. McCarn that opened this chapter and this one from Mr. Haddock using very careful language that reinforced the ideas of his supporters but without any overt racial prejudice. By the late 1960s, segregationist language was shifting to a more race-neutral tone, and as historian Dan T. Carter has argued, Wallace knew when to be more outspoken and when to be careful.[74] When writing letters that could prove difficult to explain away later, his language was not inflammatory but drew on what he claimed were medical justifications for segregation and what would be best for patients. There is no evidence that Wallace had read any of the psychiatric or psychological literature that had historically constructed this justification, but the frequency and ease with which he used this defense demonstrates how widespread and well established these thoughts were.[75] They indicate not only a "scientific" rationale for segregation but also a social one, in the context of medical facilities where the intimate closeness of bodies was cause for segregationist concern.

Wallace reiterated this point in a reply to Mr. Eugene Threadgill when he wrote, "It has always been my contention that the integration of mental patients would be very harmful to the patients themselves."[76] Wallace was no medical expert, but he did have access to members of a Mental Health Board who were not keen to overturn existing social relations in facilities where people had impaired memory, cognition, and self-control. It is entirely possible that knowing that the three Southern senators were also using "medical justifications" to find loopholes in Civil Rights Act compliance, Wallace felt he was on relatively safe and neutral ground with this repeated claim. His real concern, however, was the rhetoric of states' rights, and he followed up his comment to Threadgill with the telling statement that "this is just another area where the Federal government is trying to impose its will upon the rights of the sovereign people of a state."[77]

Some Alabamians, however, were aware that this insistence on segregation would lead to increased funding pressures, and they told Wallace so. Mrs. Alpha Corkle, a white woman, sent Wallace a petition signed by more than thirty people from Opelika. Corkle's husband was a patient at Bryce, and she understood that the refusal to integrate would mean a loss of federal funds. "Since all patients benefit from the funds," she wrote, "I would like to appeal to you to change this situation. I am sure the patients would rather associate with Negroes than have the lack of attention they need."[78] In this response, Corkle exemplified the concerns of white moderates who favored practical accommodations rather than continued resistance because they also stood to gain—what Derrick Bell has called "interest-convergence."[79]

Wallace assured her that no funds had been lost and again used the rhetoric of medical benefit to justify his actions, writing, "It is my understanding that some eminent psychologists would testify that it is very detrimental to the health and welfare of patients for them to be integrated."[80] Wallace gave no source for his information, but in these responses he was drawing on older psychiatric rhetoric that argued that segregation was necessary because the mentally ill, especially those with any kind of dementia, were liable to act out in racially motivated violence.[81] In this rationale, the fear was almost always for the white male patient, who could be the victim of (however righteous) Black anger, or the white female patient, who could be the victim of mythical Black sexual avarice.[82] Even though these ideas were becoming outdated in the medical literature, they still held sway in the popular consciousness and would prove hard to dislodge.[83]

Not everyone in Alabama's mental health system believed that segregation was necessary, however. An anonymous employee from Searcy Hospital wrote in opposition to the integration reversal, stating that there had been no problems with the original integration attempt, from either patients or staff, and that to move people again would simply add more stress to already emotionally vulnerable people. The employee called Wallace out on his blatant opportunism and accused him of adding unnecessary fuel to the fire of Alabama's resistance to integration.

"The action you have taken," the writer stated, "will only slow down the eventual complete integration and place on public display hundreds of mentally ill patients as well as endangering their lives and the lives of already underpaid, overworked employees. Trouble is already expected this weekend in the form of a demonstration. You know what this involves. If you think placing lives of incompetent persons in danger is the only way to get votes and makes you rest better at night, I feel sorry for you. Signed, one of the underpaid, overworked employees that really enjoys the work."[84] Here the writer made clear to Wallace that the only danger to patients was from the extreme violence of white supremacists, a danger borne out in LeFlore's investigation.

In fact, the state's argument that it was in the medical interests of all patients to maintain segregation had no support from anyone working within the system itself, including Tarwater. While Tarwater made no conclusions as to the medical benefits of segregation, he testified at the HEW hearing that the integration attempt had not, despite the protestations of some family members, caused any distress to or complaints from the patients themselves.[85]

At the same time as the state was playing political games, the Legal Defense Fund (LDF) was preparing to act, helped by the evidence compiled by LeFlore and the Medical Committee for Human Rights. On February 23, 1966, LeFlore received a letter from Conrad Harper at the LDF head office in New York. Harper was new to the LDF, having graduated from Howard University, then Harvard Law School in 1965. He had worked on the Civil Rights Commission during his summer internships, and the LDF was his first legal job.[86] He was handed the Alabama case by Michael Meltsner after LeFlore wrote again to James Quigley at HEW and copied in the LDF. Harper wrote to LeFlore, "Mr. Meltsner is of the opinion the only way to obtain significant action with respect to these hospitals is to file suit."[87] This meant ascertaining the status of federal funding for the hospitals and building a case from the ground up with affidavits, like the one from Mrs. Brown (see chapter 7).[88]

The LDF was building this case at the same time as the HEW investigation, and when that investigation was complete, the US surgeon general found Alabama in breach of the Civil Rights Act and ordered that all current applications for funding be suspended until compliance could be secured.[89] Rather than accept this finding and find ways to become compliant, on October 13, 1967, Alabama's attorney general MacDonald Gallion filed a complaint in US district court (Civil Action No. 2610). Instead of arguing that the state was medically justified to segregate facilities (a claim that might have held popular rather than legal sway), the complaint rested on a charge of federal overreach.[90]

Before the court had a chance to act on this complaint, the LDF launched a countercomplaint. On November 17, 1967, the complaint in *Marable v. Alabama Mental Health Board* (Civil Action No. 2615), a class action on behalf of patients, was filed in the district court by the LDF's Jack Greenberg, Michael Meltsner, and Conrad Harper, and Birmingham civil rights attorneys Orzell Billingsley and Demetrius Newton. The named plaintiffs were Loveman Marable from Bryce Hospital (a client of Newton's) and Joe Nathan Brown Jr. from Searcy Hospital (the subject of the affidavit secured by

LeFlore in August 1966).[91] The complaint rested on charges of blatant discrimination against and inferiority of services for Black patients. Their relatives were also named as Alabama taxpayers seeking to secure nondiscriminatory treatment for their relatives as patients. The original complaint listed the many ways in which the services provided were both separate and unequal, which LeFlore and Stiles had gleaned from their own investigations supporting the evidence presented in Rose's case at the administrative hearing.[92]

The two cases were filed in the Middle District court in Montgomery, Alabama, bringing them within the purview of Judge Frank M. Johnson. Given Johnson's record in continually upholding federal civil rights law in Alabama and forging new ground for the active protection of those rights, it may seem curious that Alabama even bothered to fight the case.[93] Indeed, in a memo to the other judges, Johnson noted that both sides recognized "what they consider to be inevitable, that is, an adjudication that the statutes and present practice that require segregation on the basis of race or color is illegal and in violation of Title VI of the Civil Rights Act of 1964, and the Fourteenth Amendment to the Constitution of the United States."[94] However, the performative aspect of the attorney general's political strategy dictated that Alabama's administration make a show of fighting back. The point for segregationist bureaucrats and politicians was not necessarily to win or lose but to perform Alabama's official motto—"We dare defend our rights"—and to garner popular support for doing so.[95]

Noting that the two cases now before him dealt with the same issue, and that there were constitutional implications at stake, Johnson requested the consolidation of the cases and an identical three-judge panel for both (Frank Johnson, John Godbold, and Virgil Pittman). The case from each side was built on the testimony and evidence contained in the record of the administrative proceeding, now known as Docket MCR44.[96] There was no trial. Instead, parties prepared briefs and responses, and then representatives from each side appeared in Johnson's chambers to argue their respective positions.[97] At no point in the court proceedings did the State of Alabama dispute the findings of either the investigation or the administrative hearing. There were now no references to the rhetoric of "medical justification" for segregation that had featured in Wallace's letter writing. Rather, the state's complaint was a long list of ways that the federal government had not followed correct procedure (even when it had) and demonstrated an intention to fight over loopholes rather than any substantive content about racial segregation.

The Alabama attorney general used language familiar to many white Southerners to describe the intervention of the federal government in the affairs of Alabama, including the claim that rather than out of concern for patients, "the present controversy arises because when, like the proverbial camel, HEW gets its nose under the tent in one federally supported program, it insists that all programs operated by the Alabama Mental Health Board must integrate whether or not they are supported by federal funds."[98]

This comment indicated that the state had adopted the deliberate tactic of underfunding to avoid surveillance and compliance. That is, if there were no federal funds being used in a particular facility (in this instance, Searcy Hospital), then, the state argued, it was not required to comply with Title VI. The issue for Johnson, as it had been for HEW general counsel, was moot—some parts of the state's mental health program did receive federal funding, so all parts of the program needed to be in compliance.[99]

On February 11, 1969, the court handed down its finding in what Judge Johnson described as "long and complicated litigation over a rather straightforward problem."[100] He gave officials three months to integrate the Partlow school and hospital and twelve months to integrate Bryce and Searcy's patient population and declared Sections 207, 208, 209, and 248 of Title 45 of the Alabama code, which allowed and facilitated segregation, to be in violation of the Fourteenth Amendment.[101]

For Johnson, the cases were an important part of his overall strategy of using judicial activism to fight desegregation in all areas in Alabama.[102] He likened his approach in these mental health cases to the way he had ruled in educational segregation: "that the patients were entitled to non-racial staff assignments."[103] Johnson signaled his intent to do more than just rule against the state but to demand affirmative action in the transfer of patients, the employment of staff, and the pay and conditions for employees.[104] The court also ordered that the administrators of the Alabama Mental Health System report to the court on their integration progress every six months until the court was satisfied.

Judge Johnson was also presiding over other mental health and civil rights cases during this time, which complicates our understanding of the effectiveness of this legal action in integrating mental health facilities in Alabama. The reports from the *Marable* case continued until at least 1975, even after Johnson had ruled in another extremely significant mental health case, *Wyatt v. Stickney*, about the rights of all patients. It is possible to link the *Marable* case to *Wyatt* through an expansion of the concept of civil rights to patient (or human) rights, something that historians and Johnson himself later considered when assessing the cases.[105] However, at the time, Johnson made a clear link between his affirmative action in *Marable* and another case about the rights of Black workers to equal pay, *US v. Frazer*.[106] This case was pending at the same time as Johnson was considering the evidence in the *Marable* case, and it sought to end discrimination in employment practices in federally funded grant-in-aid programs in Alabama. The Department of Mental Health was also a defendant in the *Frazer* case. Johnson saw *Marable* as a central case in his efforts to uphold federal civil rights law in both *Frazer* and the later *Wyatt* because it "is the only decision and decree which addresses across-the-board employment, by race, by the Department of Mental Health."[107]

As LeFlore had argued, the issue on which the court could unequivocally rule was the integration of personnel and the eradication of unequal pay and working conditions under the Constitution and Title VI of the 1964 Civil Rights Act. By using the *Marable* reporting requirement, Johnson was able to continue to gather data about the employment and payment practices of workers within the mental health system and continue to put pressure on the state to apply for federal funds for construction, research, and training.[108] He used the same reporting system to monitor the integration of patients, and in the later *Wyatt* and follow-up cases, he instituted a human rights commission to monitor the other constitutional protections afforded to patients.[109] The reports submitted to the court over the next eight years demonstrate a continued pattern of attempts at integration of patients and personnel, and the failure to meet even barely minimal standards.

In his final ruling in *Marable v. Alabama Mental Health Board*, Johnson noted that the record "reveals considerable expert testimony to the effect that there is no medical justification for the segregation of patients and personnel in the Alabama mental health system."[110] While he reserved the right for physicians to make medical decisions that included a patient's fears and delusions, he warned the state that "racial classifications are always suspect" and that medical justifications for segregation would not fare well in his court.[111]

In this statement, Johnson was referring to the amendment that Stennis and Co. were able to sneak into civil rights compliance for hospitals, but the judge made it clear what he thought of that loophole and called the segregationists out. He also spoke, advertently or not, to a major problem at the heart of medical and psychiatric logic: the practice of making diagnoses along racial lines. They were, and are, always suspect, and yet long after science proved otherwise, they continue to prevail.

Whether or not race was a biological fact that required different forms of diagnosis, treatment, and care, the racism that drove white people's behavior was not miraculously eradicated by the Civil Rights Act. Similarly, the court finding that there was no medical justification for separate and unequal treatment based on race did not end the practice. The idea that it was no longer acceptable to talk about racial segregation created a kind of "race-neutral language" that worked to hide continued disparities because many mental health institutions stopped recording the race of patients entirely.[112]

This was reinforced by the same "freedom of choice" rhetoric that was being used to justify continued educational segregation. In the case of mental health, families and relatives of patients were now "free" to have patients committed to any institution that they could pay for, usually private and usually the one closest to home, thereby reinforcing existing economic and geographical segregation. At the same time, the rhetoric of racial difference between the white and Black psyche found new forms of expression in the marketing of race-specific drugs dressed as science and the changing diagnostic criteria that now cast the Black man as inherently more aggressive.[113] This was not new rhetoric, merely a repackaging of much older ideas in the history of American psychiatry and medicine.[114]

None of these ideas or practices were news to Black people themselves. They knew all too well that medical spaces were not necessarily safe ones, and that the institutions that purported to care for them were in no way exempt from the rhetorical and actual violence of white supremacy.[115] Patients, relatives, and activists approached those institutions with caution yet continued to demand their rights as citizens and taxpayers. It was through these demands that activists sought to end Jim Crow in the asylum, but the state fight to maintain it came at a great cost to all people in the Southern states.

As Dr. Myers knew all too well, the "crippling preoccupation with race" meant that more money was spent on fighting the federal government than on applying for new mental health funding. Today, the three states in this book are ranked among the lowest for access to care (Mississippi is ranked 50, Alabama 47, Georgia 46), and spend more money on building new prisons than on expanding Medicaid.[116] Most of the hospitals in this book in their original form no longer exist, but the poor and people of color in the southeast continue to find themselves at the mercy of separate and unequal mental health care as white supremacy is remade beyond the asylum walls.

Aftermath
Mrs. F.'s Letter

....

May 20, 1972
Sen. Herman Talmadge
Dear Sir,
I came home from Milledgeville Hospital. . . . My mind isn't functioning too well yet but believe me I know enough to have the Hospital investigated. They are treating the colored patients much worse than white, and I don't put myself above no one regardless of color. That is no place for anyone to go. They're giving shock treatments to people who aren't half as crazy at the doctor is. . . . God knows the patients scream, especially when electricity is turned on them and especially colored ones. . . . They force mostly colored people to work in [the] kitchen. . . . If they catch patients crying they give them shock treatments. . . . Lord I can still hear the screams of those people. I can't sleep nights for being haunted by those crys [sic]. . . . I promised the patients I'd try to do something so please I beg you to try and do something before more die. It isn't fair especially to colored ones. I pray some way this brutality is stopped, so pray pray without ceasing I'd like to see equal rights for colored people. May this nation see peace.
Mrs. F.

Mrs. F. wrote her letter to the conservative senator more than seven years after Georgia had agreed to comply with the Civil Rights Act of 1964, a fact of which she seemed well aware.[1] For Mrs. F., the rights of "colored patients" were indelibly connected to the enactment of their broader civil rights. The connection between psychiatry and civil rights is not, and was never, an "on the side" cultural issue. Rather, there could be no equality for Black patients within psychiatry because psychiatry itself was indelibly racist, constituted by the racist society in which it was formed and then reinforcing and constitutive of that racism itself.

The focus in this book on segregation as one enactment of that racism—one way of performing the Jim Crow routine—has been a deliberate choice in order to show both the strengths and the limitations of the formal civil rights movement's ability to challenge the racism at the heart of medical discourses themselves. Segregation as a social or legal practice could be challenged by activists, by families, and by the court itself, but it could not eradicate the underlying anti-Blackness that has always shaped and continues to shape mental health care in the aftermath of desegregation and deinstitutionalization. In this closing chapter, therefore, I want to trace some of the long-term impacts of the legal fight to end segregation, to think about the strengths and limitations of a "civil rights" approach to psychiatry, and to explore some possible moments when psychiatry could have, and should have, made different choices.

The civil rights case in Alabama was not the end of the legal story but the beginning of a whole new one. *Marable v. Alabama Mental Health Board* was a case that set in motion a chain of events that links past to present like a trail of dominoes, one tile falling with a clink against the next, demonstrating how everything is always connected.

From *Marable*, Judge Johnson learned not just about segregation but about atrocious conditions for all patients. As someone with skin in the game not just in terms of upholding federal civil rights law but in personal experience with a mentally ill child, he went out of his way to advise local lawyers on how to make a case against the entire Alabama mental health system that would stick. In 1968, the state had finally employed an actual psychiatrist, Dr. Stonewall Stickney, as its first commissioner of the new Department of Mental Health. Stickney was pro-integration and drew the ire of Governor Wallace, who threatened to cut funding to Bryce Hospital in Tuscaloosa.

Journalist Paul Davis remembers Stickney's first impressions of Bryce Hospital: "Folding his arms across his chest, he simply said 'The thing this hospital needs is some real therapy. Bulldozer therapy. These wards look just like chicken coops. No one should have to live like that.' He was right of course."[2] When some local workers, including the aunt of patient Ricky Wyatt, decided to sue the state to halt the funding threat, Judge Johnson told their lawyers that he could not rule on a labor case, but he could rule on a patients' rights case, particularly anything that related to the newly established "right to treatment."[3]

The lawyers established a class action known as *Wyatt v. Stickney*, and in 1971, hot on the heels of his decision in *Marable v. Alabama Mental Health Board*, Judge Johnson ruled that patients being held in a so-called hospital not only had a right to treatment but were entitled to minimum standards of care.⁴ The decision in that case, rendered in a district court, was monumental and transformative, but it was not easily implemented. The minimum standards were devised by a panel of psychiatric experts from across the country and included a plan for programs that would support the release of many thousands of patients.

The potential cost was enormous, and rather than pay it, the State of Alabama again chose to litigate. There are many follow-up cases to the original—*Wyatt v. Alderholt, Lynch v. Baxley*—and the original remedies set out in *Wyatt v. Stickney* were not ruled as met, or the case dismissed, until December 2003, under Judge Johnson's immediate successor, Judge Myron Thompson. Between them, Judges Johnson and Thompson have ruled over and tried to shape Alabama's mental health policy for more than fifty years. Thompson continues to advocate for the rights of the mentally ill in his work on Alabama prison reform in cases like *Braggs v. Dunn*.⁵ In another interesting twist, Judge Thompson is from Tuskegee—born in 1947, the same year that the Mental Hygiene Clinic was established.

Wyatt v. Stickney was one of the longest and most expensive class actions ever litigated in the United States, according to one of the lead plaintiffs, Mr. James Tucker from the Alabama Disability Advocacy Program (ADAP). I have had the great pleasure of getting to know Mr. Tucker through my research for this book. His personal tour of the old grounds of Bryce Hospital, which is now the property of the University of Alabama, where the football stadium and coach's budget are multiple times the entire state's mental health budget, shaped the form and content of this book before I had even started writing. Mr. Tucker explains the consequences of *Wyatt* better than I ever could in his own writing, but I remember meeting him for the first time in the café at the back of Manna Grocery & Deli in a little strip mall on a gray, rainy day in Tuscaloosa, and asking him whether the state's continued refusal to spend money on mental health care was because of race. He hesitated for a minute and then said, "Yes, and the poor. They don't want to spend money on *those people*."⁶

The irony, of course, is that they have spent far more on litigating the federal orders in the mental health cases and the subsequent prison cases, in which Judge Thompson's assessment of Alabama's mental health care was simply, "woeful and inadequate."⁷ Beth Shelburne has covered this situation in her brilliant article and reporting related to Jamie Lee Wallace (no relation to the governor) and all the people who have died from lack of mental health care in Alabama's prisons.⁸ This belligerence occurs in the context of spending $3 billion on new prisons, which makes a total lie of the state's claim that it cannot afford to provide better mental health care.

While many historians rightly argue for nuance and tentativeness around the claim that closing large psychiatric hospitals led straight to incarceration, it is the case that for Black folks in the South, jails and prisons had always been part of the mental health system, and one immediate consequence of both deinstitutionalization and integration was the movement of more people into the prison system.[9] Was that a deliberate tactic? It is certainly a historically accepted fact that the carceral system developed after slavery as a deliberate response to Black freedom.[10] In relation to people with mental illness, it would be naive to think that Southern administrators did not know what would happen to people once they let them out of the psych hospitals with nowhere else to go.

As early as 1974, the impact was clear. In a memo dated January 16, Rob Cleland, the director of hospitals in Alabama, wrote to Judge Hawkins seeking his advice about how to handle commitment procedures given the post-Wyatt reforms. "As discussed in your chambers on Monday," he wrote, "the warden of the city jail needs relief from the number of former Bryce patients who are now his guests. Bryce needs to know how to handle these patients in light of their own personal competency, and the federal court order, which (combined) make it nearly mandatory that we release them; whereas, there do not exist appropriate statutes and appropriate facilities for the kind of behaviour they will fall into outside of an institution without a community program to enable them to maintain appropriate behaviour."[11] More than ten years after the passing of the Community Mental Health Act, all the planning, all the good ideas, all the work of dedicated mental health professionals in Alabama, were lost as the state chose to spend money instead on litigating the orders in both *Marable* and *Wyatt*.

This was not a problem unique to Alabama. In Mississippi, lawyer Barry Powell, who was the director of Community Legal Services of Mississippi (CLS) from 1975, told me that it was his goal to try to bring a comprehensive *Wyatt*-type class action against Whitfield Hospital, but he was denied every time by the ruling district court judge. Instead, he forged a Mental Health Project team, led by David Seth Michaels, who litigated individual cases against the state's institutions using the constitutional protections around due process, habeas corpus, and new "right to treatment" laws.

I met Mr. Powell in Jackson, Mississippi, in early 2020, and he told me about the arrangement he made with Dr. Jaquith to provide legal advice to patients at Whitfield from a van in the parking lot. Mr. Powell had pulled a series of boxes for me from his attic. They were dusty and littered with mouse droppings, and I sat at his dining room table, covered with a red cloth and white lace doilies, scanning page after page of case file while Mrs. Powell made tea in the kitchen and helped jog her husband's memory, college football playing on the TV over Mr. Powell's crowded desk.[12] The Powells were incredibly open and hospitable to me. They introduced me to a group of people still working on disability advocacy and prisoners' rights in the state, and helped me make the links between the state hospital, juvenile detention, and the prison system.[13]

The annual reports from the CLS are a catalog of the state's attempts to subvert or ignore patients' rights, and the impact of community legal activism to ensure that they were protected. In 1975 alone, the CLS settled or successfully litigated cases that provided a variety of relief: "State mental hospitals can no longer confine persons on criminal charges indefinitely because of incompetency to stand trial; Building 90, the most notorious of unhabitable buildings at the State Hospital at Whitfield, has been closed; the population of the maximum security unit at Whitfield has been released to residential buildings; the State Mental Hospital at Whitfield must now provide a hearing to patients who are being punished by being placed in more secure confinements or whose privileges are denied."[14]

The CLS was also involved in a long list of cases designed to test various aspects of admission and conditions at Whitfield: "whether the State Mental Hospital can apply electric shock treatments to patients not wanting such treatment; whether conditions and lack of treatment at the State Mental Retardation Annex is unconstitutional; whether the State Mental Hospital can summarily revoke a patient's trial leave without hearing; whether the State's involuntary commitment laws are constitutional; whether inmates of the State Penitentiary can be summarily transferred to the State Mental Hospital without a hearing."[15] I could go on.

The complete failure of the state of Mississippi to do anything meaningful about the abject state of mental health care, especially for young Black people, is borne out by at least two subsequent pieces of evidence, one of which points to the ambiguous role of Dr. Jaquith in the aftermath. Mr. Powell suggested that Jaquith, while maintaining his political allegiances, did at least care enough about his patients to allow the presence of the CLS on-site at Whitfield and welcomed the prosecution of cases, as he hoped they would raise awareness and concerns about conditions that might help him advocate for more funding.

Jaquith knew that things remained problematic—in his unprocessed collection at the Mississippi Department of Archives and History are a number of scrapbooks, and in one he had pasted clipping after clipping about ongoing litigation, complaints, and occasional improvements. One of the most confronting items in this collection is a series of pages cut from the magazine *Mississippi Today*—large, full-page photos from a five-part series written by Cordelia Cottingim, with photos by Wayne Cottingim.[16]

The Cottingims had been given full access to Whitfield, and they documented its aging and failing facilities, lack of staff, poor hygienic conditions, attempts at treatment and care, and everyday life for patients. The award-winning series pulled few punches but was also sympathetic to attempts by Jaquith to improve conditions and his constant pleas for more funding. *The Clarion-Ledger* and the *Delta Democrat-Times* continued to pay close attention to conditions at Whitfield and ran extensive coverage of the Mississippi CLS cases throughout the 1970s and beyond, which they also hoped would raise public awareness and political willpower.

None of that coverage made a great deal of difference, as both Whitfield and East Mississippi State Hospital continue to operate today but are now under the threat of a federal court order. In a long ruling in the case of *United States v. Mississippi*, first issued in 2019, Judge Carlton Reeves documented the many ways that the State of Mississippi had failed to meet its legal obligations under both the Civil Rights of Institutionalized Persons Act (CRIPA) and the Americans with Disability Act.[17] He wrote that "on paper, Mississippi has a mental health system with an array of appropriate community-based services. In practice however the mental health system is hospital centered and has major gaps in its community care. The result is a system that excludes adults with SMI [serious mental illness] from full integration into the communities in which they live and work, in violation of the Americans with Disabilities Act. . . . Mississippi's current mental health system—the system in effect, not the system Mississippi might create by 2029—falls short of the requirements established by law."[18]

Judge Reeves ordered various remedies, including the establishment of a monitor, but to no avail. The case, originally brought by the US Department of Justice (DOJ), has continued to bounce between the district and appellate courts as Mississippi, like its neighbor Alabama, spends money on litigation that could easily be used to apply for grants, raise wages and conditions for mental health workers, and build new facilities. In late 2023, the notoriously conservative three-judge US Court of Appeals for the Fifth Circuit overturned Reeves's original order, arguing that he "erred" in his interpretation that "institutionalization" was a form of discrimination. Now, the onus falls back to the individual to make a case unless the DOJ will appeal the most recent decision, which Mississippi will no doubt continue to fight. The state argues that it is making attempts to improve access to community-based care, but it is a fact that more than 2,000 people with mental illness are being held in jail without charge, awaiting psychiatric evaluation.[19] It is beyond frustrating, as a historian, to see this cyclical and ill-informed approach to planning and the failure to implement change at a moment when the money was readily available.

Things were also slow to improve in Georgia, despite its rapid response to the Civil Rights Act of 1964. The state did carry out its plan of regionalization and began to operate smaller in-patient units located at existing hospital facilities in places like Savannah, Albany, Thomasville, and Atlanta, but Central State Hospital remained a large regional facility until at least 2009. Too much happened in those decades for me to relate in full here, but what I do know is due to the meticulous documentation of people who used to work at Central State or the Department of Behavioral Health and Development Disabilities, which became the governing body of the state's mental health system. Over the last few years I have spoken with Mary Lou Rahn, Lynne Wright, Derril Gay, John Gates, Doug Skelton, and Susan Trueblood, who were able to help fill in some of the gaps in the official archives of what happened in the post–civil rights and post-Wyatt periods.

In the 1970s and 1980s, Georgia built eleven community mental health centers affiliated with general hospitals, and twenty-four other community programs with federal funds. The implementation of the Community Mental Health Act was complicated by the funding mechanism that required matched funds from counties that wished to participate, which meant that as late as 1972, more than a third of Georgia's 150 counties did not claim state mental health funds. The state then began to fund combined community mental health and mental retardation programs in some of the other counties, the operation of which they left to the counties themselves. This meant a sometimes-patchy approach, even further complicated by the establishment of Community Service Boards, which covered multiple counties in a region and either employed people directly or contracted out for services. In 1975, the state Medicaid program was amended to allow community mental health centers to bill for outpatient services, but this still relied on individual counties agreeing to expand Medicaid to allow for such claims.[20] This lack of direct oversight from either federal or state authorities allowed local politics to set the agenda when it came to mental health.

At the same time, the legacy of race relations in Georgia continued to impact Central State Hospital. In 1977, three social workers filed suit against the state, claiming discrimination in hiring and promotional practices at the state hospital in Milledgeville. The suit was filed in the Northern District Court by three Black social workers, Sherard Kennedy, Crawford Finley, and James White.[21] Kennedy in particular claimed that he had resigned his position at Central State Hospital because even though he had a master's degree, he was confined to performing secretarial duties instead of social work. The three men asked the court to review hiring and promotional practices at the hospital, to stop the hospital from hiring and promoting white persons unfairly, and to reinstate Kennedy as a social worker.[22] The plaintiffs named Dr. Crittenden, the superintendent at the time, as the offending party, but the case was quickly settled by the state department.[23]

At the same time, and purely by coincidence, a public scandal erupted at the discovery of patients working on local farms around Milledgeville. Originally encountered by a local voting rights education worker, the men were reported to the mayor, Maynard Jackson, as "being pressed into forced labor."[24] The mayor made a public statement about the situation before he informed the relevant state authorities, which raised hackles, but the situation was untenable and required public exposure.

The allegation initially concerned one young boy, J.D., who had been admitted to Central State Hospital seven years ago and was living in appalling conditions on a farm outside Macon, with filthy clothes and nothing to eat. The allegation caught the state department on the back foot, and a spokesman for the Department of Human Resources (DHR), the agency responsible for mental health at the time, said, "We know of no such conditions and would not put up with it for two seconds. . . . The mayor's comments make us all look like dummies. He should tell us if he has any knowledge of such activity. . . . I don't see how something like an indentured servant situation could occur."[25] That comment alone revealed how far removed state officials were from the history and the reality of life at Central State, which had been operating on one version or another of indentured servitude for over 100 years.

The department launched an immediate investigation, with reporter Beau Cutts covering the story for the *Constitution*. The main investigator and subsequent DHR spokesperson was Nick Taylor—a journalist, not a mental health worker—and what he discovered shook him profoundly. He was candid in his findings with the *Constitution*, and also when I talked to him in April 2022. He remembered undertaking a review of patients in a furlough program in which about 250 men had been placed on local farms in the 1950s and 1960s. The program had been terminated in 1971, and apparently the men were told by a social worker that they were formally discharged from Central State, but some of the men had not understood what that meant or had nowhere else to go.

Taylor's investigation led to the discovery of ten men who had been part of the program and had slipped through the cracks in the hospital reorganization. Taylor found the men, nine Black and one white, some of them deaf and mute, doing menial chores on small farms and lots owned by poor white people. Taylor told the *Constitution* that he had found six former patients "kept like animals" at one farm in Jones County. "I wouldn't expect human beings to live in conditions those men were living in. Eyewitnesses said flies buzzed around the men, who themselves were physically dirty and wore grossly soiled clothing," he reported. This farm was owned by the Chambers family, who lived in a trailer on the same site but provided no running water or toilet for the men. J.D. chose to live in a corner of the dairy barn rather than in the concrete block shelter, and he was the only one capable of independent work. One of the other men had been there for ten years, and on another farm in Baldwin County, Taylor found two other ex-patients, one of whom was eighty years old and had been on the farm for thirty-three years, doing yard work. "I asked him if he wanted to go somewhere, and he said he figured he'd just stay on there," Taylor stated.

The mental health commissioner at the time, Doug Skelton, acted quickly and had most of the men removed, examined, and prescribed necessary medication. Two of them were admitted to a state nursing home, and arrangements were made for the others to be returned to Central State if needed or to their families where possible. But some men did stay on the farm under improved conditions and monitoring.[26] Taylor told me that in his recollection, the Chambers family felt as though they were doing a service for the men, who had nowhere else to go, but that J.D.'s family in particular was upset by the whole scenario. They had visited him twice on the farm and wanted to take him home but had been dissuaded by reminders of his past violence and told that they would not be able to cope with him. While Taylor was fairly quick to rationalize the way the department dealt with the situation, he also recognized it as a legacy of past practices in which Black servitude on local farms was accepted practice, regardless of disability. Nobody questioned the practice of leasing Black men out to local white farmers because that was where they had always been.

It was into this environment and the mess left by Dr. Crittenden that Dr. John Gates became the superintendent of Central State in 1978. A New Yorker by birth, Dr. Gates had trained as a research and experimental psychologist and undertaken his master's and PhD programs at Florida State in Tallahassee. I was able to interview Dr. Gates twice before he passed away in 2022, and he told me many stories about his work and what motivated him.

After taking over as superintendent in 1978, Dr. Gates was able to achieve accreditation from the Joint Commission in 1981 through a rigorous program of setting and meeting standards. In 1980, the passage of CRIPA gave Dr. Gates more legal justification for increased improvements, but by the late 1980s, the hospital was again senselessly overcrowded and the state's system woefully underfunded.

Despite various individual cases, mental health lawyers in Georgia had not been able to bring a *Wyatt*-type class action, but this changed with the advent of the Americans with Disabilities Act. The act gave local legal activists the leverage to launch the case that has become the landmark decision known as *Olmstead v. L.C.* Brought originally by Atlanta Legal Aid, the case argued that two women with a developmental disability had completed their treatment and were considered fit to be returned to the community but were being held against their will at Georgia Regional Hospital. Much has been written about the case and its profound impact for institutionalized people with disabilities, but the prevailing principle is that people with disabilities are entitled to live in the least restrictive environment.[27] The decision also rested on a reconceptualized concept of civil rights in which segregation now meant "removal from society." In this conceptualization, civil rights became patients' rights, removing some of the racial and political complexity of the original concept.

Despite the success of cases like *Olmstead* and other "least restrictive environment" cases, continued underfunding and irrational fear of the mentally ill place undue stress on people of color because mental illness is still criminalized at the intersection with race. This is particularly egregious in the context of a country that refuses to enact meaningful gun regulation but is happy to blame mental illness for mass shootings that are actually the result of a culture of toxic masculinity and white men's race-related violence.[28] The continued problem of police involvement in mental health has led to a situation that many recognize as a national crisis.[29] Journalists and commentators spill a great deal of ink writing about the ways that this jail or that prison is now the largest mental health provider in the county/state/nation, but the reality is that they are not providing mental health care at all. They exist to lock up, seclude, remove, and kill people of color.

In September 2022, thirty-five-year-old Lashawn Thompson, a Black man with mental illness who had been arrested for sleeping in a park in Atlanta, died in the psychiatric wing of Fulton County Jail. Thompson's body was found dehydrated, malnourished, and infested with bed bugs and lice. He had also not received any treatment for his schizophrenia. An independent autopsy, paid for by former quarterback and activist Colin Kaepernick, found that he had died of neglect. On August 2, 2023, Thompson's family settled with Fulton County for $4 million and the promise of a change of policies. The family has also reached a settlement agreement with the third-party provider of mental health care services to Fulton County Jail, NaphCare. Fulton County had intended to end its agreement with NaphCare, but the county could not find a replacement provider so has given NaphCare more money instead.

Since then, at least a dozen Black men with mental illness have died in Fulton County Jail, a place notorious for keeping its mostly Black population in horrendous conditions of violence and neglect and that is now the subject of a DOJ investigation.[30] This kind of situation often leads for calls to a return to the asylum, but this book should have made clear why this is not an option. As a historian, it would be arrogant of me to suggest solutions, but I would argue that the police are not it.

Recently, Georgia passed House Bill 1013, which has been celebrated as providing insurance parity for mental health claims. The bill also provides more funding for police as first responders, which are deemed necessary to ascertain whether a crime has been committed. This is the heart of the problem though: the overlay between illness and criminality, the pathologization of disease that disproportionately effects people of color. Nowhere in HB 1013 were historical or geographic issues raised to explain the lack of care in Georgia or the problems with accessing it. Recent work by Dr. Avi Wofsy shows that the long history of structural racism in psychiatry, combined with geographic racism like redlining, has led to the current situation in Georgia.[31] This situation is exacerbated, of course, by states' refusals to expand Medicare or Medicaid in the first place, creating a bifurcated system based on who can pay and who cannot.

Understanding the historical and structural problems is only one part of the issue, however. The other looming elephant in the room is the internal racism of psychiatry itself. Literal and physical segregation in service provision was the obvious target of the medical civil rights movement, based on the argument that conditions would only improve if they were racially integrated. But this was, and is, a limited tactic—a nonreform reform. It is not simply that the mandate to integrate was avoided through a refusal to expand Medicaid or the idea of "freedom of choice" or the reliance on the prison system; there is something at the heart of psychiatric practice itself that was left untouched by the move to community mental health and medical civil rights, which has been replicated and reinforced through the science of diagnosis.

In his book *The Protest Psychosis*, Jonathan Metzl locates one key moment in the shifting diagnostic criteria related to schizophrenia, in which "aggression" was added as a symptom where it had not previously been.[32] This change was made in the revision of the *Diagnostic and Statistical Manual of Mental Disorders* (*DSM-2*) in 1974. That change had profound effects, as it led to the marketing of race-specific drugs, like the now notorious advertisements for Haloperidol aimed specifically at the angry Black man. Metzl makes the point that we cannot separate this change in diagnostic practice from the prevailing social and political context in which it occurs—that is, the long civil rights movement. (I am greatly simplifying Metzl's argument and evidence.)

Again, there is a domino effect here in that what was a deliberate and highly political change became accepted custom and practice, handed down unquestioned from one generation of psychiatrists to the next. The result is what Metzl's colleague and fellow psychiatrist Helena Hansen calls "diagnostic apartheid"—the highly discriminatory practice of differentiating both psychiatric symptomology and subsequent treatment and care options based on what is basically just skin color. This is especially problematic at the intersection with drug use and the options that become available to patients of color.[33]

As my own research has shown, diagnosis was a highly racialized and politicized practice before the changes made in the *DSM-2*. Data collected and analyzed from Central State Hospital in Milledgeville clearly show the way that schizophrenia as a diagnosis shifted away from white women to Black patients—and to Black women in particular from 1968 onward.[34] This timing is not a coincidence. Every time Black people across the South rose up to defend themselves, every technology of white supremacy was mobilized to keep them down. Schizophrenia, with its symptomology of paranoia and delusions, became a tidy bucket in which to dump legitimate grievances about the social order. It was a diagnosis that allowed and facilitated continued confinement at a time when liberty and patients' rights were high on the agenda, but those were rights and liberties that could only be allowed for some. The fear of the free Black person was magnified tenfold by the fear of the free Black person with schizophrenia. That fear allowed their continued confinement and segregation by any means, either in hospitals or in prisons.

A diagnosis of schizophrenia had, and still has, serious implications. As the most feared and serious mental illness, it carries with it the stigma and power of a dreaded label, and it is used to justify and feed public fear, leading to involuntary commitment and incarceration (ostensibly for the safety of self and others). It allows for the use of extremely strong and impactful medications like clozapine, which create irreparable physical and neurological changes and can also impact genetic makeup, rippling down generations in ways that are barely understood. But if a diagnosis can change as a result of social change or political pressure in ways that negatively impact one racial group over another, then it is not science, it is racism.

This is the internal racism of psychiatry, which permeates all the history documented in this book. There is plenty of evidence to suggest that psychiatrists themselves knew that racism itself was a problem, rather than race. Even the original debates about alleged emotional differences between Black and white patients toyed with the idea that the problems were social, not biological. While most psychiatrists did not actually believe that segregation was necessary, they tended to think that integration solved the problem—tick a box, one and done. But there have always been Black psychiatrists who knew that the problems in psychiatry, and in society, were the product of white racism, not anything biologically different about the Black patient.[35] The Black Psychiatrists of America, for example, worked to isolate racism as a problem not just for the makeup of the profession but for psychiatric practice itself, and they published their work in groundbreaking books such as *Black Rage* and the brilliant collection *Racism and Mental Health*.[36]

As a result of the civil rights movement, some psychiatrists began to consider that the problems in psychiatry ran deeper than just structural issues, taking a moment to look inward and think about their own role in creating racism and supporting oppression. As I worked through the records of the Medical Committee for Human Rights (MCHR) at the University of Pennsylvania, it struck me how many members of the executive committees and local chapters were psychiatrists. The most obvious and notable was Alvin Poussaint himself, a man who not only led the medical civil rights movement but wrote about the implications of civil rights and Black Power work on mental health.[37] Also active in MCHR leadership were psychiatrists Richard Morrill and Paul Lowinger. Morrill was the chair of the Greater Boston chapter of the MCHR, and Lowinger was national chair of the MCHR. Both of them were members of the American Psychiatric Association's "radical caucus," a group dedicated to using psychiatry for social change and considering psychiatry's role in that change.

Lucas Richert has written extensively about the caucus and its relationship to other counterculture movements, including its link to what is often called "anti-psychiatry," but my focus here is on the group's overt engagement with the internal racism of psychiatry.[38] The group held meetings at regular APA conventions, circulated petitions, and discussed issues such as "Racism: How can we define it and deal with it in our white community—the job no one ever seems to get around to" and "Black Power: implications for autonomy and identification, how does the white psychiatrist fit in?"[39]

As well as addressing the structural issues around racism in health and medicine, the group also discussed strategies for dealing with white racism as an attitude and a behavior, which remained an elusive target, as it was everywhere and nowhere at once. But they were also concerned with the role of psychiatry in perpetuating oppression. At a meeting held in Philadelphia in June 1969, a group of radical psychiatrists associated with the Medical Committee for Human Rights held a workshop titled "Psychiatry as the Instrument of the Establishment." The flyer for the workshop led with the statement, "MCHR observes psychiatry used all too often as a defender of the status quo and of standards of behavior within the narrow range defined by society as 'normal.'" The workshop agenda included items such as "peonage and mistreatment of patients in state mental health institutions; community mental health projects as colonial pacification programs; psychiatry and racism; [and] the psychiatrist as tranquillizer."[40]

At a conference in Miami in 1969, the radical caucus set a comprehensive agenda that explicitly sought to call out the hypocrisy of American psychiatry for its critique of violence overseas (e.g., the Vietnam War) while acting as a type of military within its own borders. The carceral implications of psychiatry were clear to the caucus, as was its role in the perpetuation of racial oppression. One discussion point raised questions that directed participants to look inward: "[Are] psychiatrists and other mental health professionals misusing their energies 'adjusting' people to our oppressive society? Do we serve as agents of the ruling class that . . . represses liberation struggles at home and abroad, in a blind determination to preserve its power?"[41]

Importantly, the caucus considered the psychological benefits of "participation in organized struggle against the establishment [as] a necessary condition for the achievement of personal mental health in an oppressive society."[42] These concerns stand in sharp contrast to what was happening in mainstream psychiatric practice at the time, where freedom protests and civil unrest were being framed as a form of pathology; as the "protest psychosis" that could be explained away as a failure to adjust and adapt; as unhealthy individual anger, treatable with a diagnosis of schizophrenia and a shot of Haldol.

Psychiatrist and MCHR national chair Paul Lowinger summed up the concerns of the radical caucus a few years later in an article titled "Radicals in Psychiatry." In summarizing the work of the caucus and the problems with American psychiatry, he referenced "the oppression caused by many of the traditional systems of psychiatry, the use of drugs, diagnosis, commitment, individual therapy and so on." He supported the critique of psychiatry "as a sedative-tranquillizing force, helping the survival of the social order," and issued "a challenge to psychiatry to become a liberating force in a radical and new conception of society."[43] Lowinger's vision was never realized, but the radical caucus and the legions of Black mental health professionals, civil rights and legal activists, Black patients and families and communities, and the people who supported them, should remind us that racism is always a choice, that another way is always possible.

Appendix 1

Power and Politics in the Psychiatric Archives

> In the face of the dead ends of racial justice that define our present, it is reparatory history that ought to command our attention.
> —D. Scott, "Reparatory History of the Present."

Sometimes it feels like everything in Alabama is an archive. I remember the first time I drove into Montgomery—it was October and still hot. Everything was still, the sun bouncing off the white marble buildings, shimmering up from the black tar roads. There was no one on the streets; it felt like a ghost town. A ghost town of the confederacy, a lost cause, the whitest of white supremacy. The Alabama Department of Archives and History looked like both "a temple and a cemetery," a gothic white marble building complete with columns, a heavy door, marble tiles squeaking under my sneakered feet as I perform the "quasi-magical" ritual of being granted entry.[1] Physically, the politics is laid bare from the beginning—a bronze confederate soldier dominates the foyer, surrounded by busts of mostly white men. Two Black men, George Washington Carver and Booker T. Washington, both from Tuskegee, were added in the 1990s, and recently two women—one Black, one white—were added to commemorate the struggle for voting rights. I think about these official statues again later, when I go to the National Memorial for Peace and Justice (also known as the National Lynching Memorial), just down the road from the state archive, where the first thing you see is a statue of the enslaved family, in chains, reaching out for justice. They are both the true history of Alabama, but one is marginalized while the other glorified.

In this book, my ability to say anything about the experience of Black patients in Southern asylums has required a sometimes fraught negotiation with the politics of archival power and the obfuscation and resistance with which I was met. If the Black person is not even a person in the context of Southern power in the mid-twentieth century, if the very nature of that personhood is the grounds for contestation over rights, then there is no chance that the formal archive will consider the Black "mental patient" a worthy subject of assemblage. And especially not when to do so would lay bare the blatant inequities that would challenge the myths of "separate but equal" and the benign paternalism of segregation.

But also this silence reflects that segregation. Segregation was about invisibility, and this continues into the archive, where the Black noncitizen is relegated to the margins in a kind of archival social death. If history is written by the winners, this is particularly the case when it comes to the assemblage of the psychiatric archive, in which both the formal structures of psychiatry and the governments they operate within are interested in creating a particular image of their practices—ordered, fair, procedural, rational—and these are the things deemed worth filing in the acid-free folders in the acid-free boxes, the organization of which is part of the ongoing colonial project.

In his writing on archives, Achille Mbembe argues that as "the term 'archives' first refers to a building, a symbol of a public institution," and then the "collection of documents—normally written documents—kept in this building," the "inescapable materiality of the archive" is what gives it its power "as an instituting imaginary."[2] He is not saying that this is the only form an archive can take, rather that this particular form is designed to embody and symbolize the power of the state, and that the imposing buildings deliberately give a weight and seriousness to the documents contained within, which makes them the only "legitimate" source of evidence about the past and its implications for the present.

Like Trouillot before him, Mbembe is quick to point out that these official spaces are as notable for what they leave out as for what they include.[3] For Mbembe, the act of collating an official archive, of deciding what is included and therefore what counts, is also "a ritual of forgetting," because once an item or a happening is subsumed into the official archive, it ceases to exist.[4] It is incorporated into the official corpus like a skeleton into the soil, dead to living memory until a historian comes along. These official archives, and the historians who have traditionally used them to write their official histories, are part of the process by which the archive is "transformed into a talisman," a symbol of the ideal state, where debt and accountability are buried.[5]

What is left out of these archives, what Mbembe calls the "debris," represents the way power works in the assemblage of the official archive, but this debris also represents resistance. "The destroyed archive haunts the state in the form of a spectre, an object that has no objective substance, but which, because it is touched by death, is transformed into a demon, the receptable of all utopian ideals and of all anger, the authority of a future judgement."[6] Here, historians are enjoined to do more than simply read between the lines or against the grain; we are called to look elsewhere for the debris, to take it seriously, and to use it to hold the state to account. In this sense, I have deliberately approached this book as a potential act of reparation.[7]

In Alabama, the psychiatric archival debris is everywhere, scattered across the state like shards of paper tossed from a speeding train. Trying to locate records that give me a full picture of the nature of segregation and its impact on Alabama's psychiatric hospitals has felt at times as if I am standing in a field trying to grab those shards and put them together like a jigsaw puzzle. My attempts to locate one particular document is a good example of what I mean and demonstrates some of the politics embedded in this process.

By the time of my first trip to the Alabama Department of Archives and History, I had already gathered a great deal of information from the Reynolds-Finley Historical Library at the University of Alabama at Birmingham (UAB). Here, where it seemed there was no overt political agenda other than the documenting of Alabama's medical history, I had unfettered access to an almost entire set of annual reports from the 1950s and 1960s, as well as a plethora of publications, newsletters, reports, and planning documents. But of course this is an inescapably white history. Elusive in most of these sources was any idea about how segregation actually worked, or what life was like for Black patients. The nature of the material available at this archive reflected the broader assumptions inherent to the production and cataloging of American medical history that privileged white knowledge, the white body, and the white experience. Apart from the rare mentions of the Tuskegee Mental Hygiene Clinic in *Alabama Mental Health* (see chapter 1), there was very little about the way that racial politics had affected Alabama's mental health systems. It was as if racial politics did not exist at all, as if the entire psychiatric profession was unsullied by and completely detached from one of the most foundational and divisive aspects of American society.

This was also true of the newspaper stories that appeared throughout the 1950s in Alabama. There was no single exposé like the ones we saw in Mississippi or Georgia, just hundreds of articles about the various problems at "the mental hospitals," which usually meant Bryce, the white hospital in Tuscaloosa. Sometimes Searcy, the Black hospital, was bundled in with Bryce, but usually it was not mentioned at all. Late in the 1950s, these stories mentioned a planning committee and a visit from the American Psychiatric Association, which included a series of public hearings.

In 2018 at the National Library of Medicine in Maryland, I found a copy of a document titled *A Mental Health Program for Alabama*.[8] This is a long document, running to 275 pages, which catalogs every aspect of Alabama's inpatient, community, private, and public services as they were reported to the APA's representatives. But there are no details about the nature of facilities at either Bryce or Searcy in this document. Rather, a note clearly spelled out that "this section does not include the reports on the Alabama State Hospitals which were submitted by the Central Inspection Board of the American Psychiatric Association." This comment sent me on the hunt for these reports, a search which again revealed the many layers of silence, obfuscation, gatekeeping, and political interference in the creation of the psychiatric archive.

The logical place to look for records related to Alabama's mental health institutions should be the Alabama Department of Archives and History in Montgomery. But nothing is ever as simple as that in Alabama. By the time I found this document, I was deep into the research on the court case that sought to end segregation in Alabama's psychiatric hospitals. Looking for material related to that case (of which there is very little at ADAH) had already revealed the challenges for research on the history of mental health there. The organization of the archive reflected the general organization (or lack thereof) of the state's mental health system itself, which had no single department or government entity to refer to.

The main repository for material related to the psychiatric hospitals is a record group called "State Institutions," which falls under either the Governor, Department of Health and/or Department of Public Health, and then is organized by year, rather than by type of institution. This meant pulling boxes based on years and looking for the folders related to "Mental Hospitals" in each box. These boxes also contain material relevant to each of the other institutions focused on disability, child welfare, prisons, and charity schools. This approach reflects the fact that there was simply no single government entity related to the comprehensive oversight of "mental health services"—the APA program plan listed this fact as a serious shortcoming for the state and recommended that all the various mental health services be united and consolidated under a single state agency.[9]

In none of these files did I find the APA Central Inspection Board report I was looking for. How could a report that spelled out the problems of the biggest inpatient facilities and precipitated a statewide reckoning and program overhaul not be anywhere in the official files? And if it was not there, where was it?

At first I tried to access the actual archives of the APA's Central Inspection Board itself and hit the wall of professional gatekeeping. The APA archives are in Washington, DC, and I know psychiatrist-historians have used them, but my repeated requests for help, information, and access were met with repeated denials because I was not a psychiatrist and not a member of the APA. Here, a la Trouillot, professional power creates and curates the archive, and then only gives access to those with vested interest in the mythology of the organization and the stories it tells itself.

This is particularly well illustrated by the sudden downfall of a past APA president, happening as I write, who tweeted about Blackness as a "freak of nature" and is responsible for one of the most hagiographic and one-sided books about the history of psychiatry in existence.[10] In 2021, the APA issued a statement about its past problems with racial discrimination and stereotyping, apologizing for its role in these practices without specifying exactly what that role was.[11] By limiting archival access to its own members, the APA continues to perpetuate its secrets and lies, and protects the very ideologies and practices of which Jeffrey Lieberman is just the most obvious tip of the iceberg.

Thwarted by the APA, my next step was to try to find records still in the possession of Bryce Hospital itself. While the original Bryce Hospital was sold to the University of Alabama in 2014 and is now in the process of being transformed into a visitor and arts center, the "New Bryce" hospital exists close by as a smaller inpatient unit. I was given the name of someone to contact within the Alabama Department of Mental Health who might be able to help. That person, who is the official historian for the department, wasted no time in laying out the state of play. He made it clear that anything that "even has the mention of a patient name can only be released through . . . [the] Health Information Management Department with approval of . . . [the] Legal Department."[12] He was not being vindictive, merely stating the facts.

In retrospect, I think that this exchange shaped the direction of this project immediately. It was an instant red flag, not so much as to a bull but rather as a warning about the obvious political and power relations I was wading into. It was not that I had even asked for individual patient files. Apart from this APA inspection report, what I was hoping for were operational records, policies, procedures, internal memos, notes from the superintendent, anything about the day-to-day running of this huge system that was not revealed in the annual reports that I'd already had access to. This official response, as honest and well-intentioned as it was, put me on edge about the issue of records very early in the project and let me know that I would need to proceed carefully, as not everyone would be happy to see me. It also made it very clear that my ability to tell the story of segregated psychiatry in the Deep South was going to be highly mediated by the silences, deliberate and otherwise, that structured the psychiatric archive.

My search for the APA document was hindered by the onset of the COVID-19 pandemic, but when I was ready to return to the archives, I wrote to the official historian again, and he helpfully updated me on the process of removal of various items to the Special Collections at the University of Alabama's Hoole Library. This made sense, given the fact that the library is quite literally on the site of the original Bryce Hospital campus and is now a fifteen-minute walk from the old admissions building (now known as Bryce Main on the University of Alabama campus map).[13]

I had looked at the collections listing previously but seen only material related to the first superintendent, Dr. Peter Bryce, from the 1800s. The collection listing was more extensive this time and included a record group of documents related to the operation of the hospitals. And there was the report I was looking for: APA Inspection Report, 1958. I had plans to travel to Tuscaloosa to look at this report and other items in January 2021, but the COVID Omicron variant made me wary, so I delayed again, but this time I encountered some unexpected openness.

Unable to travel but knowing I needed this document to proceed, I asked the incredibly helpful institutional records analyst at Special Collections, Kevin Ray, whether I could hire a research assistant to go and scan the document for me. There was no need for that, Kevin told me. He had someone in the library scan the document into two long PDFs, all 500 pages, and emailed it to me for free.

The contents of the document were both shocking and not surprising and revealed again the way that the Black experience is sidelined and silenced in the history of psychiatry. They also demonstrated the deeply embedded racism and complicity with white supremacy on the part of the American Psychiatric Association, particularly in the context of civil rights battles in Alabama. In the same way that Alabama "dares defend its rights," it defends its history, and this becomes defensiveness that has no logical point. But logic is not the driving force here, nor is truth.

Alabama is not alone in its approach or in its level of defensiveness, and the implications for historians trying to document the everyday experience of patients are profound. Issues with provenance, conservation, and political risk aversion have meant that the material culture possibilities for this project have been scarce and problematic. It is interesting how often I am asked about patient records and material culture, as though I am missing something obvious, but it is hard to miss something that was never created, assembled, or preserved to begin with. The repeated question about patient records has made me think long and hard about the use of them in the history of medicine and psychiatry, and why we place so much emphasis on them, as if they are somehow the benchmark of good history. I have written elsewhere about my complicated thoughts about the ethics of using patient records, so I will not repeat myself here, but even when they are not there, the possibility that they might be has caused defensive attitudes and practices from state governments that even archivists find frustrating.[14]

For example, the conservation of material from Central State Hospital (CSH) in Milledgeville, Georgia, has been the subject of a particularly tumultuous relationship between the Georgia state government, the Department of Behavioral Health and Developmental Disability (DBHDD), and the state archives, which I first encountered while trying to help the ACLU (American Civil Liberties Union). Early in the research for this project I was contacted by the capital defense team operating out of Durham, North Carolina. They had been referred to me by Mab Segrest, whose work on Central State Hospital drew on records and materials she had been able to access because of the presence of an onsite museum at CSH. But the museum was now closed, and Mab's records did not extend beyond the 1940s.

The ACLU team was looking for records related to a much younger client they were representing on death row in Florida, whose family had a long history with CSH, and they were hoping to find material that would help them bring a mitigating circumstances case. I met Sarah, the ACLU's mitigation specialist, at the state archives in Morrow, Georgia, with a list of items from the catalog that I thought might be useful in locating general information, but it was pretty clear that the records there were not straightforward. A simple search for "central state hospital" in the state archives online catalog immediately revealed that there was no single collection related to the hospital neatly arranged by chronology. Rather, documents, letters, and reports were scattered across many collections and departments, often under the name of the division director, shifting from public welfare to public health to mental health over time. None of the superintendents were represented as a distinct collection; rather, they appeared only as correspondents with the relevant department director or other mental health policymakers. And there were certainly no patient records.

The ACLU was actually looking for personal records related to their client, and had his permission to do so, but it was obvious to me that they were not listed in the catalog, only in an admissions book. The head archivist came out to chat, and she explained that if we were really serious about getting access to patient records, we would have to bring a lawsuit against the state of Georgia because they had never deposited such records in the state archives, even though they were required to do so by the state's own recordkeeping policy.

Regardless of what this meant for my own research, this practice has had serious consequences for people looking for family records. When I spoke to a contact at the Georgia DBHDD about what had happened to records like the ones Mab Segrest had had access to at the old museum onsite at Central State, he explained that what records the department now possessed were being processed for HIPAA purposes and then would be moved to the Georgia College and State University in Milledgeville.

Those records also do not contain patient information, and a link on the Special Collections listings related to Central State Hospital directs people back to the DBHDD website with instructions for family members to contact Baldwin County Probate Court for information.[15] This court, of course, only contains information related to people who died at Central State or people who were admitted to Milledgeville via that particular court, which represented only a small portion of the patient population, given that people were admitted from all over the state. These records, including death certificates, would be obtainable only if you could prove you had written permission or were a family member after paying the requisite fee. For this reason, I never tried to track down admission records via the probate courts—why go down a rabbit hole when you know it won't take you to wonderland?[16]

Issues with archives in relation to Central State did not begin and end with individual patient files. As if the organization of files scattered through multiple record groups didn't make things hard enough, there were restrictions on even seemingly innocuous boxes. Before the COVID-19 pandemic, I requested a box called "Patient Complaints." The box was delivered to my table, and I began to sort through the contents. I had not gotten very far when the reading room attendant came over and pointed to the red sticker that no one (including me) had noticed on the side of the box. "Oh, this is restricted," she said, and took the box back so they could process it.

Then COVID came along and interrupted everything. When I was allowed back to the state archives almost two years later, I requested the box again, thinking it must have been processed, and the exact same scenario occurred. This time I was more prepared, and when the reading room attendant wanted to take the box back, I asked what the rationale was, since archived patient records are not covered by HIPAA. He disappeared and returned a minute later with a copy of the Georgia Code, which contained a section on records containing "medical information." He pointed to the part that explained why the files were restricted and then flipped the page to show a paragraph that set out the process by which researchers could request access to restricted files.

From there, I worked with the general counsel at Emory University to draft a letter that addressed the relevant legislation and set out my rationale for using the records and my approach for maintaining confidentiality, then sent that off to the state archivist, who responded and said he would review my request. Sometime later I followed up and was informed that the archivist felt that the matter needed to be escalated to the Board of Trustees of the University System of Georgia (USG), the umbrella body for the state archives. I won't repeat the expletives I uttered at the time, but I was particularly frustrated because of the notoriously conservative nature of the board and the USG and was sure I would never see that box again.

I put it out of my mind and continued to work with what I had until I had reason to come to that section of the chapter about six months later. I sent another email to the state archivist just to see where things were at, and he let me know that my request had been approved subject to certain conditions, one of them being that the box would be properly processed, and any identifying information redacted. He would let me know when the box was ready. Well, that was a surprise. It took another year before the box was ready and I could get back down to Morrow to try again.

This time the box was clearly marked "restricted," and some files were now housed in red folders, which I was not allowed to take out of the box at all. The other files were mostly letters from families asking to have their family members moved or released, and any identifying information was blacked out. The only letter in the box that was of any use to me now was the one I used at the start of chapter 3, from

Dr. Olson in DC to Dr. Bush at the Department of Public Health, about a Black youth who needed to be transferred. His name was blacked out too. Without access to certain red files in the box, I have no idea what sort of complaints were being made by either patients or their family members; three years for one letter.

At this point it was painfully obvious why no one except Mab Segrest had tried to write a history of Central State, and why her own story stopped at 1940. The removal of other records from the old railway museum to the Georgia College adds a further layer of difficulty for both researchers and descendants, because they are now in a small college library three hours outside Atlanta, and not easily searchable via the library's website. However, the college has done a great job of translating some of its collections into publicly available digital exhibitions, including a general overview of the "People, Places and Progress" at CSH, which also contains a terrific story about the history of nursing at Central State.[17] Because these resources exist, I have not repeated any of the material in this book unless I used them to check dates or names.

In Mississippi, things are complicated by the fact that both Whitfield Hospital still exists and has patients on the same campus that I am writing about. At one time they did tours, and you could gawk at the horrors of psychiatry past in a small museum, but it is now closed. The person who answered my email request for any artifacts or objects wrote, "We don't keep that kind of material here" and referred me to the Mississippi Department of Archives and History, where I had already been twice.

If things had been difficult in Alabama and Georgia, they were unsurprisingly worse in Mississippi—not through any fault of the archivists themselves, who were (and continue to be) extremely efficient and helpful, but because of the paucity of records. It was frustrating to discover that there was no single official departmental record at MDAH under which records related to Whitfield were housed; if the problem in Georgia had been that there were lots of records spread across multiple departments, it was depressing to see in Mississippi how little had made it to the state archives to begin with.

In large part, this was because of the organizational structures, or lack thereof, related to mental health in Mississippi for much of the period under study in this book—it was not until the 1970s, when integration and community mental health had really forced their hand, that the Mississippi government had any formal governance structure for or oversight of the state mental health system, which was centralized at Whitfield.

I am 100 percent sure that there are in fact realms of records, letters, notes, memos, procedural manuals, and photos at the physical site halfway between Pearl and Brandon in Rankin County, and it is frustrating that my repeated emails have gone unanswered. I have made what I can out of the other items in the MDAH collection, including subject files full of newspaper clippings (I wish every archive had these!), digitized newspapers like the *Delta Democrat-Times* and *Clarion Ledger*, the board of trustee minutes on microfilm, and the items in Dr Jaquith's collections.

I found other copies of annual reports and correspondence in the special collections, in Senator Stennis's political papers library at Mississippi State University in

Starkville, and in Governor Johnson's papers at the University of South Mississippi (which had no problem with me looking at one restricted file related to Whitfield). There is one set of annual reports supposedly held at MSU that appears in the catalog but is not where it is supposed to be, and the archivists there have not been able to track it down for me, so I made do with what I could. While none of these issues are the fault of the actual front-line archivists and librarians, who have always been incredibly helpful, it is the case that state governments are intent on making these histories as obscure and inaccessible as possible, and the logical conclusion, which this book has sought to document and expose, is that state governments are hiding behind HIPAA and so-called concerns for patient privacy to shield themselves from both accountability and liability.

State archives are not alone: I was also unable to access any files related to the Department of Justice's work against Alabama in the desegregation case, or any other Civil Rights cases, and lodged a Freedom of Information Act request for access to those records which has not been processed at the time of publication.

I hope that by making these processes clear, by publishing open access, by making my sources available online, and by creating a publicly available archive of all my research materials at Emory University post-publication, families, communities, and descendants can find traces of themselves in these archives. I hope to continue the work this book has begun through a call for oral history participants, and I hope that state officials and racist psychiatrists will also see themselves in these pages and know that the people they incarcerated, abused, and neglected will not be forgotten.[18]

Appendix 2

Theorizing the History of "Black Madness"

> Without Theory, History is naught but tales,
> told by victors and moralists, signifying
> nothing beyond themselves.
> —Kleinberg et al., "Theses on Theory and History"

The argument of this book has been indelibly shaped by extensive reading in theories of bio- and necropolitics, anti-Black racism, and critical disability studies. While this admission may indeed mean I am putting the proverbial cart before the horse and committing that other great sin of bringing theory into history where it is not apparently wanted or needed, I am following Joan Scott's lead by arguing that critical history, which is what we have in fact always been doing whether we want to admit it or not, is not possible without several theoretical tools.[1] As Kleinberg, Scott, and Wilder have argued, "Critical history is theorized history. It does not treat theory as an isolated corpus of texts or bodies of knowledge. Nor does it treat theory as a separate, non-historical form of knowledge. Rather, it regards theory as a worldly practice (and historical artifact)."[2] To even attempt a history of psychiatry without theory is to ignore both the way that the history of psychiatry has always been theoretical (if not downright ideological) and the vast amount of theory about psychiatry as a practice that already exists.

In a book that is constructed around many silences in the archive by someone who is neither American nor Black, a theoretical framework is not a superfluous luxury but an ethical responsibility. In the prologue I discussed the importance of dealing with my positionality in this project, but here I want to explore the way that I am engaging various debates or schools of thought within the history of psychiatry at the intersection with race and racism. I have used theory to help me unpack questions that range from the meta to the micro.

Big-picture questions that have shaped this project include the following: To what extent do the sources demonstrate the way that psychiatry was as constitutive of racism as it was shaped by it? Is it fair to link twentieth-century psychiatric practices to the plantation South? Does the depth of the existing racism fully negate psychiatry as a discipline? How do we engage with the anti-psychiatry critique while advocating for better and more mental health services?

At the micro level I am trying to think about questions of agency and voice. These are common questions I get at conferences: What am I doing to demonstrate the ways that patients resisted oppression? How am I centering the voice of the Black patients? These are tricky questions, not simply because this resistance, or those voices, are rarely documented in the archives but because the reality of the situation for the Black disabled in Southern institutions did not in fact present a great many opportunities for resistance.

And why is there an expectation that a person should "resist," as a political act, when they have been admitted to a hospital for an illness? Maybe there is no time or space or energy for resistance. Maybe a person just wants to sleep, to be left alone, to be able to go home as soon as possible. Maybe a person knows that to resist is in itself seen as a pathology and will only make matters worse. But these are important questions to keep in mind, and they have shaped the way I have read between the lines of sources. They have helped me to unpack silences and have been essential for the way I presented material, left things out, and structured the book.

Importantly, theoretical questions have helped me shift the focus away from simply describing all the bad things that ever happened but to think in more nuanced ways about the relationships between local contexts and approaches to psychiatry. These relationships were dynamic and shifting, responding to local and racial politics that were not exceptional to the South but did play out in specific ways there.

This is an approach informed by Foucault. The lesson to learn is not that things were better or worse in the South or the North; rather, it is how psychiatric power manifested in the local context, and what that tells us about biopolitics and state power more broadly. But it is absolutely the case that in the South, this was a state power embedded in white supremacy, and it is this particular context that I sought to unpack. In other words, I was interested in thinking through how psychiatric power worked in the American South "in the wake" of slavery and as part of a broad network of confinement.[3]

This could not just be a story about "what happened," because I wanted to go beyond that moment and think about how it still happens, and how it happens at the level of ideology, not simply as a relic of the now-abandoned asylum. The problem, therefore, lies not simply in segregated spaces, which were supposedly eradicated in the late 1960s, but in the persistence of scientific ideologies that reify difference and hold race as a biological given, even when we know it is no such thing.

Theory is important here not just to make some a priori point a la Foucault about how the asylum is also a prison (even though it is) but because what was happening in psychiatry in the American South was actual theorizing about the nature of humanity itself, what constituted normalcy, and how Blackness had always been excluded from the project of American citizenship. Southern psychiatry in the postwar period was built on a theory of racial difference as inferiority, which emanated from the plantation; thus, unpacking the way that this theory was enacted into practice requires a theoretical intervention.

Of course, in the history of psychiatry, it is impossible to proceed without thinking about or through Foucault, and there are a range of concepts in his oeuvre that can be engaged in a study like this one. The central question from a Foucauldian angle asks *how* psychiatric power worked in its specific context. What was specific to that time and place that tells us something about the link between psychiatric power and social norms? At the most obvious level, Foucault argues that "psychiatric power is above all a certain way of managing, of administering, before being a cure or therapeutic intervention: it is a regime. Or rather, it is because and to the extent that it is a regime of isolation, regularity, the use of time, a system of measured deprivations, and the obligation to work, etcetera, that certain therapeutic effects are expected from it."[4]

There is much in this single quote that has resonated throughout this book. At the intersection with race, psychiatric regimes were about the management and control of the Black personality (and body) for the protection and perpetuation of white society. Techniques of isolation, deprivation, and work were not designed for any real therapeutic effect of the Black patient, who existed beyond therapy, but merely for the reproduction of the system that has always seen them as a means of production.

This conceptualization has also helped me think through questions of agency and resistance. In her use of the concept of biopolitics, Saidiya Hartman argues that the idea of productive power inherent to Foucault's theory of biopolitical relationships is useful but applicable only to scenarios in which everyone is free. That is, "There cannot be relations of power [as opposed to domination] unless subjects are free. If one were completely at the disposition of the other and became his thing, an object on which he can exercise an infinite and unlimited violence, there would not be relations of power. In order to exercise a relation of power, there must be on both sides at least a certain form of liberty."[5]

Were Black psychiatric patients in the South in the mid-twentieth century free? It can be argued that technically, no psychiatric patient is ever truly free, once admitted to the psy-system. Its very rationale is to curtail freedom that is expressed in behaviors that are seen as a threat to social order, and thus the full force of the medico-legal system is brought to bear to actively limit the movement of those deemed "mentally ill."

Involuntary commitment is the most oppressive tactic in this arsenal, but even so-called voluntary commitment is voluntary insofar as the patient really understands and has access to the legal devices needed to navigate the complex rules for admission and appeals for release. While the patients' and civil rights movements and continued disability activism have worked to ameliorate some of these problems, in the mid-twentieth century this activism was still nascent, and for Black patients committed against their will, domination was the power relation. If the very point of Jim Crow in the South was to perform relations of subservience and deference, aimed explicitly at the continued oppression of Black communities even when technically free, then the Black person suffering mental distress was subject to a form of alienation and domination akin to incarceration. This domination occurred initially at the point of contact with the psychiatric-carceral system, where commitment processes themselves were arbitrary and confusing, and continued within the institution, which barely served to keep the patient alive, let alone restore them to a state of freedom.

Even without this limit, Foucault can only get us so far in a study of psychiatry in the wake of the plantation. If social death was a driving conceptual framework for understanding the experience of patients in that system, then theoretically the flip side to the concept of biopolitics is necropolitics.[6] In his development of necropolitics, Mbembe takes us deliberately to Fanon. In a book like this one, where I am seeking to make a claim that psychiatric practice needs to be understood in the context of the Southern plantation, itself a tool of colonization, Fanon has much to offer.

While Foucault does make links between psychiatry and literal colonization, he does not do so in the context of either French colonization of Africa or slavery in the Atlantic.[7] His analysis of the tools of deprivation, labor, and so on, are largely focused on the critique of eighteenth-century moral therapy and restraint, and the impossibility of the institution as reformable.[8] Beyond the institution, his analysis is a total critique of psychiatry and psychoanalysis, which for Foucault have few if any redeeming features and are colonizing projects to the extent that they seek to normalize (and of course discipline) the human self.[9]

Reading Fanon expands this idea because he was a psychiatrist and a scholar who thought deliberately about the link between psychiatry and literal and metaphorical colonization of the Black person in particular. In fact, as theorist Chloe Taylor argues, many of Foucault's arguments were anticipated in Fanon's work.[10] But reading them together also adds the complexity of a practicing psychiatrist's point of view, a psychiatrist who believed in his practice at the same time as he was well aware of the way in which it was used to construct Blackness as otherness and as a deliberate tool of Western colonization.[11]

Fanon experienced this literal colonization firsthand in his work in North Africa, and his critiques of psychiatry are grounded in this specific experience; but it is also the case that across his body of work, he had plenty to say about the way that the specific processes he saw were generalizable to the way that psychiatry worked as a form of internal colonization with whiteness at the center.[12] It is in this sense that he is particularly useful to the way that psychiatry was complicit in the creation of race as a category of difference and in the creation of ideas that justified the continued oppression of the Black person in particular. This was an oppression that rested on the othering of the colonized. "Because it is a systemized negation of the other, a frenzied determination to deny the other any attribute of humanity, colonialism forces the colonized to constantly ask the question 'Who am I in reality?'"[13]

The "I" that the colonized thought was theirs comes under attack through colonization, which always seeks to import another "I" as justification for the colonization in the first place. At one level this is part of the general project of dehumanization, which is required to justify the violence of dispossession and genocide. Marilyn Nissim-Sabat has argued that this is a central theme in all of Fanon's work, that he "emphasized with great poignancy and power throughout his writings that the goal and consequences of colonial and other forms of oppression is dehumanization."[14]

This is not just any old "dehumanization," however. It was dehumanization forged against the alleged normal, natural, and superior humanity of whiteness. The repeated tropes in this process of dehumanization were ideas about savagery, primitivism, and idolatry. Without exception, the native state was constructed as an inferior one and colonization as a benevolence, divinely inspired and sanctified, and the rhetoric of science and medicine, which positioned whiteness as the only fully human state, was an integral part of this process.[15] These are ideas that became foundational to the practice of modern psychiatry.

The psychological consequences of this process for both the colonizer and the colonized, under Fanon, are complex. While we might not particularly care about the hurt feelings of the colonist (nor should we recenter whiteness), Fanon makes the important point that the process of creating racial difference through scientific method, especially in the twentieth century, was a fraught and ridiculous enterprise that had psychological consequences for colonial systems.

The original and actual violence of colonization, and the racism that was created by it, required a series of mental gymnastics to justify, because if the colonial cause was a righteous one, supported by a peaceful God and "civilization," that civilizing force was in fact often a violent and genocidal one. To create such violence and trauma, to dislocate people from land that was theirs, to enslave whole populations of people that you knew were people, and then to tell yourself they were not people, and that what happened to them after that was not even your fault, was to create a level of psychic denial and alienation so deep that it could not ever be faced, not ever be admitted, and not ever be repaired. This is the great hypocrisy of Western society—that "they are never done talking of Man, yet murder men everywhere they find them, at the corner of every one of their own streets, in all the corners of the globe."[16]

In the twentieth century, the European model had taken on a new, terrifying version of itself in the form of the United States. The American story was one in which "two centuries ago, a former European colony took it into its head to catch up with Europe. It has been so successful that the United States of America has become a monster where the flaws, sickness, and inhumanity of Europe have reached frightening proportions."[17] For Fanon, this new modern society, long since done with slavery, had found new ways to double down on the terror and was therefore an inherently sick society, "fractured, fragmented, split, not whole."[18]

For the "colonized," racist ideas about alleged inferiority as rationale for colonization become perpetuating and embodied, continuing long after formal colonization had ended, in a process Fanon called "sociogeny."[19] In *Black Skin, White Masks*, he wrote, "We shall see that the alienation of the Black man is not an individual question. Alongside phylogeny and ontogeny, there is also sociogeny."[20] That is, if mental illness was a problem for the colonized, it was because of the circumstances in which he was forced to live, including an ideological environment in which he was also cast as Other: "White civilization and European culture have imposed an existential deviation on the black man."[21]

The problem, of course, for Fanon, as a practicing psychiatrist, was that he saw the way these processes became internalized. The steady stream of pathologizing tropes and epistemic violence, originating from outside the culture, family, and mind of the colonized, also became embodied, worn on and seeping through the skin. That is, "The inferiority complex can be ascribed to a double process. First, economic. Then, internalization or rather epidermalization of this inferiority."[22] It was not, and is not, that the Black person was literally or actually inferior but that the stress of being told that they were manifested as both internalized self-hatred and repressed (or expressed) anger at knowing that they were not.

In this theorizing, Fanon was deliberately taking issue with Freudian psychoanalysis, which posited all pathology as rooted in the family. As this idea became more prevalent in modern psychiatry, the implications for the colonized, or for the pathologizing of Black people, were profound, because unlike with white families, this pathologization was then generalized as a characteristic of *all* Black or colonized families, especially those who struggled in the face of assimilation. For Fanon, though, this struggle was not a characteristic intrinsic to the family but to the relationship that Black families had to white society. That is, "a normal black child, having grown up with a normal family, will become abnormal at the slightest contact with the white world."[23] He spoke here from his own experience of being a Black child of white France.

Fanon, therefore, took the simple but profound step in his writing to make the point that families were in fact microcosms of the societies in which they were formed. The white child, growing up in a white family in a white society, never needed to confront the dissonance of difference. This was the gap in Freud's thinking that reflected the normalization of whiteness within a rapidly globalizing psychiatry: the lack of theorization about families as both reflective and constitutive of society.[24] If families were the problem in Freud's thinking, this did not go far enough because it failed to recognize that behind every family was society. That is, "the white family is the guardian of a certain structure. Society is the sum of all families. The family is an institution, precursor of a much wider institution, i.e. the social group or nation. . . . The white family is the educating and training ground for entry into society."[25]

If neurosis starts in the family, when the family is white, the neurosis is not seen as a signifier of anything beyond immediate interpersonal relations; it is not taken to be an extension of, or caused by, the flaws in white society more broadly. But neurosis in a Black family is almost always seen by psychiatry as a problem of Blackness, something inherent to the Blackness itself, not the fault of the colonizer or of white society, either through its actions or discourses about difference. W. E. B. Du Bois characterized this disorienting reality in his own way as double consciousness in *The Souls of Black Folk*.[26]

For Fanon, the cause of Black mental illness is obvious: "The black man is, in every sense of the word, a victim of white civilization. . . . The black problem is not about Blacks living among whites, but about the black man being exploited, enslaved, and despised by a colonialist and capitalist society that happens to be white."[27] White society, white psychiatry, justifies the violence of oppression by pathologizing Blackness, by characterizing it as inferiority, by enshrining it as the Other against which whiteness is itself defined. In a neat rhetorical shift, white psychiatry then characterizes the psychic toll of this process, the damage done to the Black person, as evidence of said pathology. A sociogenic scenario becomes a racial biology one. Case closed.

This tautological thinking also manifested in explanations for what was characterized as "Black violence" and shaped Fanon's thinking about the need for active resistance in the decolonization process.[28] If, as Richard Keller has pointed out, some historians are uncomfortable with Fanon's advocacy of violence, it is because they are not thinking about, or are actively ignoring, the lived experience of the colonized and the violence that permeates the very air they breathe.[29] That is, "you do not disorganize a society, however primitive it may be, with such an agenda if you are not determined from the very start to smash every obstacle encountered. The colonized, who have made up their mind to make such an agenda into a driving force, have been prepared for violence from time immemorial."[30]

To then claim that people seeking to decolonize should resort to something other than violence, as was so often the case in psychiatric justifications for confinement, was to actively deny the way that every agent of the colonizing state was an agent of violence, that violence in action and in language shapes and enshrouds the colonial encounter. In Fanon's words, "We have seen how the government's agent uses a language of pure violence. The agent does not alleviate oppression or mask domination. He displays and demonstrates them with the clear conscience of the law enforcer, and brings violence into the homes and minds of the colonized subject."[31]

Where that agent of colonization has been the psychiatrist, violence has also followed. There is the violence of confinement, commitment, and incarceration; the violence of diagnosis; the violence of treatment; and the psychic violence that permeates the medical encounter, which engenders only distrust.[32] Psychiatry has in fact been an act of "colonial war" through the conception of subjectivity.[33] For Fanon, decolonization cannot be complete until it takes place at the level of the self, where the colonized rejects the alienation from self that has been forced upon him and reclaims his sense of self before it was warped by colonial psychiatric practice. If "the "thing" colonized becomes a man through the very process of liberation" it is also true that this liberation needs to involve the complete destruction of the colonial world in all its forms: "to destroy the colonial world means nothing less than demolishing the colonist's sector, burying it deep within the earth or banishing it from the territory."[34] Literally and figuratively this means that decolonization can only occur not through assimilation with the dominant culture, the "psychiatrized" one, but through its complete rejection.

Yet there is necessarily a bind here, because to enact violence, as a Black person, is to be seen as intrinsically insane, if not criminal.[35] This deep imbrication between Black madness as "(in)sanity, cognitive disability, anger" is a relationship that psychiatrist and historian Jonathan Metzl has explored in *The Protest Psychosis*.[36] Black theorists like Therí Alyce Pickens and La Marr Jurelle Bruce unpack this relationship further, using the lens of disability studies to question what it means to be "mad" in the first place.[37]

For Pickens, it is not simply that Blackness and madness are posed as mutually constitutive (which they often are, either in the historical or psychiatric discourse) but that the idea of "Black madness" itself needs to be called into question. Using a disability studies approach engages the relationship between race, disability, and madness, which appears so entangled as to be taken for granted. That is, "racism and ableism are quotidian practices in which the experience of being raced and being disabled are mundane. For that reason, one cannot have race without disability, nor disability without race."[38] Pickens argues against simply "bringing race" into disability studies, but rather suggests that ideas about madness itself, what is mad and what is not, are both sanist and racist. Thinking about madness through and with a racial lens reveals the way that "madness becomes the place to engage because racism adheres to a peculiar kind of rationality," and it is at this adherence that we see the way that what is considered sane is only ever white.[39]

"To address Blackness/madness imperils the twin pillars of whiteness and sanity that uphold Western notions of intellectual enterprise," Pickens argues, and this idea is particularly important to this book because it gets to the heart of not only how psychiatry is internally racist but how it is intentionally so and how it is wielded and weaponized "at the seams" of the real material conditions of life.[40]

Picken's terrain of analysis of this imbrication is speculative fiction, but she gestures deliberately to the importance of historical context and the way that taken-for-granted ideas about sanity and what it is are problematic for the historian, who needs to be able to not take things like diagnosis at face value. Rather, she argues that madness is not a mere metaphor/substitute for Blackness, but that ideas about madness are always already racist, "steeped in discourses that have long histories, including racist antebellum pseudoscience, disability as the rationale against civil rights gains, and rhetoric that binds white racism to a series of unspeakable and unintelligible acts."[41]

Black rage and Black "excess," historically characterized as the entirety of a monolithic "Black culture," are posed as irrational and uncivilized in the same way that the enslaved person was. If this type of Black rage does exist, then it is barely considered a just and legitimate reaction to the reality of American life, at least not by the white carceral-psychiatric system, despite the fact that Black psychiatrists from Fanon to Cobbs and Grier have argued for this interpretation.[42] As is obvious every day in the United States, only the "excess" of Black rage and the violence it allegedly invokes is characterized as pathological, while the very real violence of white supremacy gets a pass.

In his work on "madness and black radical creativity," La Marr Jurelle Bruce builds on Pickens, Fanon, and Hortense Spillers, among others, to unpack the way that "antiblack psychiatry has variously engaged enslavement, colonization, institutionalization, incarceration, disenfranchisement, assimilation to whiteness, abnegation of blackness and mind-dulling or mind-destroying medical procedures as 'treatments.'"[43] He argues that the pathologization of "Black culture," either in its characterization as excessive, uncivilized, and irrational or in the supposed deprivation of the Black family, continues to be used as a weapon of devastation, underpinning practices of incarceration and violence. For Bruce, however, the very aspects of Black culture and self-expression that are seen as excessive or irrational are in fact the very logical and creative ways in which Black people have sought to make sense of their experience, to flourish, thrive, and survive despite the evils of white supremacy—beyond the reach of racist psychiatry.

While Bruce talks about the possibility of antiracist psychiatry, he is also clear that this would only be possible if we were also willing to "reckon with the pathology of white supremacy, to attend to the ongoing trauma of antiblackness, and most ambitiously, to overturn the extant racial order."[44] Following Fanon but extending him, Bruce is arguing that a true analysis of psychiatry can lead only to its abolition, because psychiatry and racism cannot be separated.[45] Racism is central to the language, ideology, and practice of psychiatry itself, so that the problem is not the Black person's "worrisome behavior [as] psychosocial alterity; instead it is white supremacist Reason laid hideously bare."[46]

The point in all of this theorizing is that psychiatry is acting as a shield for white supremacy. The focus on individual, or even group, psychopathology (a generalization rarely extended to white culture, such as it is), deflects from the actual violence of the way that white supremacy works in the wake of the plantation, the continuities of systemic violence, and the damage wrought by anti-Black racism, of which psychiatry is in fact a part. Because of this imbrication between psychiatry and white supremacy, it is barely possible to say anything about "Black madness"—the criteria themselves are so flawed, so white-centric, so normalizing.

These theoretical considerations raise a tension for this book and the analysis I am trying to do here. It is the case that Fanon was still a psychiatrist, and practiced many of its technologies, including the use of shock therapies. While he may have argued that psychopathologies of the Black person were at least partially sociogenic, he did not fully divest himself of psychiatry's role in creating or perpetuating the problem in the first place. As a psychiatrist, he held that mental illness did exist, as did many of the Black psychiatrists at Tuskegee. The issue for them was a Fanonian one—that the cause of mental illness in their communities was sociogenic, not biological.

I do not mean to claim that mental illness does not exist in Black folks, either related to or separate from the reality of racism. Demanding that psychiatry reckon with its racism does not negate the reality or lived experience of mental illness itself. But it does call psychiatry as a practice and a profession into question. I return to Foucault for a moment here. The issue is that psychiatry was a form of biopolitical power, and it was enacted on the bodies and minds of thousands of people across the South in particular ways, for reasons that cannot be separated from white supremacy. During the civil rights era, the external racism of psychiatric structures was laid bare, demonstrating the way that segregation had allowed abuse, neglect, and violence that replicated plantation ways of life. The material presented in this book aims to demonstrate the way these structures were experienced, supported, and justified by the banal racism of everyday life in the South, and how these structures were resisted. The material also demonstrates that these structures were undergirded by the far more pernicious and malevolent internal racism of psychiatry, which barely registered as the thing to be dealt with. It is this internal racism of psychiatry itself that remains a cause for concern.

Acknowledgments

This book would not exist without the support of a great many people.

First and foremost, I want to thank everyone who shared their stories and experiences of these institutions with me. I am particularly grateful to the entire Hurston family, particularly Ronald, Donald, and Pamela, who have been so open and generous with their mother's and brother's stories.

I spoke to many people who have worked in or brought legal action against these institutions and am deeply grateful for the time and courage it took to speak openly and honestly about their experiences.

From the legal perspective, I am indebted to Michael Meltsner and Conrad Harper from the Legal Defense Fund, James Tucker from the Alabama Disabilities Advocacy Program, Ira Burnam from the Bazelon Center for Mental Health Law, and Barry Powell from Community Legal Services of Mississippi.

From the administrator or clinician perspective, huge thanks to Dr. John Gates and Dr. Derril Gay from Central State Hospital in Georgia, who were incredibly forthcoming and spent many hours in person or on Zoom with me. Thank you to Mary Lou Rahn, Lynne Wright, Susan Trueblood, and Mrs. Marsha Gates for their support. Thanks also to Steve Davis from the Alabama Department of Mental Health and Greg Hoyt from the Georgia Department of Behavioral Health and Developmental Disabilities for their forthright information about the location of records, and to Jessica Whitehead for information about current processes. Thank you to Nick Taylor, Andy Miller, and Beth Shelburne for their journalistic perspectives.

Despite the challenges, this book relies heavily on several state and federal archives, and archivists have been co-creators of my knowledge from the beginning. First, thanks to Margaret (Peggy) Balch at the Reynolds-Finley Historical Library at the University of Alabama at Birmingham. Extra-special thanks to Cheryl Ferguson, Cynthia Beavers Wilson, and Dana Chandler for their support, assistance, and treasure hunting at the Tuskegee University Archives. Scotty Kirkland and Nancy Dupree from the Alabama Department of Archives and History were present at the eureka moment and then helped me locate the files for *Marable v. Alabama Mental Health Board*. I am also particularly grateful to Maureen Hill at the National Archives and Records Administration, Southeast Division, who has continued to help me navigate the case records of the US district court.

Thanks to Laura Heller and her team at the Mississippi Department of Archives and History, who helped me navigate various collections related to Whitfield and processed Dr. Jaquith's collection. Thank you to everyone at the Georgia State Archives who helped process boxes and requests, and scanned files for me. Thanks also to the archivists at special collections at Tougaloo College, Mississippi State

University, the University of Southern Mississippi, the University of South Alabama, the University of Alabama, Georgia Southern University, the Library of Congress, the National Archives and Records Administration at College Park, and the Kislak Center at the University of Pennsylvania.

I have had the intense privilege of receiving incredible support and resources from Emory University. A huge thank-you to Erica Bruchko, US history librarian, who helped me access many expensive databases and newspaper archives; to Jonathan Coulis for assistance with oral history taking; to Jennifer Doty for help with digital archiving processes; and to John David Morgenstern and Lisa Macklin for copyright and contract advice.

This book has been supported in multiple ways by the Fox Center for Humanistic Inquiry (FCHI) at Emory, as well as by Emory's Department of History and Nell Hodgson Woodruff School of Nursing, and I have many people to thank here. Thank you to the Fox Center, Emory president Greg Fenves, and dean of the nursing school Linda McCauley for supporting the award of the President's Humanities Fellowship, which gave me a precious year of thinking and writing time.

The Fox Center is also home to the Digital Publishing in the Humanities initiative, which has financially and intellectually supported this book from its inception. Thank you to Walter Mellion, Carla Freeman, Keith Anthony, and Collette Barlow for creating such a welcoming space for humanists across Emory. Thank you to Sarah McKee and Mae Velloso-Lyons for their stewardship through all the processes and decisions related to digital open access publishing. Thank you to my fellow Digital Monograph Writing Workshop members for the collegiality and inspiration: Christina Crawford, Geraldine Higgins, Patricia Cahill, Maria Montolvo, and Cocoa Williams. Thank you also to George Yancy for the generative discussion about Fanon.

The open access digital version of this book has been supported by the FCHI and the Emory Center for Digital Scholarship, particularly Yang Li and Megan Slemons, who slaved over data and GIS visualizations and asked the hard questions. Thank you to Jordan Pelkmans in the School of Nursing for the number crunching.

Thank you to colleagues across Emory for the intellectual and emotional support: Joe Crespino, Jason Morgan Ward, Danny LaChance, Carl Suddler, Yanna Yanakakis, Thomas Rogers, Judith Miller, Karen Stolley, Susan Youngblood Ashmore, Sander Gilman, William Billups, Marissa Nichols, Elizabeth Wilson, Sameena Mulla, Ben Reiss, Falguni Sheth, Mary Dudziak, Matthew Lawrence, Ani Satz, Avi Wofsy, Octavia Vogel, Gaea Daniel, Sarah Febres-Cordero, Lisa Thompson, and Whitney Wharton. Thank you to the Nell Hodgson Woodruff School of Nursing for all the work that goes into supporting an historian: to Linda McCauley, Ken Hepburn, Sandi Dunbar, Kimberley Dupree Jones, Laura Kimble, Lisa Muirhead, and Benjamin Harris.

I was lucky to present early versions of parts of this book at invited lectures and symposia, and the book was shaped and made better by that early engagement and feedback. Thanks to participants at the Johns Hopkins Institute for the History of Medicine colloquium for the generative feedback on an early version of the Tuskegee chapter. Special thanks for the thoughtful discussions at workshops and symposia, including Viral Networks at the National Library of Medicine, the Molina Symposium on Reckoning with the History of Racism in Medicine at Johns Hopkins University, and the University of Sydney History of Psychiatry Winter School.

Thank you to organizers and audiences at several guest lectures, including the Rubenstein Library and School of Medicine at Duke University, the Centre for the Social History of Health & Healthcare at the University of Strathclyde, the CF Reynolds Medical History Society at the University of Pittsburgh, the Barbara Bates Center for the Study of the History of Nursing at the University of Pennsylvania, the Center for Health Policy and Law at Northeastern University, the Art HX group at Princeton University, the Weill Cornell Medical College, and the Program in the History of Science, Medicine and Technology Center at the University of Minnesota.

A version of chapter 1 appeared as the article by Kylie M. Smith, "A Clinic for the People: Toward an Antiracist Psychiatry at the Tuskegee Institute, 1947–1965," *Bulletin of the History of Medicine* 98, no. 2 (2024): 235–65. Sections of chapters 7 and 8 appeared in the article by Kylie M. Smith, "No Medical Justification: Segregation and Civil Rights in Alabama's Psychiatric Hospitals, 1950–1972," *Journal of Southern History* 87, no. 4 (2021): 645–72. Thank you to the editors and anonymous reviews of those articles, and deep appreciation to the anonymous reviewers of this manuscript.

I am particularly grateful for all the history of medicine and psychiatry colleagues who have helped shape and refine my argument along the way: Hans Pols, Mark Micale, Jeremy Greene, Ahmed Ragab, Adam Biggs, Mary Fissell, Elizabeth Obrien, Sasha White, Rana Hogarth, Christopher Willoughby, Samuel Kelton Roberts, Jessica Adler, Udodiro Okwandu, Hannah Zeavin, Ayah Nuriddin, Mical Raz, Bradford Pelletier, Christina Ramos, Hafeeza Anchrum, Nic John Ramos, Rich McKay, Claire Clark, Jason Glenn, Mab Segrest, and many others in audiences and classrooms over the last seven years.

Special thanks to Rick Mizelle for being such a great UNC Press sibling and cheerleader. I can't wait to read yours. Huge thanks to my mentors Susan Reverby and Jonathan Sadowsky. And extra thanks to Thomas Foth, Daniel Goldberg, and Richard Keller for always pushing me to think better and harder.

For writing and personal support at various points throughout, thanks go to a collective of amazing women: Dominique Tobell, Elena Conis, Sari Altschuler, Melanie Tanielian, Aparna Nair, Cornelia Lambert, Jessica Dillard-Wright, Jane Hopkins-Walsh, Jennifer Grant, Jacqueline Antonovich, Courtney Thompson, Amanda Mahoney, Lauren MacIvor Thompson, Elizabeth Neswald, Janet Golden, Sharrona Pearl, Sarah Swedberg, Jai Virdi, and Kelly O'Donnell. Special thanks to Julie Fairman, who was there at the beginning.

I have been blessed with excellent research assistance throughout this project from Virgo Morrison, Jordan Seidman, and Leanne Jong, who helped to wrangle archives, documents, and data. Thank you so much for being part of this project.

This project has been made possible by several grants, most notably the G13 Award from the National Library of Medicine (NIH). Thank you also to the Emory University Research Committee, the Reynolds-Finley Historical Library, the

American Association for the History of Nursing, and the Barbara Bates Center for the Study of the History of Nursing for various research grants over the last seven years.

I am incredibly grateful to the team at UNC Press, especially Lucas Church, who has believed in this project since its inception in 2018. He has shepherded it through many iterations, dealt with my convoluted writing with grace and humor, and never wavered from the commitment to open access. A book could not have a better editor, or an author a better champion.

Finally, thanks to the family I chose, the Dillard-Wright clan, Lou Robinson and Bill DeLoach, our collective fur babies, and my feral ratbag Cookie. Thank you to my Aunt Jenny for support and encouragement during very difficult times. Special thanks to my sister Nardine Smith, who knows what it has taken to get here. Love you, sissy.

Notes

Abbreviations

ADAH	Alabama Department of Archives and History, Montgomery, AL
AGSIF	Alabama Governor State Institutions Files, Alabama Department of Archives and History, Montgomery, AL
Dibble Papers	Dibble Papers, Tuskegee University Archives, Tuskegee, AL
MCHR	Medical Committee for Human Rights Records, 1963–2004, Ms. Coll. 641, Kislak Center for Special Collections, Rare Books and Manuscripts, University of Pennsylvania
MCR44	Civil Action 2610, Record of Administrative Hearing Docket No. MCR-44, US District Court Case Files 74-C-0813, National Archives and Records Administration, Morrow, GA
MDAH	Mississippi Department of Archives and History, Jackson, MS
NARACP	National Archives and Records Administration, College Park, MD
NPVLP	Non-Partisan Voters League Papers, Doy Leale McCall Rare Book and Manuscript Library, University of South Alabama, Mobile, AL
Stennis Papers	John C. Stennis Collection, Mississippi Political Collections, Division of Archives and Special Collections, Mississippi State University, Starkville, MS

Prologue

1. Hurston to HEW, January 1965, Stennis Papers. I am repeating this letter verbatim, including with Mrs. Hurston's full name and address, with the express permission of her remaining family, but I acknowledge that Thomas himself, who passed away in 2018, cannot give permission for his own name to be used or his story to be told. His family has given me permission to do so.

2. K. M. Smith, "No Medical Justification."

3. K. M. Smith, "No Medical Justification."

4. See, for example, Oshinsky, *Worse Than Slavery*; Blackmon, *Slavery by Another Name*; Alexander, *New Jim Crow*.

5. K. M. Smith, "No Medical Justification." See chapters 7 and 8 for a detailed account of these investigations and the subsequent court case.

6. Sharpe, *In the Wake*; Hartman, *Scenes of Subjection*.

7. Sharpe, *In the Wake*, 14.

8. Edwards-Grossi and Willoughby, "Slavery and Its Afterlives." See also Willoughby, *Masters of Health*; Edwards-Grossi, *Mad with Freedom*.

9. Mbembe, *Necropolitics*.

10. Sharpe, *In the Wake*, 17.

11. I draw heavily on the work of disability and abolition activists here. See, for example, Ben-Moshe, *Decarcerating Disability*; Ben-Moshe et al., *Disability Incarcerated*.

12. Patterson, *Slavery and Social Death*. See also Cacho, *Social Death*; Guenther, *Solitary Confinement*; Price, *Prison and Social Death*.

13. Brown, "Social Death and Political Life."

14. Hartman, *Scenes of Subjection*, 13.

15. See Hartman, *Scenes of Subjection*; Hartman, "Venus in Two Acts." These ideas are explored in more depth in the appendices.

16. Foucault, *Psychiatric Power*; Berrey, *Jim Crow Routine*.

17. See, for example, Taggart, "'Are You Experienced?'"; Spandler and Poursanidou, "Who Is Included in the Mad Studies Project?"; Burch and Rembis, *Disability Histories*.

18. Trouillot, *Silencing the Past*, 26.

19. I discuss this more in appendix 1, but the idea that historians should push back against archival restrictions comes from Susan Lawrence's book *Privacy and the Past*. For a discussion of these issues and the ethical questions they raise, see essays in Thompson and Smith, *Do Less Harm*. See also Sadowsky and Smith, "Reflections on the Use of Patient Records."

20. I discuss the possibility of reparatory history at the end of this book (see aftermath) as well as in K. M. Smith, "Reparatory History."

21. For contact details, please see http://jimcrowintheasylum.com.

Chapter 1

1. A version of this chapter first appeared in the *Bulletin of the History of Medicine* 98, no. 2 (Summer 2024): 235–65. Copyright 2024, The Johns Hopkins University Press. Barker, "Psychoanalysis of Groups."

2. See appendix 2 for an analysis of how Fanon's work has informed my approach in this book.

3. "Tuskegee Clinic . . . Of, by and for the People," *Alabama Mental Health* 2, no. 11 (November 1950): 1, Reynolds-Finley Historical Library, University of Alabama at Birmingham.

4. "Tuskegee Clinic . . . Of, by and for the People," 3.

5. "Tuskegee Clinic . . . Of, by and for the People," 3.

6. Summers, "'Suitable Care of the African When Afflicted with Insanity'"; Summers, *Madness in the City of Magnificent Intentions*; Gambino, "'These Strangers within Our Gates'"; Doyle, *Psychiatry and Racial Liberalism in Harlem*; Mendes, *Under the Strain of Color*; Nuriddin, "Psychiatric Jim Crow." For a comprehensive overview of Black psychiatrists and their role at the Tuskegee VA Hospital, see Spurlock, *Black Psychiatrists and American Psychiatry*; Kaplan, *Tuskegee Veterans Hospital*.

7. Reverby, *Examining Tuskegee*.

8. Kirkbride, "Proceedings"; Tomes, *Art of Asylum-Keeping*; Gonaver, *Peculiar Institution and the Making of Modern Psychiatry*.

9. McCandless, *Moonlight, Magnolia and Madness*; Gonaver, *Peculiar Institution*.

10. Gamble, *Making a Place for Ourselves*.

11. Gamble, *Making a Place for Ourselves*, 78; Kaplan, *Tuskegee Veterans Hospital*.

12. Minutes of the Consultants on Hospitalization, quoted in Gamble, *Making a Place for Ourselves*, 74n216.

13. Gamble, *Making a Place for Ourselves*, 103.

14. A. C. Rose, *Psychology and Selfhood in the Segregated South*; Kaplan, *Solomon Carter Fuller*; Gamble, *Making a Place for Ourselves*; Kaplan, *Tuskegee Veterans Hospital*.

15. Spurlock, *Black Psychiatrists and American Psychiatry*; A. C. Rose, *Psychology and Selfhood in the Segregated South*.

16. Barker, Biographical Sketch, File: Correspondence Dr Prince Barker, box 18, Dibble Papers.

17. Barker, "Obscure Syphilitic Manifestations"; Barker, "Neuropsychiatry in the Practice of Medicine and Surgery."

18. Barker, "Results and Observations on Insulin Shock Therapy"; Dwyer, "Psychiatry and Race during World War II."

19. Barker, "Results and Observations on Insulin Shock Therapy."

20. Barker, "Results and Observations," 22.

21. Barker, "Psychoanalysis of Groups," 445–46.

22. Barker, "Psychoanalysis of Groups," 445–46.

23. Larson, *Sex, Race and Science*.

24. Dorr, "Defective or Disabled?," 360.

25. Partlow, "Degeneracy"; Partlow, "Annual Message of the President."

26. Partlow, "Annual Message of the President."

27. Vickery, "History of Mental Health in Alabama," Reynolds-Finley Historical Library, University of Alabama at Birmingham. See also Holley, *History of Medicine in Alabama*.

28. Holley, *History of Medicine in Alabama*, 335.

29. Larson, *Sex, Race and Science*; Dorr, "Defective or Disabled?"; Holley, *History of Medicine in Alabama*; S. M. Smith, "Eugenic Sterilization in 20th Century Georgia"; Hughes, "Labeling and Treating Black Mental Illness in Alabama"; A. C. Rose, *Psychology and Selfhood in the Segregated South*.

30. Dorr, "Defective or Disabled?," 361.

31. Felix, "Mental Hygiene and Public Health"; Kearl, "Etiology Replaces Interminability"; Meyer, "Birth and Development of the Mental Hygiene Movement"; Richardson, *Century of the Child*; Beers, *Mind That Found Itself*.

32. Richardson, *Century of the Child*; Jones, *Taming the Troublesome Child*.

33. Nuriddin, "Liberation Eugenics"; Robinson, "Battle for Respectability"; Du Bois, *Souls of Black Folk*; Moore, *Booker T. Washington, W. E. B. Du Bois, and the Struggle for Racial Uplift*; Chandler and Powell, *To Raise Up the Man Farthest Down*.

34. Nuriddin, "Liberation Eugenics"; Nuriddin, "Engineering Uplift."

35. This is also an idea that Susan Reverby explores in her work on the syphilis study, arguing that we need to understand the role of the doctors in that study at the intersection of their lives as "race men" and "science men." Reverby, *Examining Tuskegee*, 157.

36. Kardiner and Ovesey, *Mark of Oppression*; D. M. Scott, *Contempt and Pity*.

37. Nuriddin, "Engineering Uplift."

38. A. C. Rose, *Psychology and Selfhood in the Segregated South*; A. C. Rose, "Putting the South on the Psychological Map."

39. Barker, "Frontiers of Mental Hygiene."

40. Barker, "Frontiers of Mental Hygiene," 15.

41. Barker, "Frontiers of Mental Hygiene," 15.

42. Barker, "Frontiers of Mental Hygiene," 15.

43. Thomas, "Hill-Burton Act and Civil Rights"; Thomas, *Deluxe Jim Crow*; Byrd and Clayton, *American Health Dilemma*; D. B. Smith, *Health Care Divided*; Reynolds, "Hospitals and Civil Rights."

44. Memo by Sarah Howell, Tuskegee Mental Hygiene Society, September 1947, box 27, file 14, Dibble Papers.

45. Memo, Dibble to Barker, box 27, file 14, Dibble Papers.

46. Reverby, *Examining Tuskegee*.

47. Foster, report to Dibble, March 1951, box 27, file 14, Dibble Papers.

48. Foster, report to Dibble, box 27, file 14, Dibble Papers.

49. Foster to Jarvis and Dibble, Report of Activities, May 9, 1951, Dibble Papers.

50. Undated note, box 27, folder 14, 030.027, Mental Hygiene Clinic/The Tuskegee Mental Hygiene Society, 1947–1951, Dibble Papers.

51. Harvey to Barker and Dibble, box 27, file 13: Correspondence: Mental Hygiene, Dibble Papers.

52. Roberts to Barker, December 22, 1952, box 27, file 14, Dibble Papers.

53. While I am not writing specifically about industrial training or reform schools in this book, they are a large part of the broader carceral system that psychiatric hospitals inhabited. Mt. Meigs was the subject of several inspections and exposés throughout the mid-twentieth century and is still an active part of the Alabama Department of Youth Services, serving today as a juvenile correctional facility.

54. Dibble, notes, April 28, 1955, box 27, file 13: Correspondence: Mental Hygiene, Dibble Papers.

55. Dibble, notes, April 28, 1955, box 27, file 13.

56. The relationship between Tuskegee and Mt. Meigs is best documented in the Administrative Files of the State Health Officer, Public Health, box SG006303 1963, folder 019, and box SG006310, folder 03, ADAH. Alabama operated two other training schools, one for white boys in Birmingham and one for white girls in Chalkville. Mt. Meigs had both male and female Black children on site together.

57. Barker to Dibble, "Informal Comments on Dr. Menninger's Visit," April 23, 1954, box 18, file 2, Dibble Papers.

58. Menninger to Boone, April 13, 1954, box 28, folder 6: Correspondence: Dr. Karl Menninger, The Menninger Clinic Topeka Kansas 1950–1954, Dibble Papers.

59. Menninger to Boone, April 13, 1954, box 28, folder 6.

60. Dibble to Menninger, December 23, 1959, box 28, folder 7, Dibble Papers.

61. The work of the SREB is documented to some extent in K. M. Smith, *Talking Therapy*. Individual nurses from Tuskegee were sometimes part of the various ef-

forts to improve psychiatric nurse education through the SREB, but there is no evidence of Tuskegee psychiatrists present at any SREB conferences in the 1950s. See, for example, SREB, *Mental Health Training and Research in the Southern States*; SREB, *Psychiatrists for Mental Health Programs*.

62. Barker, "Psychiatry at the Tuskegee VA Hospital in Retrospect," 152.
63. Barker, "Psychiatry at the Tuskegee VA Hospital in Retrospect," 153.
64. Barker, "Psychiatry at the Tuskegee VA Hospital in Retrospect," 152.
65. Barker, "Psychiatry at the Tuskegee VA Hospital in Retrospect," 153.
66. These issues are the subject of chapters 6 and 8.

Chapter 2

1. George Schuyler to Louis T. Wright, October 2, 1935, box 5, folder 84, Louis Tompkins Wright Papers, 1879, 1898, 1909–1997, H MS c56, Harvard Medical Library, Francis A. Countway Library of Medicine. This letter was shared with me by Dr. Adam Biggs, to whom I am eternally grateful.

2. See, for example, Schuyler, *Black No More*; Schuyler, *Rac(e)ing to the Right*. For critical engagements with Schuyler's work, see Ferguson, *Sage of Sugar Hill*; Williams, *George S. Schuyler*.

3. Silver, *Mississippi: The Closed Society*; Ward, *Hanging Bridge*.

4. See appendix 1 for the extensive theoretical framework that informs my thinking here.

5. Rucker and Jubilee, "From Black Nadir to *Brown v. Board*," 151; Adams and Adams, *Just Trying to Have School*; Downs, *Sick from Freedom*; Long, *Doctoring Freedom*; Thomas, *Deluxe Jim Crow*.

6. Gamble, *Making a Place for Ourselves*; McBride, *Caring for Equality*.

7. Plessy v. Ferguson, 163 U.S. 537 (1896).

8. See Hogarth, *Medicalizing Blackness*; Savitt and Young, *Disease and Distinctiveness in the American South*; Savitt, "Use of Blacks for Medical Experimentation and Demonstration"; Owens, *Medical Bondage*; Fett, *Working Cures*; Willoughby, *Masters of Health*; Willoughby, "Running Away from Drapetomania."

9. Hughes, "Labeling and Treating Black Mental Illness in Alabama"; Willoughby, "Running Away from Drapetomania"; Edwards-Grossi, "Truth in Numbers?"; Edwards-Grossi, *Mad with Freedom*; Muhammad, *Condemnation of Blackness*.

10. Gonaver, *Peculiar Institution and the Making of Modern Psychiatry*; McCandless, *Moonlight, Magnolias, and Madness*; Segrest, *Administrations of Lunacy*.

11. Edwards-Grossi, *Mad with Freedom*.

12. Willoughby, "Running Away from Drapetomania"; Edwards-Grossi, *Mad with Freedom*.

13. Grossi, "Truth in Numbers?"; Edwards-Grossi, *Mad with Freedom*. For an in-depth exploration of the concept of "soundness," see Fett, *Working Cures*.

14. Gonaver, *Peculiar Institution and the Making of Modern Psychiatry*; Edwards-Grossi, *Mad with Freedom*.

15. Gonaver, *Peculiar Institution and the Making of Modern Psychiatry*; Tomes, *Art of Asylum-Keeping*.

16. S. M. Smith, "Eugenic Sterilization in 20th Century Georgia"; Murphy, "Inhospitable in the Hospitality State"; Dorr, "Defective or Disabled?"; Larson, *Sex, Race, and Science*. A lot of this work has focused on the eugenic practice of sterilization, but this is not my focus here, partly because it has already been covered but also because it has often been posed as the ultimate evil of institutional segregation, and my argument lies elsewhere.

17. See appendix 2 for an explanation of the difficulty around sources related to the hospitals under study here.

18. CSH was known by many different names over time, but in the 1950s and 1960s, it was increasingly referred to as Central State Hospital or just "Milledgeville," which is how I will refer to it in the rest of the book.

19. Segrest, *Administrations of Lunacy*.

20. Thomas F. Green, *Annual Report of the Milledgeville State Hospital*, 1870, cited in Segrest, *Administrations of Lunacy*, 152.

21. "Milledgeville State Hospital," RCB29742, Georgia State Archives.

22. See Segrest, *Administrations of Lunacy*, for a detailed analysis of the first 140 years at CSH and Powell's impact.

23. Personal communication from Walter Reynolds, past director of the Central State Redevelopment Authority, personal communication, July 2019. See also Segrest, *Administrations of Lunacy*, 4–9.

24. For details on the establishment and maintenance of segregation in the first 100 years of the hospital, see Segrest, *Administrations of Lunacy*. Later chapters in this book deal with the impact of newspaper reports and then the Community Mental Health Act and the Civil Rights Act on both exposing and ending segregation in the various hospitals under study here. Thank you to Mary Lou Rahn, Lynne Wright, and Walter Reynolds for their help in identifying the populations and naming origins of various buildings at CSH.

25. Information about Jasmine Ridge and the markers is from Walter Reynolds, past director of the Central State Redevelopment Authority, personal communication, July 2019. Mab Segrest has also written about her experience with the cemeteries in *Administrations of Lunacy*.

26. K. M. Smith, *Talking Therapy*.

27. D'Antonio, *American Nursing*.

28. Since I began researching this book, Georgia College and State University, inheriting collections that were once kept on-site at the hospital museum (which Segrest had access to for her book), have begun to catalog and display items relevant to aspects of the history of Central State. Much of a current digital exhibit focuses on nursing, and specific information about the Black nurses can be found at https://georgialibraries.omeka.net/s/central-state-hospital/page/african-american-nurses.

29. *Annual Report of the Milledgeville State Hospital*, 1956, 13.

30. More about the use of farms and patients as laborers would be publicly revealed later in 1959 in a scathing exposé by journalist Jack Nelson. I explore this exposé and the continuation of farm work in chapter 5.

31. Holley, *History of Medicine in Alabama*.

32. 1894 Annual Report to the Board of Trustees, quoted in Tarwater, "Alabama State Hospitals and the Partlow State School and Hospital."

33. Tarwater, "Alabama State Hospitals," 176.

34. Tarwater, "Alabama State Hospitals," 178.

35. Tarwater, "Alabama State Hospitals," 180.

36. This report is discussed in more detail in chapter 4.

37. *Report on the State Mental Hospitals of Alabama, Made by the Central Inspection Board of the American Psychiatric Association, 1958*, vol. 2, 14–16, Bryce Hospital Collection, W. S. Hoole Special Collections Library, University of Alabama, Tuscaloosa.

38. Tarwater, "Alabama State Hospitals," 180.

39. "Robert Jemison Jr.," Encyclopedia of Alabama, last updated June 14, 2023, https://encyclopediaofalabama.org/article/robert-jemison-jr/.

40. "State Hospital Farm Strides Revealed," *Jackson Daily News*, October 1938, sourced from Whitfield State Hospital Subject File, MSU Special Collections.

41. "Mississippi Hospital's Farm Cares for Patients," *Commercial Appeal*, October 9, 1938, sourced from Whitfield State Hospital Subject File, MSU Special Collections.

42. Previous directors or superintendents had been direct appointments by the state legislature, making the position, and the hospital, subject to many claims of corruption. Details of how this worked are included in chapter 3.

43. "Father of Mental Health Program Retiring," *Clarion Ledger*, November 25, 1979.

44. For more details about these students and their important work at Whitfield, see chapter 3.

45. *Laurel Leader Call*, July 20, 1955, MDAH.

46. *Biennial Report of the Mississippi State Hospital, Whitfield, Mississippi* (hereafter known as *Biennial Report*), 1951–53, MDAH.

47. Jaquith had a particular concern for alcoholic and narcotic patients, which had extra significance in Mississippi as a state that maintained alcohol prohibition at the state level until 1966, at which point individual counties were allowed to vote for alcohol repeal or supply. Jaquith, *The Mississippi State Hospital*, Whitfield Mississippi, 1951, 11.

48. *Jackson Daily News*, November 29, 1952.

49. *Biennial Report*, 1955–1957, 53.

50. *Biennial Report*, 1955–1957. The report uses the small *n* for Negro, which is how I have reproduced it here, but its use in this way reflects the lack of respect for Black people in the official sources from Mississippi, which I do not support.

51. *Biennial Report*, 1955–1957.

52. Jaquith, *The Mississippi State Hospital*, 1951, 13.

53. *Biennial Report*, 1957–1959, 37.

54. *Biennial Report*, 1955–1957, 22.

55. Treatment and therapeutic regimens are the subject of chapter 3.

56. See appendix 1 for more information about this.

57. *Admission Laws for State Mental Hospitals of Mississippi*, Mississippi State Hospital, Whitfield, 2nd printing, 1964, 374.6:196401, 2, MDAH.

58. *Admission Laws for State Mental Hospitals of Mississippi*, 3.

59. This experience was reported to me by Mr. Barry Powell, director of Mississippi Legal Services, personal communication, January 20, 2020. Mr. Powell shared insights and details from many of his cases against Whitfield with me, and I discuss these in the aftermath.

60. *Report on the State Mental Hospitals of Alabama, Made by the Central Inspection Board of the American Psychiatric Association*, 1958, 13.

61. I talked about this issue extensively with Mr. Powell in Mississippi and Dr. John Gates, superintendent of CSH in Georgia from 1974, who reported many instances of this kind of pressure brought to bear while he was in charge. Mr. Barry Powell, personal communication, January 2020; Dr. John Gates, personal communication, February 2021.

62. Segrest, *Administrations of Lunacy*, 302.

63. Georgia Health Code 1966, Public Health—Mental Health—Director's Administrative Records RCB29733, Georgia State Archives, Morrow.

64. Georgia Health Code 1966, 43–47.

65. Georgia Health Code 1966, 44.

66. Kidd to Gates, August 8, 1989, Culver Kidd Papers, Zach Henderson Library, Special Collections, University of South Georgia, Statesboro.

67. Peacock reported an average patient daily head count of around 11,844, with an additional 2,214 patients out of the hospital on furlough, or "trial visit." The use of furlough meant that people could be discharged temporarily, simplifying their readmittance if the trial visit was unsuccessful (i.e., avoiding the requirement for a full court hearing and recommitment procedure). But this process also means there is a lack of clarity in the annual reports about who exactly was being discharged and recommitted. For my purposes here, I will focus only on the total inpatient head count, which skews heavily toward white people.

68. See "1960 Census of Population: Supplementary Reports: Race of the Population of the United States, by States: 1960," September 7, 1961, www2.census.gov/library/publications/decennial/1960/pc-s1-supplementary-reports/pc-s1-10.pdf.

69. "1960 Census of Population."

70. Jaquith, *The Mississippi State Hospital*, 1951, 21; *Biennial Report*, 1953–1955, 14.

71. Berrey, *Jim Crow Routine*; Litwack, *Trouble in Mind*.

Chapter 3

1. Dr. Harding Olson to Dr. Charles Bush, Director of Hospital Services Branch, Department of Public Health, Atlanta, Georgia, November 8, 1966, RCB-29713, Central State Hospital Complaints, 1966–1969, Public Health—Mental Health—Director's Administrative Files, Georgia State Archives, Morrow, GA.

2. Dr. Olson to Dr. Bush, November 8, 1966, Georgia State Archives.

3. In relation to sources, there are discrepancies between the states in the type and amount of data that was recorded and is now available. The main sources of data are the annual and biannual reports that were compiled to report to the relevant state authorities. Georgia submitted complex tables, breaking down diagnostics

by age, race, and gender, whereas Mississippi barely reported diagnostic data at all. Georgia and Alabama created reports every year, whereas Mississippi did so every two years, and not all of Mississippi's reports are extant or discoverable. Alabama stopped reporting complex diagnostic data around 1960.

4. I have strong caveats and even some misgivings about both the writing and the reading of this section. My decision to include diagnostic data stems not from my belief in its ability to tell us anything about disease prevalence; in fact, I would argue that the data cannot possibly tell us that. That is, the data that is available cannot be taken entirely at face value—just because certain amounts or types of people were recorded as being diagnosed in a certain way does not necessarily mean that they were acually diagnosed in that way, or that recorded diagnoses are even accurate.

5. Kramer, "Long Range Studies of Mental Hospital Patients."

6. See, for example, Grob, *Mental Illness and American Society*; Hale, *Rise and Crisis of Psychoanalysis in the United States*; Harrington, *Mind Fixers*; Braslow, *Mental Ills and Bodily Cures*; Noll, *American Madness*; Horwitz, *DSM*.

7. Horwitz, *DSM*.

8. Noll, *American Madness*; Harrington, *Mind Fixers*; Metzl, *Protest Psychosis*.

9. Horwitz, *DSM*.

10. Horwitz, *DSM*, 27.

11. American Psychiatric Association, *Diagnostic and Statistical Manual of Mental Disorders*, 5. See also Horwitz, *DSM*, 112.

12. For information about the statistical methods used and more extensive data analysis, see http://jimcrowintheasylum.com.

13. Chronic brain syndrome consisted of multiple diagnoses, but the majority of people in Georgia and Alabama were recorded under two diagnostic codes: 009-516, "Chronic Brain Syndrome associated with cerebral arteriosclerosis" (CA), and 009-79x, "Chronic Brain Syndrome associated with senile brain disease" (SBD).

14. Ballenger, *Self, Senility, and Alzheimer's Disease*; Ballenger, "Beyond the Characteristic Plaques and Tangles."

15. Thank you to Dr. Ballenger for his help with clarifying this pattern, personal correspondence, March 11, 2024.

16. Obviously, the diagnosis of Alzheimer's disease was further complicated by the lack of testing procedures before the 1990s, so diagnosis was only possible postmortem. See Knopman et al., "Brief History of 'Alzheimer Disease.'"

17. Ballenger, "Beyond the Characteristic Plaques and Tangles," 84.

18. Ballenger, "Beyond the Characteristic Plaques and Tangles," 87.

19. As Ballenger states, "Other psychiatrists redoubled efforts to deal with senile dementia within the state hospitals by conceptualizing it as a treatable mental illness." Ballenger, "Beyond the Characteristic Plaques and Tangles," 87. One of the popular treatments used for SBD was electroshock therapy, and the frequent use of that technology at Searcy Hospital, which I analyze later in this chapter, may have some correlation with Dr. Rowe's tendency to diagnose his Black patients with a disease perceived as a "mental illness" rather than a natural consequence of age.

20. Grob, *From Asylum to Community*.

21. See chapter 6 for more on this.

22. American Psychiatric Association, *Diagnostic and Statistical Manual of Mental Disorders*, 5.

23. Thomas Peacock, in *Annual Report of the Milledgeville State Hospital*, 1956, 9–10.

24. Thomas Peacock, in *Annual Report of the Milledgeville State Hospital*, 1956, 8.

25. Sadowsky, *Electroconvulsive Therapy in America*; Braslow, *Mental Ills and Bodily Cures*.

26. Dr. Bradford, Medical Department Report, in *Annual Report of the Milledgeville State Hospital*, 1956, 18.

27. Dr. Branford, in *Annual Report of the Milledgeville State Hospital*, 1956, 18.

28. Sadowsky, *Electroconvulsive Therapy in America*.

29. Dr. Bradford, Medical Department Report, in *Annual Report of the Milledgeville State Hospital*, 1956, 18.

30. Dr. Bradford, Medical Department Report, in *Annual Report of the Milledgeville State Hospital*, 1956, 19. The overall rate of improvement from drugs was about comparable with that reported as improved from the use of ECT, but the rates of cure from ECT seemed much higher. For example, Dr. Bradford's numbers suggest that 21 percent of patients administered ECT therapy were reported as cured or restored, as opposed to only 6 percent of the patients who were administered tranquilizers. This discrepancy possibly signifies the different ways that efficacy was being measured as much as it reflects the more potent and noticeable effect of ECT over the new drugs that were still largely experimental.

31. John T. Rowell, Psychology Department Report, in *Annual Report of the Milledgeville State Hospital*, 1956, 98.

32. John T. Rowell, in *Annual Report of the Milledgeville State Hospital*, 1956, 98.

33. John T. Rowell, in *Annual Report of the Milledgeville State Hospital*, 1956, 98.

34. Metzl, *Prozac on the Couch*; Hirshbein, *American Melancholy*; Khanna, *Dark Continents*; Adams, "Negro Patient in Psychiatric Treatment"; Kennedy, "Problems Posed in the Analysis of the Negro Patient."

35. Superintendent Tarwater, in *Report of the Trustees of the Alabama State Hospitals*, 1956, 8.

36. Dr. Peyman, Psychology Department Report, in *Report of the Trustees of the Alabama State Hospitals*, 1956, 94–95.

37. Peyman, "Investigation of the Effects of Group Psychotherapy on Chronic Schizophrenic Patients."

38. *Biennial Report of the Mississippi State Hospital, Whitfield, Mississippi* (hereafter known as *Biennial Report*), 1955–1957, 7.

39. *Biennial Report*, 1955–1957.

40. *Biennial Report*, 1955–1957, 16–17.

41. *Biennial Report*, 1957–1959, 9.

42. *Biennial Report*, 1957–1959, 56.

43. *Biennial Report*, 1957–1959, 56.

44. *Biennial Report*, 1957–1959, 56.

45. *Biennial Report*, 1957–1959, 36.

46. *The Whit* 1, no. 7 (April 1951): 26, MDAH. I use *The Whit* more extensively in chapter 4 to tease out some themes related to everyday life at Whitfield.

47. *The Whit* 1, no. 10 (July 1951): 21.

48. *The Whit* 1, no. 9 (June 1951): 24.

49. *The Whit* 1, no. 7 (April 1951): 25.

Chapter 4

1. D. M. to NAACP, May 23, 1952, group 2, box C40, Branch File: Milledgeville GA, 1943–1953, NAACP Branch Files, Library of Congress, Washington, DC.

2. These figures are best represented on the map "Distribution of Negro Population by County 1950," available on the Library of Congress website at www.loc.gov/item/2013593062/.

3. Book and Ezell, "Freedom of Speech and Institutional Control."

4. Murphy, "Inhospitable in the Hospitality State."

5. I set out this process in appendix 1.

6. Many of the articles in *The Whit* are written by patients who identified themselves either through their first name and last initial, or initials only. Sometimes they used "A Patient." Throughout this section, I use the names that patients themselves used. *The Whit* was a publicly circulated document, often beyond the confines of the hospital, and if patients did not want to be identified, they took their own precautions. Thus, my usage here is designed to honor patients' agency in how they wished to be known publicly.

7. In his review, Willie H. referred to the book's title as *The Land Where I Was Born and Raised*. Part 2 of the book is a "report on the Delta as of 1947." Cohn was a friend of Hodding Carter, and it is possible that Carter recommended the book to *The Whit* literary club through Dr. Daly.

8. *The Whit* 1, no. 1 (November 1950): 4, 374.2/Wh1950/51, MDAH.

9. See, for example, Molina, *Fit to Be Citizens?*; Molina, "Fear and Loathing in the US-Mexico Borderlands"; S. Roberts, *Infectious Fear*.

10. *The Whit* 1, no. 1 (November 1950): 4.

11. It is particularly difficult to write about this aspect of life at Whitfield using sources in which names have been removed. There is an irony and a tension here between respecting the privacy of the psychiatric patient, a position so heavily stigmatized, and potentially reinforcing a kind of social death by not naming. My naming convention in this section thus replicates how the patients named themselves and one another in *The Whit* in order to counter some of this tension, at the same time as I wish I could reveal more about each patient as a person.

12. *The Whit* 1, no. 12 (September 1951): 17.

13. *The Whit* 2, no. 3 (December 1951): 29.

14. *The Whit* 2, no. 3 (December 1951): 29.

15. *The Whit* 2, no. 6 (March 1952): 26.

16. *The Whit* 2, no. 6 (March 1952): 26.

17. *The Whit* 1, no. 10 (July 1951): 19.

18. *The Whit* 2, no. 2 (November 1951): 22.

19. *The Whit* 2, no. 2 (November 1951): 22.
20. *The Whit* 2, no. 4 (January 1952): 27.
21. *The Whit* 2, no. 4 (January 1952): 27.
22. All quotes from *The Whit* 2, no. 7 (April 1952): 27–28.
23. *The Whit* 3, no. 1 (October 1952): 40–42.
24. *The Whit* 2, no. 7 (April 1952): 28–29.
25. *The Whit* 1, no. 2 (November 1950).
26. *The Whit* 1, no. 9 (July 1951): 19.
27. *The Whit* 1, no. 10 (July 1951): 20.
28. *The Whit* 1, no. 8 (June 1951): 23.
29. *The Whit* 1, no. 10 (July 1951): 20.
30. *The Whit* 3, no. 1 (October 1952): 42.
31. *The Whit* 1, no. 2 (November 1950): 14.
32. *The Whit* 1, no. 10 (July 1951): 19.
33. *The Whit* 1, no. 10 (July 1951): 19.
34. *The Whit* 1, no. 7 (April 1951): 24.
35. *The Whit* 1, no. 11 (August 1951): 21.
36. *The Whit* 2, no. 2 (November 1951): 24.
37. *The Whit* 2, no. 2 (November 1951): 24.
38. The role of religion in mental health care for Black communities is a complex issue; for example, Cynthia Beavers Wilson explained to me the way that an overreliance on Jesus could be a barrier to real psychiatric care. Personal communication, March 2022, Tuskegee University Archives. An excess of religion could also be cause for a psychiatric diagnosis, as Barker and colleagues at Tuskegee had written about. The role of psychiatry in the pathologization of the Black church is covered by Weisenfeld, *Black Religion in the Madhouse*.
39. *The Whit* 2, no. 2 (November 1951): 19, 28.
40. *The Whit* 2, no. 2 (November 1951): 19, 28.
41. *The Whit* 2, no. 4 (January 1952).
42. D'Antonio, *Founding Friends*; Rothman, *Discovery of the Asylum*; Murray, *Asylum Ways of Seeing*; Tomes, *Art of Asylum-Keeping*; Segrest, *Administrations of Lunacy*; McCandless, *Moonlight, Magnolias and Madness*; Gonaver, *Peculiar Institution and the Making of Modern Psychiatry*; Summers, *Madness in the City of Magnificent Intentions*; Edwards-Grossi, *Mad with Freedom*.
43. For the longer history of moral treatment in the US context, see Deutsch, *Mentally Ill in America*; Rothman, *Discovery of the Asylum*; Grob, *The Mad among Us*; D'Antonio, *Founding Friends*.
44. Deutsch, *Mentally Ill in America*.
45. Tuke to Eddy, 1815, cited in Deutsch, *Mentally Ill in America*, 101.
46. Tomes, *Art of Asylum-Keeping*.
47. Rothman, *Discovery of the Asylum*, 144.
48. Rothman, *Discovery of the Asylum*, 144.
49. Murray, *Asylum Ways of Seeing*, 1.
50. Murray, *Asylum Ways of Seeing*.
51. Rose, *No Right to Be Idle*.

52. For critical work on the political economy and extractive logic of work in asylums, see Edwards-Grossi, *Mad with Freedom*; Ernst, "Role of Work in Psychiatry." Before historians, critical theorists had plenty to say about the exploitative and normative nature of work in asylums. See, for example, Foucault, *Madness and Civilization*; Foucault, *Psychiatric Power*; Szasz, *Myth of Mental Illness*; Goffman, *Asylums*.

53. "Father of Mental Health Program Retiring," *Clarion Ledger*, November 26, 1979.

54. *The Whit* 1, no. 9 (June 1951): 23.

55. *The Whit* 1, no. 9 (June 1951): 23.

56. *The Whit* 1, no. 11 (August 1951): 24.

57. Gonaver, *Peculiar Institution and the Making of Modern Psychiatry*.

58. See Tani, *States of Dependency*.

59. *The Whit* 1, no. 11 (August 1951): 21.

60. *The Whit* 1, no. 12 (September 1951): 18.

61. *The Whit* 2, no. 4 (January 1952): 27.

62. *The Whit* 2, no. 4 (January 1952): 27.

63. *The Whit* 2, no. 4 (January 1952): 27.

64. After much deliberation, I have chosen not to reproduce the photograph or the newspaper clipping here. The women are identified by name and easily identifiable by face, and I do not have their permission to reproduce their likenesses. Given that they were patients at the hospital at the time, it is highly likely they were not asked for their permission for their images to be used in this way. I could have blacked out their faces to hide their identity, but I did not want to dehumanize them. For discussion of the ethical use of photos, see Thompson and Smith, *Do Less Harm*; Dreger, "Jarring Bodies"; Dreger, "Seeing Yourself"; Imada, "Promiscuous Signification"; Imada, *Archive of Skin*. The original of the photograph is in Scrapbook, vol. 1, Jaquith, William L., Unprocessed collection, Z/U/79.069, MDAH.

65. Undated, uncredited newspaper story, clipping, Scrapbook, vol. 1, Jaquith, William L., unprocessed collection, Z/U/79.069, MDAH.

66. See Survey Committee House Joint Resolution 1947, box SG13403, folder 6, ADAH.

67. Conference—Bryce Hospital September 22, 1948, 6, box SG13403, folder 6, ADAH.

68. Miss Clue to Senator Patterson, transcript of inspection report, September 8, 1948, 3, box SG13403, folder 6, ADAH.

69. Miss Clue to Senator Patterson, transcript of inspection report, September 8, 1948, 2, box SG13403, folder 6, ADAH.

70. Dr. Rowe to Mr. Shelton, transcript of inspection report, September 8, 1948, 8, box SG13403, folder 6, ADAH.

71. These photos are available in box SG5612: Photos.

72. Transcript of inspection report, September 8, 1948, 4, box SG13403, folder 6, ADAH.

73. Transcript of inspection report, September 8, 1948, 17.

74. Transcript of inspection report, September 8, 1948, 17.

75. Transcript of inspection report, September 8, 1948, 19.

76. White patients worked on two other smaller farms: Greystone Farm, close to Bryce, consisted of 247 acres mostly dedicated to corn, sweet potatoes, peanuts, and garden vegetables; and on the Bryce Hospital site itself was 280 acres that produced field crops like hay corn and sorghum. See transcript of inspection report, September 8, 1948, 2, box SG13403, folder 6, ADAH.

77. Transcript of inspection report, September 8, 1948, 2.

78. Transcript of inspection report, September 8, 1948, 5.

79. LeFlouria, *Chained in Silence*; Oshinsky, *Worse Than Slavery*; Haley, *No Mercy Here*; Blackmon, *Slavery by Another Name*.

80. Investigation—State Farm for Negroes, September 21, 1948, 5, box SG13403, folder 6, ADAH.

81. Tullos, *Alabama Getaway*; Flynt, *Alabama in the Twentieth Century*.

82. Paterson, "Short History of Occupational Therapy in Psychiatry."

83. *Annual Report of the Milledgeville State Hospital*, 1956, 12.

84. *Annual Report of the Milledgeville State Hospital*, 1956, 12.

85. OT Therapy Department Report, *Annual Report of the Milledgeville State Hospital*, 1956, 88–89.

86. OT Therapy Department Report, 89.

87. OT Therapy Department Report, 89.

88. Book and Ezell, "Freedom of Speech and Institutional Control."

89. Recreation Program Report, *Annual Report of the Milledgeville State Hospital*, 1956, 92.

90. Social Service Department Report, *Annual Report of the Milledgeville State Hospital*, 1956, 109.

91. For the most comprehensive account of the establishment of Central State and its use of farm labor in the nineteenth century, see Segrest, *Administrations of Lunacy*.

92. See chapter 1 and Segrest, *Administrations of Lunacy*, 155.

93. Comparative Statement of Income and Expenditures, *Annual Report of the Milledgeville State Hospital*, 1956, 140.

94. *Annual Report of the Milledgeville State Hospital*, 1956, 122.

95. *Annual Report of the Milledgeville State Hospital*, 1956, 119, 126.

96. *Annual Report of the Milledgeville State Hospital*, 1956, 125.

97. LeFlouria, *Chained in Silence*; Haley, *No Mercy Here*; Segrest, *Administrations of Lunacy*.

Chapter 5

1. Hull Watkins to NAACP LDF, December 5, 1947, NAACP LDF Papers, Subject Files, box 74, file: Hospitals, Miscellaneous Cases, 1947–1950, Library of Congress, Washington, DC.

2. I tried to track Mr. Watkins's letter to see whether it had had any impact but was immediately led on one of the wild-goose chases that has so defined the writing of this book. The letter in the NAACP file is marked as a copy and is attached to

a typed note to Reverend W. A. Bender, president of the Jackson Branch of the NAACP. The note, written on December 9, 1947, by Franklin Williams, assistant special counsel of the LDF, states, "Dear Reverend Bender, We are enclosing for your possible action a letter we have received concerning the mistreatment of Negro patients at the State Hospital for the Insane at Whitfield, Mississippi." This immediately led me to Dr. William Bender's papers, which are housed at Tougaloo College in Jackson, and a kind archivist there informed me that the exact year I was looking for was oddly missing from Bender's files, but I might try the state chapter of the NAACP. An e-mail to the state chapter of the NAACP was answered by Corey Wiggins, the executive director at the time, who referred me to Mr. Frank Figgers, the state NAACP historian. I was on the road between Starkville and Jackson, Mississippi, at the time, and I called Mr. Figgers from my Jackson hotel later that evening. Mr. Figgers was extremely helpful in that he was interested in my story, and we talked about the role of Dr. Bob Smith (who will make an appearance in chapter 7), but the NAACP itself had no papers related to Bender's tenure as president. He did connect me with Bender family members, and I was able to speak to Michael Bender, the reverend's grandson. Michael was also interested in the story but let me know that the family, as far as he knew, had not kept any of the reverend's NAACP-related papers—everything had been donated to the Tougaloo College archives. The finding aid that Mr. Bounds sent me clearly shows that there are no boxes related to any kind of correspondence for the year 1947, and no NAACP-related correspondence has been archived before 1950. While I was in Jackson on that visit, I scoured the digital versions of the relevant newspapers and found not a single mention of a Black patient being shot at Whitfield.

3. Herman, *Romance of American Psychology*; Creadick, *Perfectly Average*; Staub, *Madness Is Civilization*; Weinstein, *Pathological Family*; Menninger, *Psychiatry in a Troubled World*; Engelhardt, *End of Victory Culture*.

4. Sareyan, *Turning Point*; S. J. Taylor, *Acts of Conscience*.

5. For an in-depth analysis of the cultural representations of mental illness in the postwar period, see Halliwell, *Therapeutic Revolutions*. See also Murray, *Asylum Ways of Seeing*.

6. For a discussion of the limitation of exposés and the "reform" agenda, see Ben-Moshe, *Decarcerating Disability*.

7. Chaney's letters are available at various locations across the state of Mississippi. A large collection exists in box 2, folder: 2–27, Carter (Hodding and Betty) Papers, Division of Archives and Special Collections, Mississippi State University Libraries, Starkville. The Mississippi Department of Archives and History holds letters in various collections, including the unprocessed Jaquith papers at Z/U/1979.069: Jaquith (William L.) Collection, but the bulk of Chaney's surviving letters are located in the manuscripts archive at Z/0369.000/S/Box 1 and Z/0369.001/F/Folder 1. For a detailed discussion of Chaney's letters, see Murphy, *Inhospitable in the Hospitality State*.

8. For an excellent timeline and analysis of these events, see Murphy, *Inhospitable in the Hospitality State*.

9. Roberts and Klibanoff, *Race Beat*.

10. "Take Politics Out of State Mental Hospital," *Delta Democrat-Times* (*DDT*), January 15, 1947.

11. "Farm Group Asks Governor for State Hospital Investigation," *DDT*, January 24, 1947.

12. "Legislative Action Expected Following Whitfield Report," *DDT*, March 12, 1947.

13. "Boswell Report Still Secret after Legislators Testify on Whitfield," *DDT*, December 16, 1948, 1. Carter mentions that the legislative committee expected to hear from Dr. Boswell at its meeting on December 15, 1948, but the report was not made available.

14. "Mississippi's Snake Pit," *DDT*, January 16, 1949.

15. "Broad Picture of Abuse Uncovered at Whitfield," *DDT*, April 26, 1949.

16. "Pack Used as 'Treatment' for Punishment Purposes," *DDT*, April 28, 1949.

17. "Pack Used as 'Treatment' for Punishment Purposes."

18. "Filth and Neglect Are Rule at Hospital," *DDT*, April 27, 1949.

19. "What Is to Be Done about Whitfield? Campbell Asks Today," *DDT*, May 1, 1949.

20. "The People Are Angry," *DDT*, May 2, 1949.

21. "Filth and Neglect Are Rule at Hospital," *DDT*, April 27, 1949.

22. Material for this report and draft versions of it are held at Campbell (Hayden) papers, Z0105.000/S box 1–3, MDAH, and in folder 3.32: Correspondence: Whitfield/Hayden Campbell 11948, Hodding II and Betty Werlein Carter Papers, MSS-127, Special Collections, Mississippi State University Libraries.

23. Campbell, Draft Report, Special Collections, Mississippi State University Libraries.

24. Campbell, Draft Report, Special Collections, Mississippi State University Libraries.

25. "Enlightened Action by Circuit Jury Shows Interest of Fine Officials," *DDT*, January 26, 1947.

26. Ward, *Hanging Bridge*.

27. "Enlightened Action by Circuit Jury Shows Interest of Fine Officials."

28. "Whitfield Board Will Ask For Raise in Funds," *DDT*, September 4, 1949, 1.

29. "Whitfield Doctor Says Insane Woman Has Been Bruised," *DDT*, September 4, 1949.

30. "Whitfield Doctor Says Insane Woman Has Been Bruised."

31. "Whitfield Doctor Says Insane Woman Has Been Bruised."

32. Berrey, *Jim Crow Routine*.

33. "More Money Needed to Improve Our State Mental Hospital, Group Says," *DDT*, December 30, 1949.

34. Deutsch, *Shame of the States*, 88.

35. Deutsch, *Shame of the States*, 89.

36. Deutsch, *Shame of the States*, 90, 91–93.

37. Deutsch, *Shame of the States*, 90, 94. Here, Deutsch is probably referring to the Hill Burton Act of 1946, passed two years before the publication of *The Shame*

of the States, which doubled down on the original "separate but equal" provision established in *Plessy v. Ferguson*.

38. Deutsch, *Shame of the States*, 94.

39. Deutsch, *Shame of the States*, 94. The disparities in service expenditure before the 1940s is well documented in Segrest, *Administrations of Lunacy*.

40. Deutsch, *Shame of the States*, 91.

41. "Insanity," *Ebony*, April 1949, 19, in Stuart Rose Manuscripts and Rare Books Library, Emory University. Some of the research in this section was undertaken by BSN Honors student Jordan Seidman.

42. "Insanity," 19. See chapter 2 for an analysis of the so-called increase in insanity among Black populations and the issues with diagnostic practices.

43. "Insanity," 19.

44. "Insanity," 19.

45. "Prejudice No Cause of Insanity, but Helps Jam Asylums," *Ebony*, April 1949, 20.

46. "Prejudice No Cause of Insanity," 21.

47. "Asylum Staffs Rather Than Patients Biased," *Ebony*, April 1949, 22.

48. "Asylum Staffs Rather Than Patients Biased," 22.

49. "Asylum Staffs Rather Than Patients Biased," 22.

50. "Asylum Staffs Rather Than Patients Biased," 22.

51. "Most Big Psychiatrists Won't Accept Negroes," *Ebony*, April 1949, 24.

52. For more detail about this clinic, see Doyle, *Psychiatry and Racial Liberalism in Harlem*; Garcia, *Psychology Comes to Harlem*; Mendes, *Under the Strain of Color*.

53. "Most Big Psychiatrists Won't Accept Negroes," 24.

54. Cranford, *But for the Grace of God*, 137.

55. Cranford, *But for the Grace of God*, 9. The irony of this comment is not lost on me, given it was not until almost seventy years later that anything like this preservation was achieved. See both the aftermath and appendix 1 for an analysis of the issues around preservation of records from Central State.

56. Cranford, *But for the Grace of God*, 9.

57. Cranford, *But for the Grace of God*, 124–25, 126.

58. Cranford, *But for the Grace of God*, 165.

59. Cranford, *But for the Grace of God*, 126, 131.

60. Cranford, *But for the Grace of God*, 142.

61. Cranford, *But for the Grace of God*, 166.

62. Cranford, *But for the Grace of God*, 164.

63. J. Nelson, *Scoop*, 63–64.

64. Nelson, *Scoop*, 63.

65. Nelson, *Scoop*, 65.

66. Jack Nelson, "1916 Report on Milledgeville Reads Like It Could Be 1959," *Atlanta Constitution*, April 12, 1959. See also Nelson, *Scoop*, 64.

67. This number is based on a search of the *Atlanta Constitution* full-text database on Proquest Newspapers, using "Milledgeville" as the key word and/or Jack Nelson as the author. There could be shorter articles or commentaries that are missed in this search.

68. Roberts and Klibanoff, *Race Beat*.

69. Nelson, *Scoop*, 66. The *n*-word appears in full in Nelson's autobiography, but I have chosen not to repeat it here.

70. Roberts and Klibanoff, *Race Beat*, 30.

71. Nelson, *Scoop*, 66–67.

72. Nelson, "Increased Funds Promised for State's Mental Health," *Atlanta Constitution*, June 20, 1959.

73. Nelson "House Mental Unit Asks 5-Year Plan," *Atlanta Constitution*, June 19, 1959.

74. Nelson, "State Raises Hospital's Salary Scale," *Atlanta Constitution*, June 25, 1959.

75. Nelson "Irregularities Added to List at Milledgeville," *Atlanta Constitution*, April 5, 1959.

76. Nelson, "5 Year Mental Plan Urged by Legislators," *Atlanta Constitution*, June 19, 1959.

77. Nelson, "Vandiver Finds Hospital 'Worse Than I Thought,'" *Atlanta Constitution*, July 10, 1959.

78. Nelson, "Vandiver Shocked by Milledgeville," *Atlanta Constitution*, July 10, 1959.

79. "Vandiver Shocked by Milledgeville."

80. "Vandiver Shocked by Milledgeville."

81. "Vandiver Shocked by Milledgeville."

82. "A Bow to Legislators on Mental Health," *Atlanta Constitution*, February 22, 1960.

83. Nelson, *Scoop*, 68.

84. Mental Institutions, Board of Trustees, Minutes, Microfilm Roll 37099, MDAH.

85. Ben-Moshe, *Decarcerating Disability*.

Chapter 6

1. Harry Rowe to Ms. AGO, June 26, 1946, Alabama Governor (1947–1951, Folsom), State Institution Files: 1944–1949, SG13397, folder 17, AGSIF. In this instance, I have chosen not to use either the letter writer or the patient's full name, as this is personal correspondence from a patient to the hospital.

2. I do not doubt that more Black families wrote letters; rather, I take their absence from these files as direct evidence of archival silencing at work. See appendix 1 for more on this.

3. Ben-Moshe, *Decarcerating Disability*.

4. Lassiter, *Silent Majority*, 101.

5. Lassiter, *Silent Majority*; Lassiter and Crespino, *Myth of Southern Exceptionalism*; Bullock and Deitz, "Transforming the South."

6. NIMH, *Treatment Services for the Mentally Ill and Mentally Retarded in Georgia*.

7. NIMH, *Treatment Services*, see appendix, 106–9.

8. NIMH, *Treatment Services*, 2.

9. NIMH, *Treatment Services*, 38.
10. NIMH, *Treatment Services*, 39.
11. NIMH, *Treatment Services*, 39.
12. NIMH, *Treatment Services*, 13.
13. NIMH, *Treatment Services*, 23.
14. NIMH, *Treatment Services*, 23.
15. NIMH, *Treatment Services*, 70.
16. NIMH, *Treatment Services*, 71.
17. Ben-Moshe et al., *Disability Incarcerated*.
18. These plans are all available at NARACP. They are located in RG511: National Institute for Mental Health, under "State Comprehensive Mental Health Plans." The plan for Alabama is in box 002 and takes up the whole box. Georgia's plan is in box 008 and is relatively compact, stored in the same box as the plans from Florida to Idaho (alphabetically). The Mississippi plan is in box 013.
19. "A Comprehensive Mental Health Plan for Georgia," i, 1965, RG511, box 008, Georgia Department of Public Health, Division of Mental Health, NARACP.
20. "Comprehensive Mental Health Plan for Georgia," 40.
21. Bureau of the Census, *Negro Population, by County*, 12.
22. Bureau of the Census, *Negro Population, by County*, 13.
23. "Comprehensive Mental Health Plan for Georgia," 5–7.
24. "Comprehensive Mental Health Plan for Georgia," 7.
25. "Comprehensive Mental Health Plan for Georgia," 7.
26. "Comprehensive Mental Health Plan for Georgia," 8.
27. "The Mississippi Plan: A Guide for Mental Health Action," October 26, 1965, 1, RG511, box 13, NIMH, Comprehensive Community Mental Health Plans, NARACP.
28. "Mississippi Plan," 28.
29. "Mississippi Plan," 25.
30. "Mississippi Plan."
31. "Mississippi Plan," 29.
32. "Mississippi Plan."
33. "Mississippi Plan," 55.
34. Ward, *Hanging Bridge*; Adams and Adams, *Just Trying to Have School*; Folwell, *War on Poverty in Mississippi*.
35. W. Arsene Dick to Governor, January 7, 1963, Paul Johnson Papers—Correspondence 1963, box 58, folder 6, University of Southern Mississippi (USM). Interestingly, Johnson was not in fact governor at this time—Ross Barnett was. It is not clear why this letter is in Johnson's papers and addressed to "Dear Governor."
36. See Cunningham, "Shades of Anti-Civil Rights Violence."
37. Dick to Governor, January 7, 1963, USM.
38. While I am not going to trace the development of community mental health services in any of these states (an enterprise beyond the scope of this book), it is worth pointing out that to this day, Mississippi's community mental health system is almost nonexistent, as noted by US district court Judge Carlton Reeves in his ruling in United States of America v. State of Mississippi, 400 F. Supp. 3d 546

(S.D. Miss. 2019). This order has been appealed by the state of Mississippi and the case is still ongoing.

39. Memo by John McKee to All Clinic Directors, October 19, 1959, box 24, folder 14, Dibble Papers.

40. State Comprehensive Mental Health Plans, Alabama, 1.01-2, RG11, box 002, NARACP.

41. State Comprehensive Mental Health Plans, Alabama.

42. State Comprehensive Mental Health Plans, Alabama, 1.1.0-9.

43. State Comprehensive Mental Health Plans, Alabama, 2.1.0-3.

44. State Comprehensive Mental Health Plans, Alabama, fig. 2.2.3.

45. This also tracks with the way that future Office of Economic Opportunity and War on Poverty programs and funding disputes would play out in the next few years. See Ashmore, *Carry It On*.

46. The method for determining relative need was set out in chap. 2, sec. 4, pp. 2.4.0-1 to 2.4.0-5, Alabama CCMH Plan.

47. State Comprehensive Mental Health Plans, Alabama, 2.4.0-4.

48. State Comprehensive Mental Health Plans, Alabama, 1.1.0-13.

49. State Comprehensive Mental Health Plans, Alabama, 2.2.5.

50. Supplement to Alabama Mental Health Plan, March 31, 1966, section 5, Alabama State Hospital System. 2.5.1 State Comprehensive Mental Health Plans, Alabama, 1.01-2, RG11, box 002, NARACP.

51. Supplement to Alabama Mental Health Plan.

52. Alabama is still in court about its failure to provide adequate mental health services in its prison system, which has become a de facto mental health system. I discuss this further in the Aftermath.

53. These processes are the subject of chapters 7 and 8.

54. Smith, *Health Care Divided*; Smith, *Power to Heal*; Reynolds, "Federal Government's Use of Title VI and Medicare"; Quadagno, "Promoting Civil Rights through the Welfare State"; Thomas, "Hill-Burton Act and Civil Rights"; Beardsley, "Goodbye to Jim Crow."

55. D. B. Smith, *Power to Heal*; D. B. Smith, *Health Care Divided*; Harcourt, "From the Asylum to the Prison"; Quadagno, "Promoting Civil Rights through the Welfare State"; Reynolds, "Federal Government's Use of Title VI and Medicare to Racially Integrate Hospitals in the United States 1963 through 1967."

56. William Burleigh to Office of General Counsel, PHS, November 17, 1965, RG235, file 6, container 7, PD 6000, Office of the General Counsel Opinion Files, NARACP.

57. Rourke to Nash, May 5, 1965, RG235, file 6, container 7, PD 6000, Office of the General Counsel Opinion Files, NARACP.

58. Rourke to Nash, May 5, 1965, NARACP.

59. Memo to Edward Rourke from Donald Young, November 8, 1965, RG235, file 6, container 7, PD 6000, Office of the General Counsel Opinion Files, NARACP.

60. Young to Rourke, November 8, 1965, NARACP.

61. Rourke to Martin Kramer, November 22, 1965, RG235, file 6, container 7, PD 6000, Office of the General Counsel Opinion Files, NARACP.

Chapter 7

1. LeFlore to Persons, October 5, 1953, folder 4, FY1954, SG12529, AGSIF.
2. Gamble, *Making a Place for Ourselves*; Dittmer, *Good Doctors*; Thomas, *Deluxe Jim Crow*; McBride, *Caring for Equality*.
3. Kirkland, "Mobile and the Boswell Amendment"; Kirkland, *Pink Sheets and Black Ballots*; Verney, "'Every Man Should Try'"; Nelson, "Organized Labor and the Struggle for Black Equality."
4. Kirkland, "Pink Sheets and Black Ballots"; Verney, "Every Man Should Try."
5. LeFlore's papers related to the NPVL demonstrate this breadth of work (see NPVLP). When I visited the University of South Alabama, I was given only access to the microfilmed scans of the papers, but the following citations refer to the box and folder locations as per the official finding aids.
6. John LeFlore to Luther Terry, June 18, 1965, box 3: Casework, Public Accommodations, folder 57: Bryce Mental and Searcy Medical Hospitals, 1966–1967, NPVLP.
7. John LeFlore to Luther Terry, June 18, 1965, box 3, folder 57, NPVLP.
8. Robert M. Nash to John LeFlore, July 13, 1965, box 3, folder 57, NPVLP.
9. See chap. 6. Carl Harper to John LeFlore, July 22, 1965, box 3, folder 57, NPVLP.
10. Henry Stiles to Ruth Adams, July 21, 1965, box 3, folder 57, NPVLP.
11. Letters were sent to Quigley on August 3, Meltsner on August 4, and Harry Rowe, along with the petition, on August 6, 1965. On August 9 and 10, LeFlore also sent a copy of the petition to James Quigley at HEW and Michael Meltsner at the LDF; box 3, folder 57, NPVLP.
12. The copy of the petition in the NPVL Papers does not have actual signatures, as these would have been on the original, which was distributed. The LDF Papers at the Library of Congress themselves do not contain any material related to this correspondence. The named signatories in the preamble at the beginning of the petition are Richard Brewer, J. C. Dotch, W. T. Smith, John L. Finley, Essley Moody, James H. Finley, and LeFlore himself. Petition to James Tarwater and Harry Rowe, August 6, 1965, box 3, folder 57, NPVLP.
13. Petition, August 6, 1965, box 3, folder 57, NPVLP.
14. Handwritten notes, February 22, 1966, box 4, folder 57A, NPVLP.
15. Affidavit, box 3, folder 57, NPVLP.
16. "Klan Terrorists Hit in Mobile County," *Mobile Beacon*, August 6, 1966.
17. "Skirmish at Searcy Hosp. Causes Stir," *Mobile Beacon*, August 13, 1966.
18. All quotes from "Skirmish at Searcy Hosp. Causes Stir," *Mobile Beacon*, August 13, 1966.
19. Harry Rowe to John LeFlore, August 18, 1965, box 3, folder 57, NPVLP.
20. Dittmer, "Medical Committee for Human Rights"; Dittmer, *Good Doctors*. See MCHR.
21. See Robert Smith, Oral History, April 2000, Digital Collections at the University of Mississippi, https://usm.access.preservica.com/uncategorized/IO_62d42568-bf00-4715-889f-daeaa5854805.
22. More about this in the aftermath.

23. Coles, "Social Struggles and Weariness."

24. Dittmer, "Medical Committee for Human Rights."

25. Memo, "Front Line Psychiatry for Civil Rights Workers," Josephine Martin MD, undated, box 29, folder 318, MCHR Records.

26. Memo, "Front Line Psychiatry for Civil Rights Workers."

27. Report on H.S., December 12, 1964, box 31, folder F335, MCHR.

28. Israel Zwerling to Robert Smith, December 23, 1964, box 31, folder 335, MCHR.

29. Robert Smith to Bob Moses, January 8, 1965, box 31, folder 335, MCHR.

30. Report on H.S., December 12, 1964, box 31, folder F335, MCHR.

31. Greenwood Report, August 1-2 1964, box 31, folder 339, MCHR.

32. Greenwood Report, August 1-2 1964.

33. Dittmer, *Local People*.

34. Charles Meyer, report from Greene County, Alabama, July 18, 1966, box 29, folder 323, MCHR.

35. Obviously, this is a different Dr. Smith than Dr. Bob Smith!

36. Charles Meyer, report from Greene County, Alabama.

37. Letter from Dr. H., February 3, 1965, box 29, folder 323, MCHR.

38. Dr. William Sykes, *Psychiatric Facilities Available in and around Clarksdale and Mound Bayou*, 8-29-64, box 31, folder 337, MCHR.

39. Sykes, *Psychiatric Facilities*.

40. Sykes, *Psychiatric Facilities*.

41. Sykes, *Psychiatric Facilities*, 2.

42. Mildred Beldoch and Clarice Whelan, "Visit to the East Mississippi State Hospital," August 12, 1964, box 31, folder 338, MCHR.

43. Beldoch and Whelan, "Visit to the East Mississippi State Hospital."

44. For the extent of Klan violence in East Mississippi, see, for example, Billups, "Martyred Women and White Power since the Civil Rights Era."

45. Beldoch and Whelan, "Visit to the East Mississippi State Hospital."

46. Memo, "Suggested Guide for Complaints on Health Facilities Receiving Federal Funds," August 1965, box 29, folder 317, MCHR.

47. "Suggested Guide for Complaints on Health Facilities Receiving Federal Funds."

48. For in-depth detail about this long and complex campaign, see D. B. Smith, *Health Care Divided*; D. B. Smith, *Power to Heal*; Quadagno, "Promoting Civil Rights through the Welfare State"; Reynolds, "Federal Government's Use of Title VI and Medicare"; Dittmer, *Good Doctors*.

49. Pouissant to Congressman, May 23, 1966, box 30, folder 328, MCHR. This looks to have been a generic letter sent to many "congressmen" not to one in particular.

50. Pouissant to Congressman.

51. Pouissant to Congressman.

52. Information about all editions of the newspaper are available online at http://southerncourier.org.

53. Box 10, file "Area Reports and Contacts," *Southern Courier* Collection, Tuskegee University Archives.

54. *Southern Courier*, January 23, 1966.

55. *Southern Courier*, January 23, 1966, 4.

56. *Southern Courier*, January 23, 1966.

57. *Southern Courier*, January 23, 1966.

58. "Sick Lady Committed to Searcy: If They Keep This Up, I'm Going to End Up Crazy," *Southern Courier*, June 3-4, 1967.

59. *Southern Courier*, June 3-4, 1967.

60. *Southern Courier*, June 3-4, 1967.

61. *Southern Courier*, June 3-4, 1967.

62. *Southern Courier*, June 3-4, 1967.

63. "Mobile Lady Released from Searcy: Gave Her 3 Shock Treatments Against Her Will," *Southern Courier*, June 24-25, 1967, 1.

64. *Southern Courier*, June 24-25, 1967.

65. *Southern Courier*, June 24-25, 1967.

66. *Southern Courier*, June 24-25, 1967.

67. "'If You Have Your Sanity, You Will Lose It': Former Patient Tells What Life Is Like Inside Searcy State Mental Hospital," *Southern Courier*, August 5-6, 1967.

68. *Southern Courier*, August 5-6, 1967, 4.

69. *Southern Courier*, August 5-6, 1967.

70. *Southern Courier*, August 5-6, 1967.

71. See, for example, Crespino, *In Search of Another Country*; Dittmer, *Local People*; Irons, *Reconstituting Whiteness*; McMillen, *Citizen's Council*; Katagiri, *Mississippi State Sovereignty Commission*; Silver, *Mississippi*.

72. Laws of the State of Mississippi, 1956 Regular Session, 512, cited in Katagiri, *Mississippi State Sovereignty Commission*, 6.

73. Erle Johnston to Governor Paul Johnson, memo, November 23, 1966. Cited in Katagiri, 200.

74. For the purposes of this book, I am using the now digitized records that were made publicly available as a result of prolonged court action by the ACLU. This may not be a comprehensive record, as it has been subject to redaction and appeal, so any materials that are the subject of ongoing court cases are not included. For the series description, see https://da.mdah.ms.gov/sovcom/colldesc.php.

75. Memo from Albert Jones (Director of the Sovereignty Commission) to Dr. William Jaquith, January 6, 1961, SCRID 2-37-1-55-1-1-1, SovComm Files Online, MDAH, https://da.mdah.ms.gov/sovcom.

76. Investigation of Reverend Wallace Carr, SCRID 2-37-1-43-1-1-1, SovComm Files Online.

77. Investigation of Reverend Wallace Carr.

78. Investigation of Reverend Wallace Carr.

79. Investigation of Reverend Wallace Carr.

80. For references to both, see chapter 4 and the sections on *The Whit* patient newsletter.

81. Negro Employees at Mississippi State Hospital, Whitfield, Mississippi, SCRID 2-37-1-94-1-1-1, SovComm Files Online.

82. Negro Employees at Mississippi State Hospital, 2.

83. Negro Employees at Mississippi State Hospital, 2.

84. See Cunningham, "Shades of Anti-Civil Rights Violence," 183.

85. Cunningham, "Shades of Anti-Civil Rights Violence."

86. The timing of this document is most likely to be post-1966, as it makes references to the "compliance pledge" with the federal government. See *Your Children's Future Is Being Made Today, What Are YOU Doing?*, United Klans of America pamphlet, box 142, folder 1: Ku Klux Klan, Paul Johnson Papers, Sovereignty Commission, USM.

87. *Your Children's Future Is Being Made Today.*

88. John LeFlore to James Quigley, January 10, 1966, box 4, folder 57A, NPVL.

89. John LeFlore to Quigley, January 10, 1966, box 4, folder 57A, NPVL.

90. A copy of this telegram was sent to Johnny Parham, national director of the MCHR, on June 10, 1965, box 34, folder 380, MCHR.

Chapter 8

1. McCarn to Wallace, April 22, 1966, box SG021597, folder 1, AGSIF. All typos and punctuation in the original.

2. K. M. Smith, "No Medical Justification."

3. Memo, Stephenson to Venable, January 4, 1965, Public Health—Mental Health—Director's Administrative Records, Civil Rights Compliance Unit 1965, RCB29713, Georgia State Archives, Morrow.

4. Memo, Bush to Venable, January 6, 1965, Public Health—Mental Health—Director's Administrative Records, Civil Rights Compliance Unit 1965, RCB29713, Georgia State Archives, Morrow.

5. Memo, Bush to Venable, January 6, 1965.

6. Memo, Bush to Venable, January 6, 1965.

7. Memo, Bush to Venable, January 6, 1965.

8. "Governor Carl Sanders Today Announced," undated, RCB29713, Georgia State Archives, Morrow.

9. Statement of Compliance with the Department of Health, Education, and Welfare Regulation under Title VI, Civil Rights Act of 1964.

10. Statement of Compliance.

11. Statement of Compliance, 9–10.

12. Statement of Compliance, 10.

13. "Governor Carl Sanders Today Announced."

14. Telex, Graning to Regional Office DHEW, March 18, 1965, Public Health—Mental Health—Director's Administrative Records, Civil Rights Compliance Unit 1965, RCB29713, Georgia State Archives, Morrow.

15. Memo, Richard Lyle to John Venable, May 17, 1965, Public Health—Mental Health—Director's Administrative Records, Civil Rights Compliance Unit 1965, RCB29713, Georgia State Archives, Morrow.

16. All material in this section comes from the Stennis Papers.

17. Fowler to Stennis, April 26, 1965, series 29, box 5, file: "Hill Burton Funds Compliance," Stennis Papers.

18. Fowler to Stennis, April 26, 1965, 2.

19. Fowler to Stennis, April 26, 1965, 3.

20. Most of these letters are collected in series 29, box 4, file: Hospitals, 1966–1970, and file: Hospital Guidelines, 1966–1969, Stennis Papers.

21. Dr. W. K. Purks to Stennis, April 11, 1966, series 29, box 4, file: Hospitals, 1966–1970, Stennis Papers.

22. Augustus Street to Stennis, April 11, 1966, series 29, box 4, file: Hospitals, 1966–1970, Stennis Papers.

23. Statement by the Executive Committee of the Association of Citizens' Councils, June 1966, series 29, box 4, file: Hospital Guidelines, 1966–1969, Stennis Papers.

24. Statement by the Executive Committee of the Association of Citizens' Councils.

25. Statement by the Executive Committee of the Association of Citizens' Councils.

26. Memo from Wilbur Cohen to Lister Hill, October 7, 1966, HEW Subseries PHS 1961–1965, box 2, file 31, PHS 1965, Stennis Papers.

27. John Gardner to Lister Hill and John Fogarty, October 11, 1966, HEW Subseries PHS 1961–1965, box 2, file 31, PHS 1965, Stennis Papers.

28. D. B. Smith, *Power to Heal*; D. B. Smith, *Health Care Divided*.

29. D. B. Smith, *Health Care Divided*, 148–49.

30. D. B.Smith, *Health Care Divided*, 149.

31. There are no official extant records currently available from the office of OEHO. Archivists at the National Archives and Records Administration at College Park, Maryland, in February 2020 advised that these have been destroyed. Federal records related to the activity of both the general counsel of HEW and the Department of Justice in Alabama in 1966–67 housed at NARA are currently restricted, and I have submitted a FOIA request to have the records released. David Barton Smith's work on the OEHO relies largely on personal testimony from ex-employees. The testimony from Marilyn Rose is from an interview she conducted with Smith, who provided the transcript to Michael Meltsner from the NAACP LDF for my use. I want to thank them both here for their generosity of time and spirit in helping me to flesh out this story.

32. Marilyn Rose, interview by David Barton Smith, October 3, 1997, transcript, personal correspondence.

33. Report attached to letter from Peter Libassi, Director, Office of Civil Rights (HEW), to Senator Stennis, December 22, 1967, series 29, box 4, folder 10: Hospital Guidelines, 1966–1969, Stennis Papers.

34. Report attached to letter from Peter Libassi.

35. Report attached to letter from Peter Libassi, 2.

36. Rose, interview, 10.

37. Rose, interview.

38. Rose, interview.

39. Rose, interview, 3.

40. Rose, interview, 10.

41. Rose, interview, 11.
42. See the aftermath for more on the current situation in Mississippi.
43. Rose, interview.
44. Rose, interview.
45. Rose, interview.
46. General Counsel Brief for HEW, 15–25, Civil Action 2610, Record of Administrative Hearing Docket No. MCR-44.
47. General Counsel Brief for HEW, 15–25, MCR44.
48. General Counsel Brief for HEW, 15–25, MCR44.
49. General Counsel Brief for HEW, 15–25, MCR44.
50. General Counsel Brief for HEW, MCR44.
51. Defendant's Response, MCR44.
52. Dr. Robert C. Hunt, April 11, 1967, HEW Administrative Hearing, 42, MCR44.
53. Dr. James E. Carson, April 12, 1967, HEW Administrative Hearing, 180–83, MCR44.
54. Dr. James E. Carson, April 12, 1967, HEW Administrative Hearing, 191, MCR44.
55. Dr. Patrick Linton, April 12, 1967, HEW Administrative Hearing, 175–76, MCR44.
56. Dr. James Folsom, April 12, 1967, HEW Administrative Hearing, 156–59, MCR44.
57. Dr. James Folsom, HEW Administrative Hearing, 160, MCR44.
58. Dr. John Carter, HEW Administrative Hearing, 166–73, MCR44.
59. Staub, *Mismeasure of Minds*; Summers, *Madness in the City of Magnificent Intentions*.
60. Carter, *Politics of Rage*; Carter, *From George Wallace to Newt Gingrich*; Frederick, *Stand Up for Alabama*.
61. Harvey, "'Wallaceism Is an Insidious and Treacherous Type of Disease.'"
62. George Wallace to James Tarwater, June 4, 1965, folder 18, box SG021951, AGSIF.
63. These memos are contained in Docket No. MCR-44, box 149, 021-74-C-0813.
64. Robert Brown to James Tarwater, July 30, 1965, GC3, MCR44.
65. William Page to James Tarwater, January 14, 1966, GC5, MCR44.
66. Tom Macklin, "Mental Facilities Desegregated," *Montgomery Advertiser*, March 15, 1966.
67. *Montgomery Advertiser*, March 15, 1966.
68. Dr. Carl Chamblee, April 12, 1967, HEW Administrative Hearing, MCR44.
69. "Bryce, Searcy, Inmates Swapped in Forced Integration Attempt," *Montgomery Advertiser*, April 27, 1966, box SG021597, folder 1, AGSIF.
70. James Tarwater to Public Health Service, June 20, 1966, General Counsel Summary, MCR44.
71. J. S. Haddock to James Tarwater and George Wallace, April 4, 1966, box SG021597, folder 1, AGSIF.
72. Crespino, *In Search of Another Country*.
73. J. S. Haddock to George Wallace, April 4, 1966, box SG021597, folder 1, AGSIF.

74. Carter, *From George Wallace to Newt Gingrich*. For explorations of the shifting language of segregation, see Crespino, *In Search of Another Country*; Berrey, *Jim Crow Routine*.

75. Along with much older writing about the "problem" of the Black psyche, Wallace or the Mental Health Board could have been drawing on more recent ideas that reified racial difference in psychology and psychiatry, such as Adams, "Negro Patient in Psychiatric Treatment"; Kennedy, "Problems Posed in the Analysis of the Negro Patient"; Lewis and Hubbard, "Manic Depressive Reactions in Negroes"; Maltzberg, "Mental Disease among Negroes in New York State." Anne Rose has shown that this obsession with difference was purely ideological—it was simply used to justify a lack of treatment for Black patients. See Rose, *Psychology and Selfhood in the Segregated South*. This therapeutic indifference was reinforced by the idea that Black culture itself was already "crazy." See Pickens, *Black Madness*; Summers, *Madness in the City of Magnificent Intentions*.

76. George Wallace to Mr. Threadgill, March 23, 1966, box SG021597, folder 1, AGSIF.

77. George Wallace to Mr. Threadgill, March 23, 1966, box SG021597, folder 1, AGSIF.

78. Alpha Corkle to George Wallace, July 14, 1966, box SG021597, folder 1, AGSIF.

79. Bell, *Silent Covenants*.

80. George Wallace to Mrs. Corkle, July 18, 1966, box SG021597, folder 1, AGSIF.

81. Summers, "'Suitable Care of the African When Afflicted with Insanity'"; Gambino, "'These Strangers within Our Gates'"; Summers, *Madness in the City of Magnificent Intentions*.

82. Summers, *Madness in the City of Magnificent Intentions*; Willoughby, "Running Away from Drapetomania"; Gonaver, *Peculiar Institution*.

83. Pride, *Political Use of Racial Narratives*; Adams and Adams, *Just Trying to Have School*.

84. Anonymous to George Wallace, April 27, 1966, box SG021597, folder 1, AGSIF.

85. Dr. James S. Tarwater, HEW Administrative Hearing, 119, MCR44.

86. Conrad K. Harper, in discussion with the author, January 6, 2020, New York City.

87. Conrad Harper to John LeFlore, February 23, 1966, box 4, folder 57A, NPVL.

88. John LeFlore to Conrad Harper, February 25, 1966; John LeFlore to Michael Meltsner, October 10, 1966, box 4, folder 57A, NPVL. These letters refer to repeated phone calls between LeFlore and the LDF. Personal correspondence with Mr. Meltsner (NAACP Legal Defense Fund, first asst. counsel 1961–70) and Mr. Conrad Harper throughout 2018 confirmed this correspondence and the LDF's communication with Mr. Billingsley and Mr. Newton.

89. Robert Nash to Dr. Tarwater, January 27, 1967, GC22, MCR44.

90. Petition for Declaratory Judgment and Further Necessary or Proper Relief, State of Alabama (Petitioner) v. John W. Gardner et al., Civil Action 2610-N, October 13, 1967, box 149, 021-74-C-0813.

91. There are several letters in the NPVL Papers detailing the organization of the named plaintiffs, which mention Mr. Marable being a client of Newton's, but searches to date for the original papers from the offices of Billingsley and Newton have been unsuccessful.

92. Complaint, Marable v. Alabama Mental Health Board, November 17, 1967, box 149, 021-74-C-0813.

93. Bass, *Taming the Storm*; Yarbrough, *Judge Frank Johnson and Human Rights in Alabama*.

94. Memo by Judge Frank M. Johnson, January 19, 1968, box 45, folder 7, 2615-N Marable v. Alabama Mental Health Board, The Papers of Frank M. Johnson, Library of Congress, Washington, DC.

95. Court proceedings took place while Lurleen Wallace and then Albert Brewer was governor, Brewer taking over for Wallace, who had died in office. Lurleen had taken over as governor in January 1967, after George had not been able to run for a third consecutive term. George Wallace became governor again in January 1971.

96. Decision, Marable v. Alabama Mental Health Board, box 149, 021-74-C-0813.

97. Personal correspondence with Mr. Conrad Harper and Mr. Michael Meltsner, January 16, 2018.

98. Brief of the Alabama Mental Health Board, March 14, 1968, 10, box 149, 021-74-C-0813.

99. Decision, Marable v. Alabama Mental Health Board, box 149, 021-74-C-0813.

100. Decision, Marable v. Alabama Mental Health Board, box 149, 021-74-C-0813.

101. Decision, Marable v. Alabama Mental Health Board, box 149, 021-74-C-0813.

102. Johnson, "In Defense of Judicial Activism," *Emory Law Journal* 28 (1979): 901–12.

103. Johnson, June 9, 1975: Response of the United States to the Court's Show Cause order of May 22, 1975, Alabama v. Gardner, box 43, folder 1, Judge Frank M. Johnson Papers.

104. Decision, Marable v. Alabama Mental Health Board, Box 149, 021-74-C-0813.

105. Johnson, "Observation"; Johnson, "In Defense of Judicial Activism"; Bass, *Taming the Storm*; Yarbrough, *Judge Frank Johnson and Human Rights in Alabama*.

106. United States v. Frazer, 297 F. Supp. 319. M.D. Ala. 1968. https://law.justia.com/cases/federal/district-courts/FSupp/297/319/2147499/.

107. Johnson, June 9, 1975: Response of the United States to the Court's Show Cause Order of May 22, 1975, box 43, folder 1, Alabama v. Gardner, Judge Frank M. Johnson Papers, Library of Congress.

108. Extensive data about patient movements and staff hiring are contained in both the official court records in the US District Court files at NARA Atlanta and in Johnson's papers in the Library of Congress.

109. The impact of the Wyatt case has been profound but was not race-specific. For further information, see Davis, "*Wyatt v. Stickney*"; Drake, "Drafting the Case"; Perlin, "'Abandoned Love'"; Slaten, "1995 Wyatt Litigation."

110. Decision, Marable v. Alabama Mental Health Board, box 149, 021-74-C-0813.

111. Decision, Marable v. Alabama Mental Health Board, box 149, 021-74-C-0813.

112. Doyle, *Psychiatry and Racial Liberalism in Harlem*, 27. This book provides a nuanced discussion of the impact of race-neutral language in psychiatry.

113. Metzl, *Protest Psychosis*.

114. Willoughby, "Running Away from Drapetomania"; Hughes, "Labeling and Treating Black Mental Illness in Alabama."

115. Washington, *Medical Apartheid*.

116. Ranking according to Mental Health America as of June 5, 2025, https://mhanational.org/the-state-of-mental-health-in-america/data-rankings/access-to-care/.

Aftermath

1. Mrs. F to Sen. Herman Talmadge, May 20, 1972, RCB-27394, 026-24-035, CSH Patients 1972, Georgia State Archives, Morrow.

2. Davis, "*Wyatt v. Stickney*," 147.

3. This right was established in Judge Bazelon's ruling in Rouse v. Cameron, 373 F.2d 451 (DC Cir. 1966).

4. Wyatt v. Stickney, 344 F. Supp. 373 (M.D. Ala. 1972), https://law.justia.com/cases/federal/district-courts/FSupp/344/373/2303083/.

5. See Braggs v. Dunn, 257 F. Supp. 3d 1171 (M.D. Ala. 2017).

6. See Tucker, "*Wyatt v. Stickney*."

7. The original order in this case can be found in Braggs v. Dunn, 257 F. Supp. 3d 1171 (M.D. Ala. 2017). The anecdote about levels of spending on litigation comes from personal correspondence with Mr. Ira Burnam from the Bazelon Mental Health Center, 2018, Washington, DC.

8. Beth Shelton, "What Happened to Jamie Lee Wallace?," July 5, 2017, www.bethshelburne.com/what-happened-to-jamie-lee-wallace-1.

9. Parsons, *From Asylum to Prison*; Harcourt, "From the Asylum to the Prison."

10. Alexander, *New Jim Crow*; LeFlouria, *Chained in Silence*; Haley, *No Mercy Here*.

11. Rob Cleland to Judge Hawkins, SG27: Mental Health and Mental Retardation, Administrative Files of Carl V. Bretz, container SG02776, File Admission Procedures, 1968–1972, ADAH.

12. I cannot thank the Powells enough for their help in understanding the long history of mental health justice work in Mississippi. Mr. Powell was diagnosed with Parkinson's disease not long before I met him, but he was determined to tell me everything he could.

13. These links, and the cases they spurred, are too numerous to list here but are the subject of my ongoing research.

14. Director's Report, Community Legal Services of Mississippi, 1975, personal correspondence, private collection of Mr. Barry Powell, Jackson, MS.

15. Director's Report, Barry Powell, 1975.

16. See William L. Jaquith, scrapbook, vol. 4, unprocessed collection, Z/U/79.069, MDAH. The Cottingims were reporters with the *Delta Democrat-Times*, and their five-part series was first published in magazine format in *Mississippi Today*, then

replicated in various newspapers including the *DDT*, which had a long history of publishing about Whitfield.

17. Most of the documents related to this case are located at the Civil Rights Litigation Clearinghouse, https://clearinghouse.net/case/15449/.

18. Judge Carlton Reeves, Memorandum Opinion and Order, United States of America v. State of Mississippi, 400 F. Supp. 3d 546 (S.D. Miss. 2019), 2–3.

19. Isabelle Taft, "Mississippi Chose to Fight': Court Overturns Justice Department Efforts to Overhaul State's Mental Health System," *Mississippi Today*, September 21, 2023, https://mississippitoday.org/2023/09/21/federal-court-overturns-efforts-to-revamp-mental-health-system/.

20. All of this information comes from the "MHDDAD Service System Time Line Prior to Passage of HB498": Prepared for the Georgia Department of Audits and Accounts, by the Division of Mental Health, Development Disabilities, and Addictive Diseases, November 2003. Shared with me by Mary Lou Rahn.

21. Kennedy et al v. Crittenden et al., No. CIV-77–01573, Filed 9/23/1977, Terminated 11/30/77, United States District Court Records, NARA Southeast, Morrow, GA.

22. Kennedy et al. v. Crittenden et al., No. CIV-77–01573, Filed 9/23/1977, Terminated 11/30/77.

23. Dough Skelton, personal correspondence. See also Kennedy et al. v. Crittenden et al., No. CIV-77–01573, Filed 9/23/1977, Terminated 11/30/77, United States District Court Records, NARA Southeast, Morrow, GA.

24. "Farms Using Forced Labor, Mayor Claims," *Atlanta Constitution*, November 5, 1977.

25. "Farms Using Forced Labor."

26. "State Will Examine Ex-Mental Patients," *Atlanta Constitution*, November 18, 1977.

27. The literature here is extensive; for the best summary of *Olmstead v. L.C.*, see https://archive.ada.gov/olmstead/olmstead_about.htm and www.olmsteadrights.org.

28. Metzl et al., "Mental Illness, Mass Shootings, and the Future of Psychiatric Research into American Gun Violence." See also Metzl, *What We've Become*.

29. Wahbi and Beletsky, "Involuntary Commitment as 'Carceral-Health Service'"; Roth, *Insane*.

30. US Office of Public Affairs, "Justice Department Announces Investigation into Conditions in Fulton County, Georgia Jail," press release, July 13, 2023, www.justice.gov/opa/pr/justice-department-announces-investigation-conditions-fulton-county-georgia-jail.

31. See Wofsy, "Policing Mental Health"; Wofsy and Smith, "Racism and Redlining in the History of Psychiatric Policy and Practice in Atlanta."

32. Metzl, *Protest Psychosis*.

33. Hansen, "Substance-Induced Psychosis."

34. Data visualization available at http://jimcrowintheasylum.com.

35. I started this book with an analysis of the work of the psychiatrists at Tuskegee for exactly this reason. For excellent documentation of the impact of many more Black psychiatrists, see Spurlock, *Black Psychiatrists and American Psychiatry*.

36. Grier and Cobbs, *Black Rage*; Willie et al., *Racism and Mental Health*.

37. Poussaint, "Stresses of the White Female Worker in the Civil Rights Movement in the South"; Poussaint, "Black Power."

38. Richert, "'Therapy Means Change, Not Peanut Butter'"; Richert, *Break on Through*.

39. American Psychiatric Association, box 36, file 393, MCHR.

40. Psychiatry as Instrument of the Establishment, box 42, file 479, MCHR.

41. Psychiatry as Instrument of the Establishment, box 42, file 479, MCHR.

42. American Psychiatric Association 1969, box 62, folder 745, MCHR.

43. Lowinger, "Radicals in Psychiatry," SS-195.

Appendix 1

1. Mbembe, "Power of the Archive and Its Limits," 19–26.
2. Mbembe, "Power of the Archive and Its Limits," 19.
3. Trouillot, *Silencing the Past: Power the Production of History*.
4. Mbembe, "Power of the Archive and Its Limits," 24.
5. Mbembe, "Power of the Archive and Its Limits," 24.
6. Mbembe, "Power of the Archive and Its Limits," 24.
7. K. M. Smith, "Reparatory History."
8. Ross, *Mental Health Program for Alabama*.
9. Ross, *Mental Health Program for Alabama*, 5.
10. I am referring to Jeffrey Lieberman, who was removed as chair of psychiatry at Columbia University in New York City. (See "Jeffrey Lieberman, Columbia Psychiatry Chair, Is Suspended," *New York Times*, February 23, 2022, www.nytimes.com/2022/02/23/nyregion/columbia-jeffrey-lieberman.html.) See also Lieberman, *Shrinks*. In relation to accessing the APA archives, I stopped asking a couple of years ago, when even pleas from colleagues who are members came to nothing.
11. For the APA non-apology, see "APA's Apology to Black, Indigenous and People of Color for Its Support of Structural Racism in Psychiatry," January 18, 2021, www.psychiatry.org/newsroom/apa-apology-for-its-support-of-structural-racism-in-psychiatry.
12. Steve Davis, email, November 7, 2017.
13. University of Alabama campus map, accessed May 29, 2025, www.ua.edu/map/.
14. Sadowsky and Smith, "Reflections on the Use of Patient Records."
15. The special collections listing related to CSH is here: https://libguides.gcsu.edu/c.php?g=396210&p=2692086. The link to the "family records" query redirects here: https://dbhdd.georgia.gov/genealogy-information-faqs#field_related_links-119-1.
16. Sarah was eventually able to find a death certificate related to an aunt of the ACLU client, and we found his father's name in the large leatherbound admission book. Ongoing conversations with Sarah indicated that the bulk of records had been moved, unprocessed, or sent to the records storage facility outside Atlanta (run by Iron Mountain), where a security guard told Sarah that she shouldn't even know they

existed. Other anecdotal evidence exists, including that reported by journalist Andy Miller from the *Georgia Health News*, that at one point patient records were scattered across abandoned buildings, ripe for theft by urban scavengers (personal correspondence). For a discussion of the consequences of this lack of record preservation, see Aparna Nair and Kylie M. Smith, "We're Historians of Disability. What We Just Found on eBay Horrified Us," *Slate*, July 21, 2022, https://slate.com/technology/2022/07/vintage-asylum-records-found-on-ebay-history-of-disability.html.

17. See "Central State Hospital, Milledgeville, GA," https://georgialibraries.omeka.net/s/central-state-hospital/page/introduction.

18. If you would like to tell me your story, please see contact details at http://jimcrowintheasylum.com.

Appendix 2

1. J. W. Scott, *On the Judgement of History*.
2. Kleinberg et al., "Theses on Theory and History," 162.
3. Sharpe, *In the Wake*.
4. Foucault, *Psychiatric Power*, 173.
5. Hartman, *Scenes of Subjection*, 55. Hartman is quoting Foucault from "Ethic of Care for the Self as a Practice of Freedom," 12, 18.
6. Mbembe, *Necropolitics*, Duke University Press, 2020.
7. C. Taylor, "Fanon, Foucault, and the Politics of Psychiatry."
8. Taylor, "Fanon, Foucault, and the Politics of Psychiatry."
9. Taylor, "Fanon, Foucault, and the Politics of Psychiatry"; Robcis, *Disalienation*.
10. Taylor, "Fanon, Foucault and the Politics of Psychiatry," 56.
11. See Shatz, *Rebel's Clinic*.
12. For works in the history of psychiatry that explore or employ Fanon and his theory and practice, especially in the context of the colonization of Africa, see Robcis, *Disalienation*; Keller, *Colonial Madness*; Sadowsky, *Imperial Bedlam*; Abi-Rached, *Asfuriyyeh*; Jackson, *Surfacing Up*; Khanna, *Dark Continents*.
13. Fanon, *Wretched of the Earth*, 182. Citations refer to the 2004 edition.
14. Nissim-Sabat, "Fanonian Musings."
15. The literature on the intersection between colonialism and the history of medicine is vast, but I am thinking primarily of Bashford, *Imperial Hygiene*; Anderson, *Cultivation of Whiteness*; Chaplin, *Subject Matter*.
16. Fanon, *Wretched of the Earth*, 311. Citations refer to the 1965 edition.
17. Fanon, *Wretched of the Earth*, 236–37. Citations refer to the 2004 edition.
18. Nissim-Sabat, "Fanonian Musings," 40.
19. Fanon developed this concept in Fanon, *Black Skin, White Masks*.
20. Fanon *Black Skin, White Masks*, xv. All citations refer to the 2008 edition.
21. Fanon, *Black Skin, White Masks*, xviii.
22. Fanon, *Black Skin, White Masks*, xiv–xv.
23. Fanon, *Black Skin, White Masks*, 122.
24. It could be argued that Freud picked up some of these themes in his later writing, for example in *Civilization and Its Discontents*, in which he considered

some of the ways that social pressures related to industrial modernity could be considered legitimate causes of mental illness, and that resistance to the same was not necessarily a sign of pathology.

25. Fanon, *Black Skin, White Masks*, 127.
26. Du Bois, *Souls of Black Folk*. Citations refer to the 2018 edition.
27. Fanon, *Black Skin, White Masks*, 162, 179.
28. Fanon articulates his thoughts most directly on this issue in the essay "On Violence" in Fanon, *Wretched of the Earth*.
29. Keller, *Colonial Madness*, 163.
30. Fanon, *Wretched of the Earth*, 3. Citations refer to the 2004 edition.
31. Fanon, *Wretched of the Earth*, 4.
32. Fanon's thoughts on distrust in the colonial medical encounter are particularly well articulated in the essay "Medicine and Colonialism" in Fanon, *A Dying Colonialism*.
33. Fanon, *Wretched of the Earth*, 181.
34. Fanon, *Wretched of the Earth*, 2, 6.
35. The long history of the processes of criminalization of Blackness is explored in works such as Muhammad, *Condemnation of Blackness*; LeFlouria, *Chained in Silence*; Haley, *No Mercy Here*; Suddler, *Presumed Criminal*. Some of these scholars make reference to overlap between psychology and criminalization.
36. Metzl, *Protest Psychosis*.
37. Pickens, *Black Madness*; Bruce, *How to Go Mad without Losing Your Mind*.
38. Pickens, *Black Madness*, 11.
39. Pickens, *Black Madness*, 14.
40. Pickens, *Black Madness*, 15.
41. Pickens, *Black Madness*, 13.
42. Grier and Cobbs, *Black Rage*.
43. Bruce, *How to Go Mad without Losing Your Mind*, 26.
44. Bruce, *How to Go Mad without Losing Your Mind*, 26.
45. Of course, plenty of people have called for the abolition of psychiatry for a variety of reasons, complaining of its dubious science and methodology, its function as a form of ableism, and its link to incarceration, especially for people of color, but I am using Bruce and Pickens here because they are making the case for abolition specifically because of its internal racism. See, as just a sample, Ben-Moshe, *Decarcerating Disability*; Ben-Moshe et al., *Disability Incarcerated*; Szasz, *Myth of Mental Illness*; Szasz, *Ideology and Insanity*; Szasz, *Law, Liberty and Psychiatry*; Goffman, *Asylums*.
46. Bruce, *How to Go Mad without Losing Your Mind*, 26, 28.

Bibliography

Primary Sources

Archives
Atlanta, GA
   Stuart Rose Manuscripts and Rare Books Library, Emory University
Birmingham, AL
   Reynolds-Finley Historical Library, University of Alabama at Birmingham
College Park, MD
   National Archives and Records Administration
Hattiesville, MS
   McCain Library and Archives, University of Southern Mississippi,
      Special Collections
Jackson, MS
   Mississippi Department of Archives and History
     Manuscripts and Special Collections
Mobile, AL
   Doy Leale McCall Rare Book and Manuscript Library, University of
      South Alabama
Montgomery, AL
   Alabama Department of Archives and History
     Manuscripts and Special Collections
Morrow, GA
   Georgia State Archives
     Manuscripts and Rare Books
   National Archives and Records Administration, Southeast Division
Philadelphia, PA
   Penn Libraries, Kislak Center for Special Collections, Rare Books and
      Manuscripts, University of Pennsylvania
Starkville, MS
   Mississippi State University Libraries, Division of Archives and Special
      Collections
     Special Collections—Subject Files
     Mississippi Political Collections and Manuscripts
       John C. Stennis Collection
Statesboro, GA
   Zach S. Henderson Library, Georgia Southern University
     Special Collections
       Culver Kidd Papers

Tuscaloosa, AL
    W. S. Hoole Special Collections Library, University of Alabama
        Bryce Hospital Collection
Tuskegee, AL
    Tuskegee University Archives
        Dibble Papers
Washington, DC
    Library of Congress Manuscripts Collection

Periodicals

Alabama Mental Health
Atlanta Daily World
Atlanta Journal Constitution
Clarion Ledger
Commercial Appeal
Delta Democrat-Times
Ebony
Jackson Daily News
Laurel Leader Call
Mobile Beacon
Mobile Press Register
Montgomery Advertiser
Southern Courier
The Whit

Books

Cranford, Peter G. *But for the Grace of God: The Inside Story of the World's Largest Insane Asylum.* 2nd ed. 1952. Milledgeville, GA: Old Capital Press, 2008.
Deutsch, Albert. *The Mentally Ill in America: A History of Their Care and Treatment from Colonial Times.* New York: Columbia University Press, 1962.
———. *The Shame of the States.* New York: Harcourt, 1948.

Secondary Sources

Books

Abi-Rached, Joelle M. *Asfuriyyeh: A History of Madness, Modernity, and War in the Middle East.* Cambridge, MA: MIT Press, 2020.
Adams, Natalie G., and James H. Adams. *Just Trying to Have School: The Struggle for Desegregation in Mississippi.* Jackson: University Press of Mississippi, 2018.
Alexander, Michelle. *The New Jim Crow: Mass Incarceration in the Age of Colorblindness.* New York: New Press, 2010.
American Psychiatric Association. *Diagnostic and Statistical Manual of Mental Disorders.* Washington, DC: American Psychiatric Association, 1952.
Anderson, Warwick. *The Cultivation of Whiteness: Science, Health and Racial Destiny in Australia.* New York: Basic Books, 2003.
Ashmore, Susan Youngblood. *Carry It On: The War on Poverty and the Civil Rights Movement in Alabama 1964–1972.* Athens: University of Georgia Press, 2008.
Ballenger, Jesse. "Beyond the Characteristic Plaques and Tangles: Mid-Twentieth Century U.S. Psychiatry and the Fight Against Senility." In *Concepts of Alzheimer's Disease: Biological, Clinical, and Cultural Perspectives*, edited by P. K. Whitehouse, Konrad Maurer, and Jesse Ballenger. Baltimore, MD: John Hopkins University Press, 2000.

———. *Self, Senility, and Alzheimer's Disease in Modern America: A History.* Baltimore, MD: Johns Hopkins University Press, 2006.
Bashford, Alison. *Imperial Hygiene: A Critical History of Colonialism, Nationalism and Public Health.* London: Palgrave Macmillan, 2004.
Bass, Jack. *Taming the Storm: The Life and Times of Judge Frank M. Johnson and the South's Fight over Civil Rights.* Athens: University of Georgia Press, 1993.
Beers, Clifford Whittingham. *A Mind That Found Itself.* New York: Longmans, Green, 1910.
Bell, Derrick. *Silent Covenants:* Brown v. Board of Education *and the Unfulfilled Hopes of Racial Reform.* Oxford: Oxford University Press, 2004.
Ben-Moshe, Liat. *Decarcerating Disability: Deinstitutionalization and Prison Abolition.* Minneapolis: University of Minnesota Press, 2020.
Ben-Moshe, Liat, Chris Chapman, and Allison C. Carey, eds. *Disability Incarcerated: Imprisonment and Disability in the United States and Canada.* New York: Palgrave Macmillan, 2014.
Berrey, S. A. *The Jim Crow Routine: Everyday Performances of Race, Civil Rights and Segregation in Mississippi.* Chapel Hill: University of North Carolina Press, 2015.
Blackmon, Douglas. *Slavery by Another Name: The Re-Enslavement of Black Americans from the Civil War to World War II.* New York: Anchor Books, 2008.
Braslow, Joel. *Mental Ills and Bodily Cures: Psychiatric Treatment in the First Half of the Twentieth Century.* Berkeley: University of California Press, 1997.
Bruce, La Marr Jurelle. *How to Go Mad without Losing Your Mind: Madness and Black Radical Creativity.* Durham, NC: Duke University Press, 2021.
Bullock, Charles, and Jenna Deitz. "Transforming the South: The Role of the Federal Government." In *The American South in the Twentieth Century*, edited by Craig S. Pascoe, Karen Trahan Leathem, and Andy Ambrose. Athens: University of Georgia Press, 2005.
Burch, Susan, and Michael Rembis, eds. *Disability Histories.* Champaign: University of Illinois Press, 2014.
Bureau of the Census. *Negro Population, by County: 1960 and 1950.* Washington, DC: Government Printing Office, 1966. www2.census.gov/library/publications/decennial/1960/pc-s1-supplementary-reports/pc-s1-52.pdf.
Byrd, W. M., and L. A Clayton. *An American Health Dilemma.* Vol. 2, *Race, Medicine and Health Care in the United States.* London: Routledge, 2002.
Cacho, Lisa Marie. *Social Death: Racialized Rightlessness and the Criminalization of the Unprotected.* New York: New York University Press, 2012.
Carter, Dan T. *From George Wallace to Newt Gingrich: Race in the Conservative Counterrevolution, 1963–1994.* Baton Rouge: Louisiana State University Press, 1996.
———. *The Politics of Rage: George Wallace, the Origins of the New Conservatism, and the Transformation of American Politics.* Baton Rouge: Louisiana State University Press, 2000.
Chandler, Dana R., and Edith Powell. *To Raise Up the Man Farthest Down: Tuskegee University's Advancements in Human Health, 1881–1987.* Tuscaloosa: University of Alabama Press, 2018.

Chaplin, Joyce. *Subject Matter: Technology, the Body, and Science on the Anglo-American Frontier, 1500–1676*. Cambridge, MA: Harvard University Press, 2009.

Creadick, Anna. *Perfectly Average: The Pursuit of Normality in Postwar America*. Amherst: University of Massachusetts Press, 2010.

Crespino, Joseph. *In Search of Another Country: Mississippi and the Conservative Counterrevolution*. Princeton, NJ: Princeton University Press, 2007.

Cunningham, David. "Shades of Anti-Civil Rights Violence: Reconsidering the Ku Klux Klan in Mississippi." In *The Civil Rights Movement in Mississippi*, edited by Ted Ownby. Jackson: University Press of Mississippi, 2013.

D'Antonio, Patricia. *American Nursing: A History of Knowledge, Authority, and the Meaning of Work*. Baltimore, MD: Johns Hopkins University Press, 2010.

———. *Founding Friends: Families, Staff and Patients at the Friends Asylum in Early Nineteenth-Century Philadelphia*. Bethlehem, PA: Lehigh Press, 2006.

Dittmer, John. *The Good Doctors: The Medical Committee for Human Rights and the Struggle for Social Justice in Health Care*. Jackson: University Press of Mississippi, 2009.

———. *Local People: The Struggle for Civil Rights in Mississippi*. Chicago: University of Illinois Press, 1995.

Downs, Jim. *Sick from Freedom: African American Illness and Suffering during the Civil War and Reconstruction*. Oxford: Oxford University Press, 2012.

Doyle, Dennis. *Psychiatry and Racial Liberalism in Harlem, 1936–1968*. Rochester, NY: University of Rochester Press, 2016.

Du Bois, W. E. B. *The Souls of Black Folk*. Chicago: A. C. McClurg, 1903. Reprint, New York: Penguin Books, 2018.

Edwards-Grossi, Elodie. *Mad with Freedom: The Political Economy of Blackness, Insanity, and Civil Rights in the U.S. South, 1840–1940*. New Orleans: Louisiana State University Press, 2022.

Engelhardt, Tom. *The End of Victory Culture: Cold War America and the Disillusioning of a Generation*. Amherst: University of Massachusetts Press, 2007.

Fanon, Frantz. *A Dying Colonialism*. New York: Grove Press, 1994.

———. *Black Skin, White Masks*. 1952. Translated by Richard Philcox. Reprint, New York: Grove Press, 2008.

———. *The Wretched of the Earth*. 1965. Translated by Richard Philcox. Reprint, New York: Grove Press, 2004.

Fett, Sharla. *Working Cures: Healing, Health and Power on Southern Slave Plantations*. Chapel Hill: University of North Carolina Press, 2002.

Ferguson, Jeffrey B. *The Sage of Sugar Hill: George S. Schuyler and the Harlem Renaissance*. New Haven, CT: Yale University Press, 2008.

Flynt, Wayne. *Alabama in the Twentieth Century*. Tuscaloosa: University of Alabama Press, 2004.

Folwell, Emma J. *The War on Poverty in Mississippi: From Massive Resistance to New Conservatism*. Jackson: University Press of Mississippi, 2020.

Foucault, Michel. "The Ethic of Care for the Self as a Practice of Freedom." In *The Final Foucault*, edited by James Bernauer and David Rasmussen. Cambridge: MIT Press, 1994.

———. *Madness and Civilization: A History of Insanity in the Age of Reason*. London: Routledge Classics, 2002.

———. *Psychiatric Power: Lectures at the Collège de France*. New York: Picador, 2003.

Frederick, Jeff. *Stand Up for Alabama: Governor George Wallace*. Tuscaloosa: University of Alabama Press, 2007.

Gamble, Vanessa Northington. *Making a Place for Ourselves: The Black Hospital Movement 1920–1945*. New York: Oxford University Press, 1995.

Garcia, Jay. *Psychology Comes to Harlem: Rethinking the Race Question in Twentieth-Century America*. Baltimore, MD: Johns Hopkins University Press, 2012.

Goffman, Irving. *Asylums: Essays on the Social Situation of Mental Patients and Other Inmates*. New York: Anchor Books, 1961.

Gonaver, Wendy. *The Peculiar Institution and the Making of Modern Psychiatry, 1840–1880*. Chapel Hill: University of North Carolina Press, 2018.

Grier, William H., and Price M. Cobbs. *Black Rage: Two Black Psychiatrists Reveal the Full Dimensions of the Inner Conflicts and the Desperation of Black Life in the United States*. 2nd ed. New York: Basic Books, 1968.

Grob, Gerald N. *From Asylum to Community: Mental Health Policy in Modern America*. Princeton, NJ: Princeton University Press, 1991.

———. *The Mad among Us: A History of the Care of America's Mentally Ill*. London: Free Press, 1994.

———. *Mental Illness and American Society*. Princeton, NJ: Princeton University Press, 1983.

Guenther, Lisa. *Solitary Confinement: Social Death and Its Afterlives*. Minneapolis: University of Minnesota Press, 2013.

Hale, Nathan. *The Rise and Crisis of Psychoanalysis in the United States: Freud and the Americans, 1917–1985*. Oxford: Oxford University Press, 1995.

Haley, Sarah. *No Mercy Here: Gender, Punishment, and the Making of Jim Crow Modernity*. Chapel Hill: University of North Carolina Press, 2016.

Halliwell, Martin. *Therapeutic Revolutions: Medicine, Psychiatry and American Culture, 1945–1970*. New Brunswick, NJ: Rutgers University Press, 2013.

Harrington, Anne. *Mind Fixers: Psychiatry's Troubled Search for the Biology of Mental Illness*. New York: Norton, 2019.

Hartman, Saidiya. *Scenes of Subjection: Terror, Slavery, and Self-Making in Nineteenth-Century America*. New York: Oxford University Press, 1997.

Harvey, Gordan E. "'Wallaceism Is an Insidious and Treacherous Type of Disease': The 1970 Alabama Gubernatorial Election and the 'Wallace Freeze' on Alabama Politics." In *History and Hope in the Heart of Dixie: Scholarship, Activism and Wayne Flynt in the Modern South*, edited by Gordon E. Harvey, Richard D. Starnes, and Glenn Feldman. Tuscaloosa: University of Alabama Press, 2006.

Herman, Ellen. *The Romance of American Psychology: Political Culture in the Age of Experts*. Berkeley: University of California Press, 1995.

Hirshbein, Laura D. *American Melancholy: Constructions of Depression in the Twentieth Century*. New Brunswick, NJ: Rutgers University Press, 2014.

Hogarth, Rana A. *Medicalizing Blackness: Making Racial Difference in the Atlantic World*. Chapel Hill: University of North Carolina Press, 2017.
Holley, Howard. *The History of Medicine in Alabama*. Birmingham: University of Alabama School of Medicine, 1982.
Horwitz, Allan V. *DSM: A History of Psychiatry's Bible*. Baltimore, MD: Johns Hopkins University Press, 2021.
Imada, Adria L. *An Archive of Skin, an Archive of Kin: Disability and Life-Making during Medical Incarceration*. Vol. 62 of American Crossroads. Oakland: University of California Press, 2022.
Irons, Jennifer. *Reconstituting Whiteness: The Mississippi State Sovereignty Commission*. Nashville: University of Tennessee Press, 2010.
Jackson, Lynette. *Surfacing Up: Psychiatry and Social Order in Colonial Zimbabwe, 1908–1968*. Ithaca, NY: Cornell University Press, 2005.
Jones, Kathleen. *Taming the Troublesome Child: American Families, Child Guidance, and the Limits of Psychiatric Authority*. Cambridge, MA: Harvard University Press, 1999.
Kaplan, Mary. *Solomon Carter Fuller: Where My Caravan Has Rested*. Lanham, MD: University Press of America, 2005.
———. *The Tuskegee Veterans Hospital and Its Black Physicians*. Jefferson, NC: McFarland, 2016.
Kardiner, Abram, and Lionel Ovesey. *The Mark of Oppression: A Psychosocial Study of the American Negro*. New York: W. W. Norton, 1951.
Katagiri, Yashuhiro. *The Mississippi State Sovereignty Commission: Civil Rights and State's Rights*. Jackson: University Press of Mississippi, 2001.
Keller, Richard. *Colonial Madness: Psychiatry in French North Africa*. Chicago: University of Chicago Press, 2007.
Khanna, Ranjana. *Dark Continents: Psychoanalysis and Colonialism*. Durham, NC: Duke University Press, 2007.
Larson, Edward J. *Sex, Race, and Science: Eugenics in the Deep South*. Baltimore, MD: Johns Hopkins University Press, 1996.
Lassiter, Matthew D. *The Silent Majority: Suburban Politics in the Sunbelt South*. Princeton, NJ: Princeton University Press, 2006.
Lassiter, Matthew D., and Joseph Crespino, eds. *The Myth of Southern Exceptionalism*. New York: Oxford University Press, 2010.
Lawrence, Susan C. *Privacy and the Past*. New Brunswick, NJ: Rutgers University Press, 2016.
LeFlouria, Talitha L. *Chained in Silence: Black Women and Convict Labor in the New South*. Chapel Hill: University of North Carolina Press, 2015.
Lewis, Nolan, and L. D Hubbard. "Manic Depressive Reactions in Negroes." In *Manic Depressive Psychoses*. Baltimore, MD: Williams and Wilkins, 1931.
Lieberman, Jeffrey A. *Shrinks: The Untold Story of Psychiatry*. New York: Little, Brown, 2015.
Litwack, Leon F. *Trouble in Mind: Black Southerners in the Age of Jim Crow*. New York: Vintage, 1999.

Long, Gretchen. *Doctoring Freedom: The Politics of African American Medical Care in Slavery and Emancipation.* Chapel Hill: University of North Carolina Press, 2012.

Mbembe, Achille. *Necropolitics.* Durham, NC: Duke University Press, 2020.

———. "The Power of the Archive and Its Limits." In *Refiguring the Archive,* edited by Carolyn Hamilton, Verne Harris, Jane Taylor, Michele Pickover, Graeme Reid, and Razia Saleh. Dordrecht: Kluwer Academic, 2002.

McBride, David. *Caring for Equality: A History of African American Health Care.* London: Rowman and Littlefield, 2018.

McCandless, Peter. *Moonlight, Magnolias, and Madness: Insanity in South Carolina from the Colonial Period to the Progressive Era.* Chapel Hill: University of North Carolina Press, 1996.

McMillen, Neil R. *The Citizen's Council: Organized Resistance to the Second Reconstruction, 1954-1964.* Urbana: University of Illinois Press, 1971.

Mendes, Gabriel N. *Under the Strain of Color: Harlem's Lafargue Clinic and the Promise of an Antiracist Psychiatry.* Ithaca, NY: Cornell University Press, 2015.

Menninger, William C. *Psychiatry in a Troubled World: Yesterday's War and Today's Challenge.* New York: Macmillan, 1948.

Metzl, Jonathan M. *The Protest Psychosis: How Schizophrenia Became a Black Disease.* Boston: Beacon Press, 2010.

———. *Prozac on the Couch: Prescribing Gender in the Era of Wonder Drugs.* Durham, NC: Duke University Press, 2003.

———. *What We've Become: Living and Dying in a Country of Arms.* New York: Norton, 2024.

Molina, Natalia. *Fit to Be Citizens? Public Health and Race in Los Angeles, 1879-1939.* Vol. 20. Oakland: University of California Press, 2006.

Moore, Jacqueline M. *Booker T. Washington, WEB Du Bois, and the Struggle for Racial Uplift.* London: Rowman & Littlefield, 2003.

Muhammad, Khalil Gibran. *The Condemnation of Blackness: Race, Crime and the Making of Modern Urban America.* Cambridge MA: Harvard University Press, 2010.

Murray, Heather. *Asylum Ways of Seeing: Psychiatric Patients, American Thought and Culture.* Philadelphia: University of Pennsylvania Press, 2022.

Nelson, Jack. *Scoop: The Evolution of a Southern Reporter.* Jackson: University Press of Mississippi, 2013.

NIMH. *Treatment Services for the Mentally Ill and Mentally Retarded in Georgia, 1964: A Survey Report to the Governor's Commission for Efficiency and Improvement in Government.* Bethesda MD: National Institute of Mental Health, 1964.

Nissim-Sabat, Marilyn. "Fanonian Musings: Decolonizing/Philosophy/Psychiatry." In *Fanon and the Decolonization of Philosophy,* edited by Elizabeth Hoppe and Tracey Nicholls. Lanham, MD: Lexington Books, 2010.

Noll, Richard. *American Madness: The Rise and Fall of Dementia Praecox.* Cambridge, MA: Harvard University Press, 2011.

Nuriddin, Ayah. "Engineering Uplift: Black Eugenics as Black Liberation." In *Nature Remade: Engineering Life, Envisioning Worlds*, edited by Luis A. Campos, Michael R. Dietrich, Tiago Saraiva, and Christian C. Young. Chicago: University of Chicago Press, 2021.

Oshinsky, David. *Worse Than Slavery: Parchman Farm and the Ordeal of Jim Crow Justice*. New York: Simon and Schuster, 1996.

Owens, Deirdre Cooper. *Medical Bondage: Race, Gender, and the Origins of American Gynecology*. Athens: University of Georgia Press, 2017.

Parsons, Anne E. *From Asylum to Prison: Deinstitutionalization and the Rise of Mass Incarceration after 1945*. Chapel Hill: University of North Carolina Press, 2018.

Paterson, Catherine. "A Short History of Occupational Therapy in Psychiatry." In *Occupational Therapy and Mental Health*, edited by Jennifer Creek and Leslie Lougher. London: Elsevier, 2011.

Patterson, Orlando. *Slavery and Social Death: A Comparative Study*. 2nd ed. Cambridge, MA: Harvard University Press, 2018.

Pickens, Theri Alyce. *Black Madness: Mad Blackness*. Durham, NC: Duke University Press, 2019.

Price, Joshua M. *Prison and Social Death*. New Brunswick, NJ: Rutgers University Press, 2019.

Pride, Richard A. *The Political Use of Racial Narratives: School Desegregation in Mobile, Alabama, 1954–97*. Champaign: University of Illinois Press, 2002.

Reverby, Susan. *Examining Tuskegee: The Infamous Syphilis Study and Its Legacy*. Chapel Hill: University of North Carolina Press, 2009.

Richardson, Theresa. *The Century of the Child: The Mental Hygiene Moment and Social Policy in the United States and Canada*. New York: Suny Press, 1989.

Richert, Lucas. *Break on Through: Radical Psychiatry and the American Counterculture*. Cambridge, MA: MIT Press, 2020.

Robcis, Camille. *Disalienation: Politics, Philosophy and Radical Psychiatry in Postwar France*. Chicago: University of Chicago Press, 2021.

Roberts, Gene, and Hank Klibanoff. *The Race Beat: The Press, the Civil Rights Struggle, and the Awakening of a Nation*. New York: Vintage, 2007.

Roberts, Samuel. *Infectious Fear: Politics, Disease, and the Health Effects of Segregation*. Chapel Hill: University of North Carolina Press, 2009.

Rose, Anne C. *Psychology and Selfhood in the Segregated South*. Chapel Hill: University of North Carolina Press, 2009.

Rose, S. F. *No Right to Be Idle: The Invention of Disability, 1840–1930*. Chapel Hill: University of North Carolina Press, 2017.

Ross, Matthew. *A Mental Health Program for Alabama: Survey of the Mental Health Needs and Resources of Alabama*. Washington, DC: American Psychiatric Association, 1959.

Roth, Alisa. *Insane: America's Criminal Treatment of Mental Illness*. New York: Basic Books, 2018.

Rothman, David J. *The Discovery of the Asylum: Social Order and Disorder in the New Republic*. New Brunswick, NJ: Aldine, 1990.

Sadowsky, Jonathan. *Electroconvulsive Therapy in America: The Anatomy of a Medical Controversy*. New York: Taylor and Francis, 2016.

———. *Imperial Bedlam: Institutions of Madness in Colonial Southwest Nigeria*. Los Angeles: University of California Press, 1999.

Sareyan, Alex. *The Turning Point: How Persons of Conscience Brought About Major Change in the Care of America's Mentally Ill*. Harrisonburg, VA: Herald Press, 1994.

Savitt, Todd, and James Harvey Young. *Disease and Distinctiveness in the American South*. Knoxville: University of Tennessee Press, 1988.

Scott, Daryl Michael. *Contempt and Pity: Social Policy and the Image of the Damaged Black Psyche, 1880–1996*. Chapel Hill: University of North Carolina Press, 1997.

Scott, Joan Wallach. *On the Judgement of History*. New York: Columbia University Press, 2020.

Schuyler, George Samuel. *Black No More: Being an Account of the Strange and Wonderful Workings of Science in the Land of the Free,* A.D. *1933–1940*. New York: Penguin, 2018.

———. *Rac(e)ing to the Right: Selected Essays of George S. Schuyler*. Knoxville: University of Tennessee Press, 2001.

Segrest, Mab. *Administrations of Lunacy: Racism and the Haunting of American Psychiatry at the Milledgeville Asylum*. New York: New Press, 2020.

Sharpe, Christina. *In the Wake: On Blackness and Being*. Durham, NC: Duke University Press, 2016.

Shatz, Adam. *The Rebel's Clinic: The Revolutionary Lives of Frantz Fanon*. New York: Farrar, Straus and Giroux, 2024.

Silver, James. *Mississippi: The Closed Society*. Jackson: University Press of Mississippi, 1964.

Smith, David Barton. *Health Care Divided: Race and Healing a Nation*. Ann Arbor: University of Michigan Press, 1999.

———. *The Power to Heal: Civil Rights, Medicare, and the Struggle to Transform America's Health Care System*. Nashville: Vanderbilt University Press, 2016.

Smith, Kylie M. "Reparatory History." In *Do Less Harm: Ethical Questions for Health Historians*, edited by C. T. Thompson and K. M. Smith. Baltimore, MD: Johns Hopkins University Press, 2025.

———. *Talking Therapy: Knowledge and Power in American Psychiatric Nursing*. New Brunswick, NJ: Rutgers University Press, 2020.

Spurlock, Jeanne. *Black Psychiatrists and American Psychiatry*. Washington, DC: American Psychiatric, 1999.

SREB. *Mental Health Training and Research in the Southern States*. Atlanta, GA: Southern Regional Education Board, 1954.

———. *Psychiatrists for Mental Health Programs: Report of a Conference Held under the Southern Regional Program in Mental Health Training and Research, August 1–3, Daytona Plaza Hotel, Dayton Beach, Florida*. Atlanta, GA: Southern Regional Education Board, 1956.

Staub, Michael E. *Madness Is Civilization: When the Diagnosis Was Social, 1948–1980*. Chicago: University of Chicago Press, 2011.

———. *The Mismeasure of Minds: Debating Race and Intelligence between Brown and The Bell Curve*. Chapel Hill: University of North Carolina Press, 2018.

Suddler, Carl. *Presumed Criminal: Black Youth and the Justice System in Postwar New York*. New York: New York University Press, 2019.

Summers, Martin. *Madness in the City of Magnificent Intentions: A History of Race and Mental Illness in the Nation's Capital*. Cambridge: Oxford University Press, 2019.

Szasz, Thomas S. *Ideology and Insanity: Essays on the Dehumanization of Man*. New York: Syracuse University Press, 1970.

———. *Law, Liberty and Psychiatry: An Inquiry into the Social Uses of Mental Health Practices*. London: Routledge & Kegan Paul, 1974.

———. *The Myth of Mental Illness: Foundations of a Theory of Personal Conduct*. New York: Harper, 1974.

Taggart, Danny. "'Are You Experienced?': The Use of Experiential Knowledge in Mental Health and Its Contribution to Mad Studies." In *The Routledge International Handbook of Mad Studies*. New York: Routledge, 2021.

Tani, Karen M. *States of Dependency: Welfare, Rights, and American Governance, 1935–1972*. Cambridge: Cambridge University Press, 2016.

Taylor, Chloe. "Fanon, Foucault, and the Politics of Psychiatry." In *Fanon and the Decolonization of Philosophy*, edited by Elizabeth Hoppe and Tracey Nicholls. Lanham, MD: Lexington Books, 2010.

Taylor, Stephen J. *Acts of Conscience: World War II, Mental Institutions, and Religious Objectors*. Syracuse, NY: Syracuse University Press, 2009.

Thomas, Karen Kruse. *Deluxe Jim Crow: Civil Rights and American Health Policy, 1935–1954*. Athens: University of Georgia Press, 2011.

Thompson, C. T., and K. M. Smith, eds. *Do Less Harm: Ethical Questions for Health Historians*. Baltimore, MD: Johns Hopkins University Press, 2025.

Tomes, Nancy. *The Art of Asylum-Keeping: Thomas Story Kirkbride and the Origins of American Psychiatry*. Philadelphia: University of Pennsylvania Press, 1984.

Trouillot, Michel-Rolph. *Silencing the Past: Power the Production of History*. Boston: Beacon Press, 1995.

Tullos, Allen. *Alabama Getaway: The Political Imaginary and the Heart of Dixie*. Athens: University of Georgia Press, 2011.

Ward, Jason Morgan. *Hanging Bridge: Racial Violence and America's Civil Rights Century*. Oxford: Oxford University Press, 2016.

Washington, Harriet A. *Medical Apartheid: The Dark History of Medical Experimentation on Black Americans from Colonial Times to the Present*. New York: Doubleday Books, 2006.

Weinstein, Deborah. *The Pathological Family: Postwar America and the Rise of Family Therapy*. Ithaca, NY: Cornell University Press, 2013.

Weisenfeld, Judith. *Black Religion in the Madhouse: Race and Psychiatry in Slavery's Wake*. New York: New York University Press, 2025.

Williams, Oscar Renal. *George S. Schuyler: Portrait of a Black Conservative*. Knoxville: University of Tennessee Press, 2007.

Willie, Charles V., Bernard M. Kramer, and Bertam S. Brown, eds. *Racism and Mental Health*. Pittsburgh, PA: University of Pittsburgh Press, 1973.

Willoughby, Christopher D. E. *Masters of Health: Racial Science and Slavery in U.S. Medical School*. Chapel Hill: University of North Carolina Press, 2022.

Yarbrough, Tinsley. *Judge Frank Johnson and Human Rights in Alabama*. Tuscaloosa: University of Alabama Press, 1981.

Journal Articles and Dissertations

Adams, Walter. "The Negro Patient in Psychiatric Treatment." *American Journal of Orthopsychiatry* 20, no. 2 (1950): 305–10.

Barker, Prince P. "Frontiers of Mental Hygiene." *Journal of the National Medical Association* 38, no. 1 (1946): 14–16.

———. "Neuropsychiatry in the Practice of Medicine and Surgery." *Journal of the National Medical Association* 23, no. 2 (1930): 109–16.

———. "Obscure Syphilitic Manifestations." *Journal of the National Medical Association* 21, no. 2 (1929): 57–61.

———. "Psychiatry at the Tuskegee VA Hospital in Retrospect." *Journal of the National Medical Association* 54, no. 2 (1962): 152–53.

———. "Psychoanalysis of Groups." *Journal of the National Medical Association* 44, no. 6 (November 1952): 455–56.

———. "Results and Observations on Insulin Shock Therapy in Negro Ex-Service Men." *Journal of the National Medical Association* 35, no. 1 (1943): 16–24.

Beardsley, Edward H. "Good-bye to Jim Crow: The Desegregation of Southern Hospitals, 1945–70." *Bulletin of the History of Medicine* 60, no. 3 (1986): 367–86.

Billups, Willam Robert. "Martyred Women and White Power since the Civil Rights Era: From Kathy Ainsworth to Vicki Weaver." *Journal of American History* 109, no. 4 (March 2023): 804–27.

Book, Constance Ledoux, and David Ezell. "Freedom of Speech and Institutional Control: Patient Publications at Central State Hospital, 1934–1978." *Georgia Historical Quarterly* 85, no. 1 (2001): 106–26.

Brown, Vincent. "Social Death and Political Life in the Study of Slavery." *American Historical Review* 114, no. 5 (December 2009): 1231–49.

Coles, Robert. "Social Struggles and Weariness." *Psychiatry* 27, no. 308 (1964).

Davis, Paul. "*Wyatt v. Stickney*: Did We Get It Right This Time?" *Law and Psychology Review* 35 (2011): 143.

Dittmer, John. "The Medical Committee for Human Rights." *AMA Journal of Ethics* 16, no. 9 (2014): 745–48.

Dorr, Gregory M. "Defective or Disabled? Race, Medicine, and Eugenics in Progressive Era Virginia and Alabama." *Journal of the Gilded Age and Progressive Era* 5, no. 4 (2006): 359–92.

Drake, Jack. "Drafting the Case: The Parallel Legacies of Wyatt V. Stickney and Lynch V. Baxley." *Law and Psychology Review* 35 (2011): 167–77.

Dreger, Alice Domurat. "Jarring Bodies: Thoughts on the Display of Unusual Anatomies." *Perspectives in Biology and Medicine* 43, no. 2 (2000): 161–72.

———. "Seeing Yourself." *Perspectives in Biology and Medicine* 47, no. 2 (2004): 160–64.
Dwyer, Ellen. "Psychiatry and Race during World War II." *Journal of the History of Medicine and Allied Sciences* 61, no. 2 (2006): 117–43.
Edwards-Grossi, Elodie. "Truth in Numbers? Emancipation, Race and Federal Census Statistics in the Debates over Black Mental Health in the United States, 1840–1900." *Endeavour* 45 (2021): 1–10.
Edwards-Grossi, Èlodie, and Christopher D. E. Willoughby. "Slavery and Its Afterlives in US Psychiatry." *American Journal of Public Health* 114, no. S3 (2023): S250–S257.
Ernst, Waltraud. "The Role of Work in Psychiatry: Historical Reflections." Supplement, *Indian Journal of Psychiatry* 60, no. S2 (2018): S248–S252.
Felix, Robert H. "Mental Hygiene and Public Health." *American Journal of Orthopsychiatry* 18 (1948): 679–84.
Gambino, Matthew. "'These Strangers within Our Gates': Race, Psychiatry and Mental Illness among Black Americans at St. Elizabeth's Hospital in Washington DC, 1900–1940." *History of Psychiatry* 19, no. 4 (2008): 387–400.
Hansen, Helena. "Substance-Induced Psychosis: Clinical-Racial Subjectivities and Capital in Diagnostic Apartheid." *Ethos* 47, no. 1 (2019): 73–88.
Harcourt, Bernard E. "From the Asylum to the Prison: Rethinking the Incarceration Revolution." *Texas Law Review* 84 (June 2006): 1751–86.
Hartman, Saidiya. "Venus in Two Acts." *Small Axe* 26 (June 2008): 1–14.
Hughes, John S. "Labeling and Treating Black Mental Illness in Alabama, 1861–1910." *Journal of Southern History* 58, no. 3 (August 1992): 435–60.
Imada, Adria L. "Promiscuous Signification: Leprosy Suspects in a Photographic Archive of Skin." *Representations* 138, no. 1 (2017): 1–36.
Johnson, Frank M., Jr. "In Defense of Judicial Activism." *Emory LJ* 28 (1979): 901.
———. "Observation: The Constitution and the Federal District Judge." *Texas Law Review* 54, no. 5 (June 1976): 903–16.
Kearl, Benjamin. "Etiology Replaces Interminability: A Historiographical Analysis of the Mental Hygiene Movement." *American Educational History Journal* 41, no. 1/2 (2014): 285.
Kennedy, Janet. "Problems Posed in the Analysis of the Negro Patient." *Psychiatry* 15, no. 3 (1952): 313–27.
Kirkbride, Thomas S. "Proceedings for the Tenth Annual Meeting of the Association of Medical Superintendents of American Institutions for the Insane." *American Journal of Insanity* 12, no. 43 (1855): 89.
Kirkland, Scotty E. "Mobile and the Boswell Amendment." *Alabama Review* 65 (July 2012): 205–49
———. "Pink Sheets and Black Ballots: Politics and Civil Rights in Mobile, Alabama 1945–1985." Master's thesis, University of South Alabama, 2009.
Kleinberg, Ethan, Joan Wallach Scott, and Gary Wilder. "Theses on Theory and History." *History of the Present* 10, no. 1 (April 2020): 157–65.

Knopman, David S., Ronald C. Petersen, Clifford R. Jack Jr. "A Brief History of 'Alzheimer Disease': Multiple Meanings Separated by a Common Name." *Neurology* 92, no. 22 (May 2019): 1053–59.

Kramer, Morton. "Long Range Studies of Mental Hospital Patients: An Important Area of Research in Chronic Disease." *Milbank Memorial Fund Quarterly* 31, no. 3 (July 1953): 253–64.

Lowinger, Paul. "Radicals in Psychiatry." *Canadian Psychiatry Association Journal* 17, no. SS-II (1972): SS-193–96.

Maisel, Albert. "Bedlam 1946: Most U.S. Mental Hospitals Are a Shame and a Disgrace." *Life* (May 6, 1946): 102–18.

Maltzberg, B. "Mental Disease among Negroes in New York State." *Human Biology* 7 (1935): 471–513.

Metzl, Jonathan M., Jennifer Piemonte, and Tara McKay. "Mental Illness, Mass Shootings, and the Future of Psychiatric Research into American Gun Violence." *Harvard Review of Psychiatry* 29, no. 1 (2021): 81–89.

Meyer, Adolf. "The Birth and Development of the Mental Hygiene Movement." *Mental Hygiene* 19 (1935): 29–37.

Molina, Natalia. "Fear and Loathing in the US-Mexico Borderlands: The History of Mexicans as Medical Menaces, 1848 to the Present." *Aztlán: A Journal of Chicano Studies* 41, no. 2 (2016): 87–112.

Murphy, Michael Thomas. "Inhospitable in the Hospitality State: The Mississippi State Hospital in the Jim Crow South, 1865–1966." PhD diss., Mississippi State University, 2018.

Nelson, Bruce. "Organized Labor and the Struggle for Black Equality in Mobile during World War II." *Journal of American History* 80 (December 1993): 952–88.

Nuriddin, Ayah. "Liberation Eugenics: African American and the Science of Black Freedom Struggles 1890–1970." PhD diss., Johns Hopkins University, 2021.

———. "Psychiatric Jim Crow: Desegregation at the Crownsville State Hospital 1948–1970." *Journal of the History of Medicine and Allied Sciences* 74, no. 1 (2019): 85–106.

Partlow, William Dempsey. "Annual Message of the President." *Transactions of the Medical Society of the State of Alabama (TMASA)*, 1918: 10.

———. "Degeneracy." *Transactions of the Medical Society of the State of Alabama (TMASA)*, 1907, 229.

Perlin, Michael L. "'Abandoned Love': The Impact of Wyatt v. Stickney on the Intersection between International Human Rights and Domestic Mental Disability Law." *Law and Psychology Review* 35 (2011).

Peyman, D. A. R. "An Investigation of the Effects of Group Psychotherapy on Chronic Schizophrenic Patients." *Group Psychotherapy* 9, no. 1 (April 1956): 35–39.

Poussaint, Alvin F. "Black Power: A Failure for Integration within the Civil Rights Movements." *Archives of General Psychiatry* 18, no. 4 (1968): 385–91.

———. "The Stresses of the White Female Worker in the Civil Rights Movement in the South." *American Journal of Psychiatry* 123, no. 4 (1966): 401–7.

Quadagno, Jill. "Promoting Civil Rights through the Welfare State: How Medicare Integrated Southern Hospitals." *Social Problems* 47, no. 1 (February 2000): 68-89.

Reynolds, P. Preston. "The Federal Government's Use of Title VI and Medicare to Racially Integrate Hospitals in the United Sates 1963 through 1967." *American Journal of Public Health* 87, no. 11 (1997): 1850-58.

———. "Hospitals and Civil Rights, 1945-1963: The Case of Simkins v. Moses H. Cone Memorial Hospital." *Annals of Internal Medicine* 126, no. 11 (June 1997): 898-906.

Richert, Lucas. "'Therapy Means Change, Not Peanut Butter': American Radical Psychiatry, 1968-1975." *Social History of Medicine* 27, no. 1 (2014): 104.

Robinson, Bridgette Trinise. "The Battle for Respectability: The Black Bourgeoisie's Use of Eugenic Rhetoric in Racial Uplift Politics, 1895-1940." PhD diss., Morgan State University, 2018.

Rose, Anne C. "Putting the South on the Psychological Map: The Impact of Region and Race on the Human Sciences during the 1930s." *Journal of Southern History* 71, no. 2 (2005): 321-56.

Rucker, Walter C., and Sabriya Kaleen Jubilee. "From Black Nadir to *Bown v. Board*: Education and Empowerment in Black Georgian Communities—1865 to 1954." *Negro Educational Review* 58, no. 3/4 (2007): 151.

Sadowsky, Jonathan, and Kylie M. Smith. "Reflections on the Use of Patient Records: Privacy, Ethics and Reparations in the History of Psychiatry." *Journal of the History of the Behavioral Sciences* 6, no. 1 (2023): e22260. 10.1002/jhbs.22260.

Savitt, Todd. "The Use of Blacks for Medical Experimentation and Demonstration in the Old South." *Journal of Southern History* 48 (August 1982): 331-48.

Scott, David. "A Reparatory History of the Present." *Small Axe* 21, no. 1 (March 2017): vii-x.

Slaten, Clifton. "The 1995 Wyatt Litigation: Beginnings, Trial Strategies, and Results." *Law and Psychology Review* 35 (2011): 179-91.

Smith, Kylie M. "No Medical Justification: Segregation and Civil Rights in Alabama's Psychiatric Hospitals 1952-1972." *Journal of Southern History* 87, no. 4 (November 2021): 645-72.

Smith, Stephen Michael. "Eugenic Sterilization in 20th Century Georgia: From Progressive Utilitarianism to Individual Rights." Master's thesis, Georgia Southern University, 2010.

Spandler, Helen, and Dina Poursanidou. "Who Is Included in the Mad Studies Project?" *Journal of Ethics in Mental Health* 10 (2019).

Summers, Martin. "'Suitable Care of the African When Afflicted with Insanity': Race, Madness and Social Order in Comparative Perspective." *Bulletin of the History of Medicine* 84, no. 1 (2010): 58-91.

Tarwater, James Sidney. "The Alabama State Hospitals and the Partlow State School and Hospital: A Brief History." *Alabama Journal of Medical Sciences* 2, no. 1 (January 1965): 168-81.

Thomas, Karen Kruse. "The Hill-Burton Act and Civil Rights: Expanding Hospital Care for Black Southerners, 1939–1960." *Journal of Southern History* 72, no. 4 (November 2006): 823–70.

Tucker, James A. "*Wyatt v. Stickney*: Due Process, Confusion, and Consequences." *Law and Psychological Review* 46 (2021): 241

Verney, Kevern. "'Every Man Should Try': John L. Leflore and the National Association for the Advancement of Colored People in Alabama, 1919–1956." *Alabama Review* 66, no. 3 (2013): 186–210.

Vickery, Katherine. "A History of Mental Health in Alabama." Master's thesis, University of Alabama at Birmingham, no date.

Wahbi, Rafik, and Leo Beletsky. "Involuntary Commitment as 'Carceral-Health Service': From Healthcare-to-Prison Pipeline to a Public Health Abolition Praxis." *Journal of Law, Medicine and Ethics* 50, no. 1 (2022): 23–30.

Willoughby, Christopher D. E. "Running Away from Drapetomania: Samuel Cartwright, Medicine and Race in the Antebellum South." *Journal of Southern History* 84, no. 3 (August 2018): 579–614.

Wofsy, Avi. "Policing Mental Health: A Historical and Geographic Analysis of Mental Health Policy in Atlanta, Georgia." PhD diss., Emory University, 2023.

Wofsy, Avi, and Kylie M. Smith. "Racism and Redlining in the History of Psychiatric Policy and Practice in Atlanta: Implications for Nursing." *Policy, Politics, and Nursing Practice* 26, no. 1 (2025): 16–23.

Index

Adams, Ruth, 183
Alabama, 25, 63, 166, 207, 211, 214–15, 228, 238, 249–50; Bryce Hospital, 48, 94, 114; and Civil Rights Act, 17, 224; community mental health in, 158, 160; and dementia, 74; Demopolis, 219; Department of Archives and History, 30, 157, 205; Department of Public Health, 29; and *Diagnostic and Statistical Manual (DSM-1)*, 68; Disability Advocacy Program (ADAP), 235; and electroconvulsive therapy (ECT), 82, 84; extractive labor practices in, 117; federal funds for, 204; Greene County, 189; institutions in, 12; involuntary commitment in, 62; Jemison Center farm, 123; Jim Crow in, 64; labor relations in, 119; and J. L. LeFlore, 180; and Lister Hill, 28, 213; Macon County, 14; and MCHR, 190–91; mental deficiency in, 77–78; mental health associations in, 173; Mental Health Board, 222–24; mental health facilities in, 22, 49, 61, 204, 251; mental health funding in, 231; mental health services in, 172, 175, 178, 206, 219, 230, 235; mental hospitals in, 52; Montgomery, 22, 33, 174, 190, 221, 228, 249; Montgomery County, 150–51, 173; Montgomery VA, 35; NAACP in, 181; OEHO in, 218; prisons in, 235; psychiatric facilities in, 39, 184; and psychotic disorders, 72–73; and schizophrenia, 73; Searcy Hospital, 83–84, 88, 114, 124, 153, 168; segregation in, 8, 42–43, 50, 52, 71, 75, 82, 175, 195, 221, 226, 251, 257; state government of, 30, 36; state hospitals, 21, 76, 157, 222; and states' rights, 221, 225, 229; Tuskegee Institute, 17, 33; Tuskegee Veterans Administration Hospital (TVAH), 34, 36; University of Alabama, 118, 220, 252–53
Alabama Comprehensive Community Mental Health Plan (CCMH Plan), 172, 174, 205
Alabama Disability Advocacy Program (ADAP), 235
Alabama Industrial School for Negro Children, 33, 50
Alabama Mental Health Magazine, 18, 20
alienation, 99, 261, 263, 265
American Psychiatric Association (APA), 24, 36, 39, 50, 61, 139, 187, 246, 251, 253
Americans with Disability Act, 238
anti-Blackness, 9, 234
asylum reform, 48
Atlanta (GA), 6–7, 121, 165–66, 183, 188, 195, 217, 221–22, 239; Emory University, 35; Fulton County, 91; Grady Memorial Hospital, 167, 210; newspapers, 78, 167; Public Health Service, 160
Atlanta Constitution, 128, 147–48
Atlanta Legal Aid, 242
Atlanta Mental Hygiene Association, 138–39
Atlanta University, 190
Augusta (GA), 43, 144, 149, 161, 210

Baldwin County (GA), 91, 123, 147, 149, 241
Barker, Prince, 17, 19, 21, 23–25, 27–37
Berrey, Stephen, 11
Black bodies, 33, 39, 88, 150
Black mental health, 25, 27, 146, 247
Blackness, 8–9, 18, 26, 33, 70, 134, 167, 203, 234, 252, 260, 262, 264–66
Black psyche, 17, 21, 27, 39, 78, 87, 92, 125, 231
Brookhaven group home, 5
Bryce Hospital, 94, 118, 174, 183–84, 196, 219, 225, 235–36, 251–53; annual report of, 83; and asylum reform, 48; and cerebral arteriosclerosis (CA), 75; electroconvulsive therapy (ECT) in, 83–84; funding for, 234; and incarceration, 158; and integration, 229; and Jemison Center, 117; and Robert Jemison Jr., 51; and Loveman Marable, 227; and OEHO, 218; psychology program, 82; as public mental health facility, 22; white patients in, 71, 77, 199; and Albert L. Patterson, 114; and Al Payman, 195; and James Sidney Tarwater, 50, 82, 223

Cartwright, Samuel, 41
Central State Hospital (CSH), 46, 62–63, 67, 122–23, 162, 166–67, 207–8, 210, 240–41; and arteriosclerosis, 76; Black patients in, 22, 77–78, 81, 161; and *Builder*, 94; and Civil Rights Act, 239; committed patients in, 61; and Comprehensive Community Mental Health Plan (CCMHP), 165; and corruption, 160; and *Ebony*, 164; and John Gates, 242; and *Golden Star*, 94; and insulin coma therapy, 80; and malpractice, 160; and occupational therapy, 120–21; and Thomas Peacock, 78–79; and progressivism, 44; and Public Welfare Department, 47; and racial difference, 76; and schizophrenia, 244; and segregation, 44; therapeutic environment of, 81; and therapy, 78; white patients in, 43, 71, 82, 121
Chaney, Fred, 128, 130, 138
civil rights, 17, 138, 158–60, 170, 172, 175–76, 178, 189–90, 200, 217, 224, 232–33, 242, 266; abuses, 186; and Hodding Carter, 128; compliance, 207, 230, 257; groups, 180; law, 228, 234; medical, 206; and mental health, 195; networks, 195; and newspapers, 148, 193; workers, 186–88, 191–92
Civil Rights Act (1964), 7–8, 17, 39, 158–59, 161–62, 175–76, 180, 183–84, 194, 204, 206, 210–11, 213–14, 219, 222–25, 227–28, 231–32, 239
civil rights activism, 3, 8, 187, 218, 220, 247, 253
civil rights movement, 4, 6, 59, 94, 152, 180, 189, 199, 203, 244–45, 261, 267; in Mississippi, 11, 126
Civil Rights of Institutionalized Persons Act (CRIPA), 238
Cohn, David, 95
colonial pacification, 246
colonial project, 13, 17, 250
colonization, 14, 262–66
Community Mental Health Act (CMHA), 158–60, 175–76, 178
Cranford, Peter, 128, 144–49, 152
criminality, 6, 8, 25, 128, 243
Cunningham, David, 202

Delta Democrat-Times (DDT) (newspaper), 129–30
Department of Health, Education, and Welfare (HEW), 1–2, 8, 160, 168, 176, 180, 183, 186, 193–95, 204, 209–11, 213–14, 216–17, 219, 222, 227, 229
desegregation, 36, 176, 178, 183, 195–96, 199, 216, 222, 234, 257
Deutsch, Albert, 127–28, 138–42, 144, 149
Diagnostic and Statistical Manual (DSM-1), 67–74, 77–78, 87, 244
Dibble, Eugene, 18, 29–31, 33, 35–36

disability, 26, 58, 107, 120, 141, 196, 208, 241, 252; advocacy, 237; and Blackness, 8, 18, 30, 125; conceptualization of, 6, 25; developmental, 161, 165, 242; intellectual, 134; mental, 22, 79; and poverty, 172; services, 6
discrimination, 142–44, 164, 179, 181, 184–85, 208, 210–11, 219, 223, 228, 230, 239, 240, 252
Division of Mental Hygiene, 172
Division of Public Welfare, 79

Ebony (magazine), 128, 141–44, 152, 164
electroconvulsive therapy (ECT), 36, 79–80, 82–84, 192, 199
electroshock therapy, 31–34, 79, 83–85, 88, 146, 197
Ellisville State Hospital, 1
Ellisville State School, 4–6, 129, 134, 215–17
Emory University, 35
Equal Employment Opportunity Commission, 4
eugenics, 21, 25–26, 34, 39–40, 49, 61, 77, 92, 128, 200; confinement, 125; positive, 27, 32; and thinking, 42; threat of, 65; and white supremacy, 172, 203

Ferguson, Charles, 133–34, 137
Foucault, Michel, 11–12, 260–62, 267
French, David, 204

Georgia, 12, 59, 62–64, 75, 78, 138, 163, 165, 209, 213, 243, 251, 254–56; access to care in, 231; admission process, 61; Black patients in, 22, 77, 91, 123; Black population of, 166; and Civil Rights Act, 17, 239; community mental health in, 158, 178; Consumer Council, 144; Department of Corrections, 46; Department of Public Welfare, 43, 47; and Albert Deutsch, 128; diagnostic practices in, 68, 71–73; electroconvulsive therapy (ECT) in, 84; Hospital Services Branch, 66; institutional nonreform in, 159–60; Jim Crow in, 124, 140; legislature, 7, 44; Mental Health Institute, 207; mental health services in, 160–61, 242; and National Institute of Mental Health (NIMH), 206; Nurses Association, 46; prisons in, 139; psychiatric facilities in, 39, 168; race relations in, 240; regionalization in, 168–69; segregation in, 42–43, 173; service utilization in, 192; social problems in, 145; state hospitals in, 21, 76, 142; State Welfare Department, 139, 148–49; and James Sidney Tarwater, 82; and Title VI, 206, 210; white women in, 83. *See also* Central State Hospital (CSH)
Gilbert, Mark, 3
Green, Thomas F., 43–44

Hill-Burton Act, 28, 176, 194, 207, 210–12, 215
Hinds Community College, 4
Hurston, Claudette, 1–4, 6–8, 168, 190, 192
Hurston, Deacon, 3–5
Hurston, Ronald, 3–5
Hurston, Thomas Hobart, 3–6, 134

incarceration, 11, 21, 59, 107, 115, 158, 170, 206, 236, 245, 261, 265–66
industrial capitalism, 108
industrial therapy, 123, 163–64, 167
integration, 21, 46, 142, 158–59, 163, 168, 171, 177–78, 197, 201, 203, 207–10, 220, 238, 245; and Black patients, 193; and Black psychiatrists, 55; educational, 200; hospital, 7, 176, 180, 199, 215–18, 222; medical, 2, 204, 213, 222, 229–30, 256; and Medical Committee for Human Rights (MCHR), 194; prison, 236; psychiatric, 206; and Public Health Service, 212; resistance to, 205–6, 224, 226; and Whitfield Hospital, 202

Index   325

Jackson, George, 151
Jackson, Maynard, 240
Jackson Daily News (newspaper), 56
Jaquith, William, 53–60, 63, 70, 84–86, 94, 96, 104, 106, 109, 113–14, 128–29, 137, 200–203, 206, 216, 237–38
Jemison, Robert, Jr., 51–52
Jemison Center, 51, 117, 119, 123, 174, 184, 219
Jim Crow, 39, 78, 126, 128, 136, 221; in asylum, 7, 231; laws, 40, 125, 140, 146; in Mississippi, 52, 64, 70, 200; relations, 38, 92; routine, 9, 11, 68, 88, 92–94, 99, 101, 106, 109–10, 114, 119, 124, 137, 168, 188–90, 200, 211, 213, 234; and segregation, 20, 139; and social death, 9–10; and social relations, 93, 101
John A. Andrew Memorial Hospital, 18, 22, 28
Johnson, Frank M., 206, 228–30, 234–35
Johnson, Lyndon B., 224
Johnson, Simon Overton, 23

Kardiner, Abram, 24
King's Daughters Medical Center, 5
Kirkbride, Thomas, 21, 42, 48, 52, 108
Ku Klux Klan, 100, 171–72, 185, 192, 202–3

LeFlore, John, 8, 179–81, 183–86, 195, 197, 204, 218, 226–28, 230

Marable v. Alabama Mental Health Board, 8, 227, 230, 234
Mays, Willie, Jr., 185
Medicaid, 7, 76, 159, 175–76, 212, 231, 239, 243–44. *See also* Medicare
Medicaid Act of 1965, 7, 176
Medical Association of Georgia (MAG), 149, 151
Medical Committee for Human Rights (MCHR), 180, 186–87, 189–91, 193–94, 204, 245–47

Medicare, 2, 7, 76, 152, 159, 175–76, 194, 202, 204, 212–13, 216, 243
Menefee, Allen, 2
Menninger, Karl, 35, 151, 160
mental hygiene, 25–27, 32, 172
mental-hygiene conscious, 19
mental illness, 6, 62, 141, 166, 191, 195, 239, 263, 267; in Black patients, 41, 43, 99, 243, 264; and Central State Hospital, 161; in *DSM*, 69; effects of, 174; and environmental stressors, 26; and eugenic thinking, 26; hospitalization programs for, 32; and Jim Crow, 128; and prison system, 236; and senile brain disease, 74; serious, 238, 245; stigmatization of, 58, 86, 242; studies of, 72; and violence, 107; and *The Whit*, 87; and Whitfield Hospital, 71
Meridian (MS), 52, 129, 134, 169–70, 192, 215, 217
Metzl, Jonathan, 244, 265
Michaels, David Seth, 236
Milledgeville (GA), 209; and Charles Bush, 207–8; Central State Hospital, 22, 43–44, 63, 67, 78, 123, 161, 244, 254; and Joe Combs, 149; and Community Mental Health Act (CMHA), 160; and Peter Cranford, 144–46, 150; and Albert Deutsch, 128, 140; elderly people in, 76; insulin shock therapy in, 85; NAACP in, 91–92; and Jack Nelson, 147–48, 152; scandals of, 138; segregation in, 43–48; State Hospital, 141–42, 147, 207, 240; and State Welfare Department, 139; voluntary patients in, 62; white patients in, 71; women prisoners in, 162
Mississippi, 2, 11–12, 58, 63–64, 102, 114, 132, 171–72, 188, 207, 213–14; access to care in, 231; admission process in, 59; Black patients in, 54, 106, 129, 133, 137–38, 152, 168, 187, 189–90; Black women in, 111; and

civil rights, 126, 178; and Civil Rights Act, 17; and Commission on Hospital Care, 211–12; and Community Legal Services, 236; community mental health in, 158; and Department of Archives and History, 238; and Department of Health, Education, and Welfare (HEW), 222; East Mississippi State Hospital, 4, 52, 94, 103, 122, 169, 192, 203, 238; and Freedom Summer, 186; hospital integration in, 7; Jackson (MS), 3, 6, 22, 52, 188, 192, 193–94, 202, 215, 236; Jim Crow in, 70, 99; and Ku Klux Klan, 202; and Medicare, 212; mental health lawyers in, 61; mental health services in, 53, 128; mental health system in, 6; Mississippi Delta, 95; occupational therapy in, 109; and OEHO, 214–16, 218; psychiatric facilities in, 39; and race, 52; segregation in, 42–43, 160, 175, 206; therapeutic practices in, 84; and Title VI, 194; and white supremacy, 38, 203; Whitfield Hospital, 22, 84, 94, 124
Mississippi Medical Center, 5, 85, 170
Mississippi River, 161
Mississippi State Extension Service, 52
Mississippi State Sovereignty Commission (SovComm), 200
Mississippi State University, 2, 256
Mobile Beacon (newspaper), 185
Montgomery Advertiser (newspaper), 223–24
Moore, Dorothy, 2
Mount Vernon, 48–49, 63, 75, 83, 114, 117, 150, 158, 185
Mt. Meigs (Alabama Industrial School for Negro Children), 33, 50

natal alienation, 99
National Association for the Advancement of Colored People (NAACP), 8, 22–23, 91–92, 126, 179–81, 204

National Institute of Mental Health (NIMH), 28, 160, 162–65, 177–78, 183, 193, 206, 208, 217
National Medical Association (NMA), 22
"Negro insane," 21–22, 27
"Negro personality," 17, 24
Nelson, Jack, 128, 147–52
nondiscrimination, 7, 158, 168, 176–78, 193–94, 211, 214
nonreform reform, 128, 159, 169, 244

occupational therapy, 47, 54, 79, 81, 88, 93, 107–9, 112, 114, 120–21, 123–25, 134, 143, 196
Office of Equal Health and Opportunity (OEHO), 206, 214–18
outpatient clinics, 28, 33
outpatient health care, 30, 32, 34, 163, 169–70, 172, 174, 177, 191, 239
Ovesey, Lionel, 24

Partlow, William Dempsey, 25, 49–50, 114, 157
Partlow School and Hospital, 22, 205, 218, 229
Patterson, Albert L., 50, 114–15, 117, 119
Patterson, Orlando, 10
Peacock, Thomas, 46–47, 61, 63, 78–79, 82, 120–21, 145, 147–48, 151
plantations, 260; and asylums, 9–10, 18, 92; and Black Belt, 166; and Black patients, 107; and holdings, 52; and labor, 40, 93, 119, 124; and melodies, 101; and "Negro insane," 21; and prisons, 8, 119; and psychiatry, 41, 261; and racial capitalism, 109; relations, 14, 88, 106; Southern, 118, 165, 218, 259, 262; systems, 47; and white supremacy, 6, 267
Plessy v. Ferguson, 40, 42
Posser, Bruce, 122
poverty, 161, 166, 167, 172–73, 191; War on Poverty, 171

Index   327

prisons, 6, 44, 137, 151, 158, 199, 242–45, 252, 260; in Alabama, 235; and asylums, 65; construction of, 231; in Georgia, 139; inmates in, 25, 123, 188; as plantation system, 8; and prisoners' rights, 237; and prison farms, 119, 123, 133–34; and prison reform, 235; and psychiatric systems, 10, 26; and school-to-prison pipeline system, 33; and women, 162
Pruitt, Inez, 196–97
psychiatric reform, 42, 128, 144, 147–49
psychotherapy, 25, 27, 32, 35, 81–84, 86
Public Health Service (PHS), 2, 176–77, 183, 195, 210, 212, 219, 222. *See also* US Public Health Service (USPHS)
public welfare, 71, 254

racial capitalism, 40, 109
racism, 9, 27, 93, 142–43, 169, 186, 232–33, 247, 253, 263; and American Psychiatric Association, 36; anti-Black, 259; harms of, 13; and internal racism of psychiatry, 11, 14, 21, 39, 59, 65, 67–68, 74, 87, 92, 144, 152, 203, 243–46, 267; and mental health, 206; and segregation, 144, 168; structural, 243; and Tuskegee, 36; and white supremacy, 159, 213, 231, 266
reform movements, 21, 43, 97, 107–8, 136, 138, 140, 151–52, 236
rehabilitation, 25, 82, 86, 131, 143, 162, 170; programs, 164–65, 215–16
resegregation, 224
rights, 10; access to, 92; of citizenship, 39, 184; contestation over, 12; of patients, 162, 164–65, 229, 233–34, 237, 242, 245, 261; of prisoners, 237; of states, 178, 221, 224–25; voting, 180, 200, 240, 249; of workers, 230
Rothman, David, 108

Schaefer, Bruce, 149
schizophrenia, 71, 73, 79–80, 83–84, 87, 196, 219, 243–45, 247

schizophrenic reactions, 68, 70, 72–73, 80
Schuyler, George, 38, 52
Searcy, James T., 48–49
Searcy Hospital, 22, 50, 75, 114–15, 117, 157–58, 168, 183, 185–86, 191, 197, 206, 227, 251; Black patients in, 71, 77, 94, 173, 184, 196, 199, 219, 223–24; committed patients in, 32, 34; conditions of, 153, 174; construction of, 116; electroconvulsive therapy (ECT) in, 84; and Medical Committee for Human Rights (MCHR), 190; and OEHO, 218; segregation in, 124, 177, 226; and therapeutic technology, 83; and Title VI, 229; and tuberculosis, 179; and white supremacy, 88
segregation, 6, 35, 38, 41, 87, 141, 146, 149, 177, 183–84, 200, 210, 215, 224–28; in Alabama, 8, 36, 50, 71, 175, 229–30, 251; in asylums, 64–65; and Black codes, 26; of Black patients, 93, 96, 140, 148, 150, 201; and Black psyche, 21; of Black workers, 208; and Central State Hospital, 43–44; and civil rights, 242; and Community Mental Health Act (CMHA), 175; and confinement, 152; de facto, 142–44, 159, 169, 209; educational, 171, 229, 231; effects of, 37; and federal funding, 202; fights against, 152–53, 180, 204; geographical, 163, 173–74, 231; in Georgia, 160, 169; hospital, 211, 245; impacts of, 39–40, 59, 97, 139, 143, 158, 162, 186, 267; and integration, 21; and invisibility, 13; and William Jaquith, 54; justifications of, 40, 49, 206, 213, 217, 221; and Medical Committee for Human Rights (MCHR), 193; and mental health services, 166–68; in Mississippi, 64; and nurses, 46; operationalization of, 43; paternalism of, 13, 249; physical, 244; of psychiatric institutions, 42, 78, 153; and public welfare, 71; in South,

20, 214; structures of, 11, 56, 96; and Tuskegee Mental Hygiene Clinic, 22; and Tuskegee VA Hospital, 22–23; violence of, 18, 52; and Whitfield Hospital, 55, 105, 124
Segrest, Mab, 122, 254, 256
Sharpe, Christina, 9
slavery, 9–10, 12, 18, 41–43, 92, 111, 119, 127, 236, 260, 262–63
Smith, David Barton, 214–15
Smith, Fred, 132–33
Smith, Robert, 187–88, 190
Smith, Rubye, 201–2
social death, 9–10, 13, 99, 249, 261
social hierarchy, 56
social justice, 175
social norms, 260
social order, 244, 247, 261
social relations, 40, 93, 110, 114, 225
Social Security Amendments, 7
social welfare programs, 6
social workers, 19, 29–32, 37, 85, 133, 139, 197, 199, 240–41
Stennis, John Calhoun, 2, 211–13, 216–17, 230, 256
Stickney, Stonewall, 234–35

Tarwater, James Sidney, 49–50, 82–83, 114, 222–24, 227
Taylor, Chloe, 262
Taylor, Nick, 240
Thompson, Lashawn, 7, 243
Thompson, Myron, 235
Tuscaloosa (AL), 22, 48–49, 51, 75, 82–83, 117–18, 158, 174, 183–84, 218–19, 234–35, 251, 253
Tuskegee Institute, 17–18, 20–21, 29–31, 40, 79, 172–73, 177, 190, 221
Tuskegee Mental Hygiene Clinic, 20, 22, 33, 251
Tuskegee Mental Hygiene Society, 28–29, 32
Tuskegee Veterans Administration Hospital (TVAH), 14, 19, 22, 26, 142, 221; Black physicians at, 23–24; Black psychiatrists at, 27–28, 50, 141, 146, 153, 267; physicians at, 33–36; psychiatrists at, 31, 36, 38; soldiers at, 24

US Public Health Service (USPHS), 29

veterans, 127; Black, 22, 24
Vicksburg (MS), 1, 3, 6, 191, 212
Vicksburg Hospital, 212
violence, 59, 107, 130, 133, 137, 186, 196–97, 218, 265; and asylum, 10; Black, 264, 266; and Black patients, 39, 99–100, 131; and Black women, 84; and eugenics, 42; and Jim Crow, 94; Klu Klux Klan, 192; and Jack Nelson, 147; police, 7; prison, 242; and psychiatrists, 42; racial, 143, 171, 185, 226, 242; and segregation, 18, 52; and slavery, 9; systemic, 267; threat of, 187, 204, 216; white, 38, 44, 216; and white supremacy, 8, 17, 88, 126, 184, 231

"the wake," 9–10, 260
Wallace, George, 175, 205, 222–26, 228, 234
Wallace, Jamie Lee, 235
Washington, Booker T., 33, 249
Washington, Charles, 54, 86
Washington, DC, 23, 217, 220, 252
Washington, Margaret Murray, 33
Washington Building (CSH), 44, 121
Washington County, 136, 202
Watkins, Hull, 126–27, 131–32, 137
welfare, 42, 61–62, 186, 226; assistance, 196, 217; child, 252; departments, 170, 196–97, 204; regulations, 194
white patients, 11, 47, 54, 129, 142, 152, 192, 220, 245; in Alabama, 173; and Black doctors, 209; in Bryce Hospital, 22, 71, 75, 77, 94, 199; and *Builder*, 94; and Cedar Lane, 46; in Central State Hospital, 43; and Community Mental Health Act (CMHA), 193;

white patients (*continued*)
    in East Mississippi State Hospital (EMSH), 52; and electroconvulsive therapy (ECT), 82; and hierarchy, 106; and integration, 56, 212, 215; and Jim Crow, 64, 124; and MCHR, 193; and occupational therapy, 114, 121; in Searcy Hospital, 115; and segregation, 55, 65, 122-23, 137, 139-40, 143-44, 149, 195; and Tuskegee, 35-36, 221; and *The Whit*, 95, 105, 128; and Whitfield Hospital, 57, 86, 102, 128, 169; and Emma Wright, 136
white supremacy, 6, 189-91, 213, 249, 253, 260; and asylums, 10; and civil rights movements, 199; and CMHA, 159; critics of, 38; and educational integration, 200; and eugenics, 26, 172; and integration, 180; and Ku Klux Klan, 203; and mental health care, 231; and occupational therapy, 125; and plantation relations, 14, 106; and psychiatric institutions, 39; and psychiatry, 13, 17, 267; and race, 78; and racial capitalism, 40; and segregation, 38, 65; technology of, 244; violence of, 8, 88, 126, 171, 184, 226, 231, 266; and white saviorism, 113

Whitfield Hospital, 1, 5-6, 64, 86, 103, 113, 171, 203, 215-17, 236, 238, 256-57; and Black illness, 70; Black patients in, 22, 57, 60, 98-100, 110-11, 169; and Black students, 87; and Hayden Campbell, 131-33; and Hodding Carter, 128-30; and Fred Chaney, 128-30, 138; conditions at, 128; desegregation of, 4; doctors, 60; establishment of, 52; and farming, 53; and Deacon Hurston, 4; and William Jaquith, 53-54, 85, 114, 128-29, 200-202, 206, 216, 237; and law enforcement, 61; life at, 55; and male patients, 71; and patient labor, 109; and racial diagnosis, 70; and racial power, 101; and segregation, 52, 124; and Robert Smith, 187; and therapeutic practices, 84, 107; and *The Whit*, 94-95, 98, 101-2, 105-6; and Hull Watkins, 126; and Emma Wright, 134, 136-37

Wright, Emma, 134, 136-37
Wright, Louis T., 38, 52, 129
Wright, Lynne, 239
Wyatt v. Stickney, 229-30, 234-36